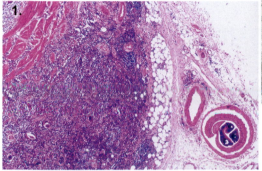

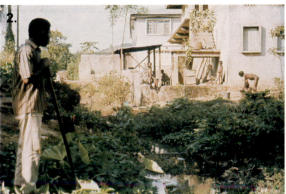

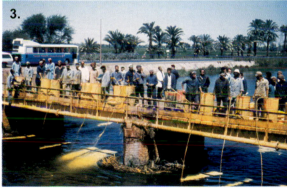

D0421283

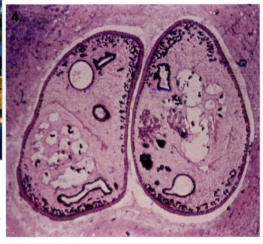

Plate 1. Tissues surrounding the colon. On the left are eggs surrounded by a tissue reaction with many leucocytes and on the right there is a cross-section of a male of *Schistosoma mansoni* surrounding a female in a branch of the lower mesenteric veins.

Plate 2. Small stream running through the centre of the city of Ibadan, Nigeria. The water contains snails, *Biomphalaria pfeifferi*, infected with *Schistosoma mansoni*. The area of bare earth around the house has numerous eggs of *Ascaris lumbricoides* and *Trichuris trichiura*, while the vegetation near the stream provides an ideal shaded environment for infective larvae of hookworms and *Strongyloides stercoralis*.

Plate 3. A large irrigation canal in Egypt containing *Biomphalaria* infected with *Schistosoma mansoni* and being treated with the molluscicide Bayluscide.

Plate 4. Section of lung with a pair of adult *Paragonimus westermani* in a cyst that has a thick fibrous wall. The two gut caeca and uterus containing numerous eggs can be seen in each fluke.

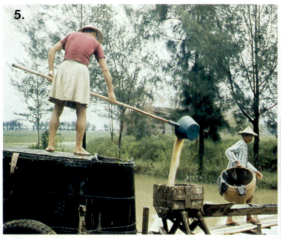

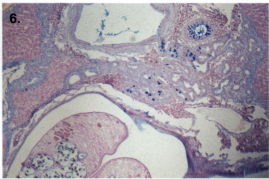

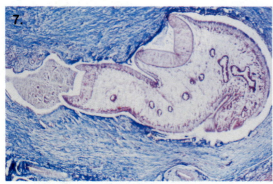

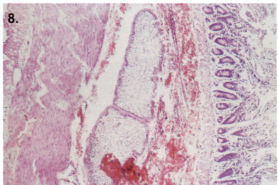

Plate 5. Emptying untreated 'night-soil' into a fish-pond in Taipeh, Taiwan. The pond contains intermediate host snails of *Clonorchis sinensis* and provides the ideal conditions for its transmission.

Plate 6. Section of liver stained for mucin with an adult *Opisthorchis viverrini* in a bile-duct and showing metaplasia of the blue-staining goblet cells.

Plate 7. Liver of sheep with adult of *Fasciola hepatica* in a bile-duct. Stained with Martius scarlet to show extensive fibrosis (stained blue). Both suckers of the fluke and the multiple gut branches are visible.

Plate 8. *Spirometra theileri*: sparganum (plerocercoid) larva migrating through the submucosa of the ileum of a monkey and causing extensive haemorrhage, oedema of the muscularis and loss of visceral peritoneum.

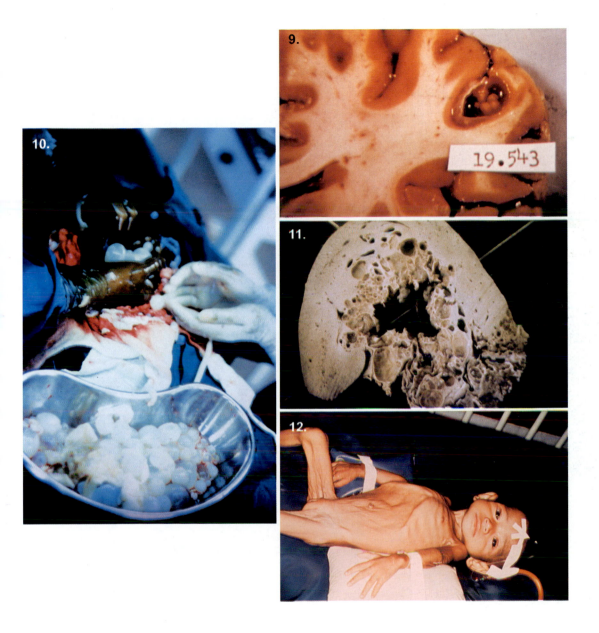

Plate 9. A cysticercus of *Taenia solium* in the brain of a fatal case in Costa Rica.

Plate 10. *Echinococcus granulosus*: operating on a liver hydatid with numerous translucent daughter cysts being removed in northern Kenya.

Plate 11. *Echinococcus oligarthrus*: liver from a fatal case in Panama cut across to show that much of the liver tissue is replaced by a polycystic hydatid.

Plate 12. An infant in Thailand showing extreme emaciation from the malabsorption syndrome caused by strongyloidiasis.

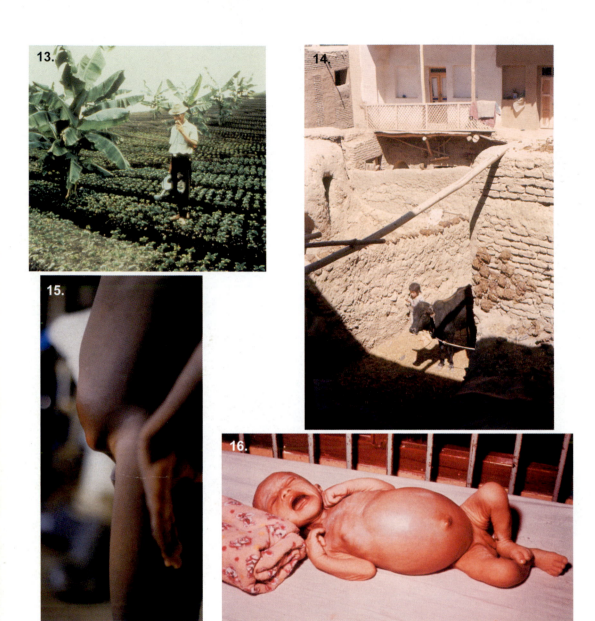

Plate 13. A young coffee plantation (finca) in Colombia providing the ideal conditions for hookworm (and strongyloidiasis) transmission. Note the bare feet of the coffee worker.

Plate 14. Backyard of a house in central Iran in which cattle are kept and dung is dried on the wall for fuel. These conditions have resulted in a high prevalence of human trichostrongyliasis.

Plate 15. *Oesophagostomum bifurcum*: characteristic 'Dapaong tumour' below the umbilicus in a boy in Burkina Faso.

Plate 16. An infant in Thailand suffering from intestinal obstruction caused by *Ascaris* infection.

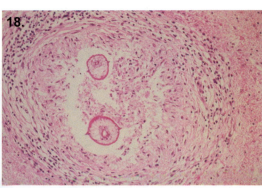

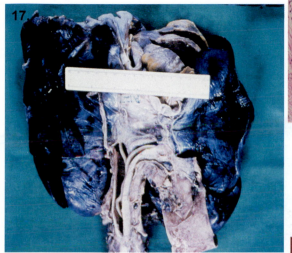

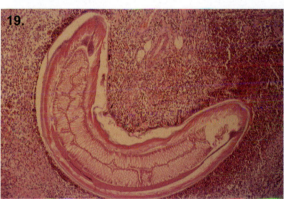

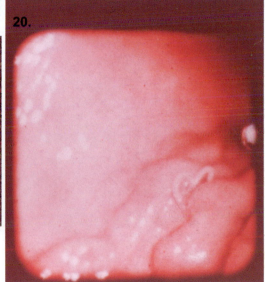

Plate 17. *Ascaris lumbricoides* in bronchi. Fatal case in a woman in the West Indies.

Plate 18. Larvae of *Bayliscaris procyonis* within a granuloma in human brain. Note ventral alae.

Plate 19. *Anisakis* sp. larva in submucosa of ileum of a woman. There is an acute eosinophilic inflammatory reaction which is destroying the larva. A layer of shed cuticle indicates that the larva has moulted within the patient's tissues.

Plate 20. Gastroscopy view of *Pseudoterranova* sp. in the wall of the stomach of a man in Japan. Worms can often be removed with biopsy forceps.

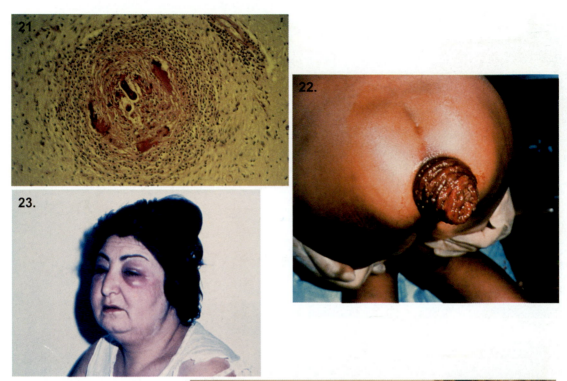

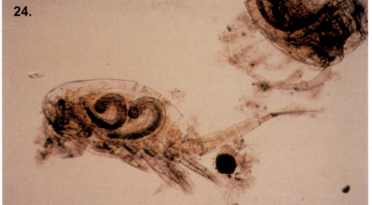

Plate 21. *Toxocara canis*: degenerating larva in the centre of a granuloma in the brain of a 3-year-old boy in England.
Plate 22. Heavy infection with *Trichuris trichiura* causing prolapse of the rectum in a child.
Plate 23. Periorbital swelling in a woman in Lebanon caused by *Trichinella spiralis* infection.
Plate 24. *Gnathostoma spinigerum*: cyclops infected with third-stage infective larvae (compare Figs 31 and 116).

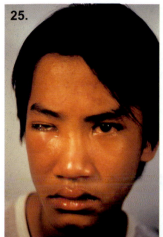

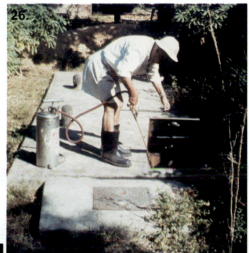

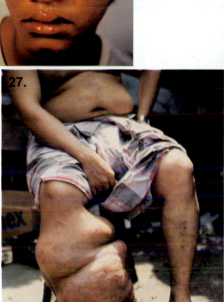

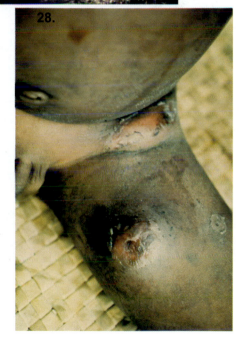

Plate 25. *Gnathostoma spinigerum*: larva migrating through subcutaneous tissues of face causing swelling in woman in Thailand.

Plate 26. Treating a breeding place of *Culex quinquefasciatus*, vector of *Wuchereria bancrofti*, with larval insecticide. This would also be an ideal location for the use of polystyrene beads.

Plate 27. Elephantiasis of leg caused by *Brugia malayi* in a man in Malaysia.

Plate 28. *Brugia timori*: abscess on the thigh of a boy in Timor caused by the presence of adult filariae in inguinal lymph gland and vessels.

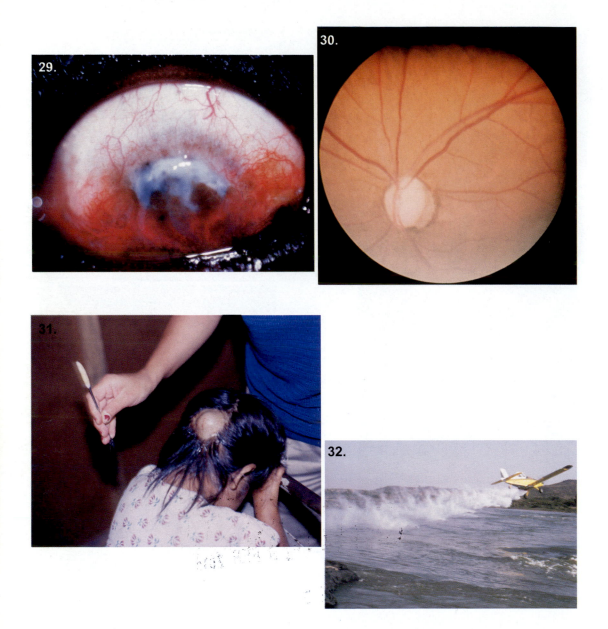

Plate 29. *Onchocerca volvulus*: eye of patient in savannah region of Cameroon with sclerosing keratitis causing complete blindness (anterior lesion).

Plate 30. *Onchocerca volvulus*: view of retina in which all elements have vanished except for the choroidal vessels, which show marked sclerosis (posterior lesion).

Plate 31. Removal of a nodule containing adults of *Onchocerca* from the head of a girl in Guatemala (nodulectomy).

Plate 32. Onchocerciasis Control Programme (OCP). Fixed wing aircraft spraying the upper Volta River with the *Simulium* larvicide, Temephos. Helicopters were also widely used in this campaign.

Worms and Human Disease

2nd Edition

_____

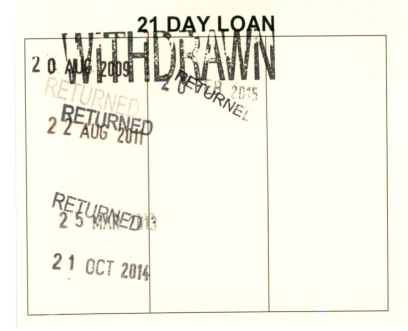

Dedicated to the memory of Annie

Worms and Human Disease

2nd Edition

_____

Ralph Muller, DSc, PhD, FIBiol

Department of Infectious and Tropical Diseases
London School of Hygiene and Tropical Medicine
University of London, UK

and

Former Director
International Institute of Parasitology
St Albans, Hertfordshire, UK

With contributions and the chapter on Immunology of Helminths from

Derek Wakelin, DSc, PhD, FRCPath

School of Life and Environmental Sciences
University of Nottingham, UK

CABI *Publishing*

CABI *Publishing* is a division of CAB *International*

CABI Publishing
CAB International
Wallingford
Oxon OX10 8DE
UK
Tel: +44 (0)1491 832111
Fax: +44 (0)1491 833508
Email: cabi@cabi.org
Web site: www.cabi-publishing.org

CABI Publishing
10 E 40th Street
Suite 3203
New York, NY 10016
USA
Tel: +1 212 481 7018
Fax: +1 212 686 7993
Email: cabi-nao@cabi.org

A catalogue record for this book is available from the British Library, London, UK.

Library of Congress Cataloging-in-Publication Data
Muller, Ralph, 1933-
  Worms and human disease / Ralph Muller ; with contributions and the chapter on immunology from Derek Wakelin.-- 2nd ed.
      p. ; cm.
  Rev. ed. of: Worms and disease / Ralph Muller. c1975.
  Includes bibliographical references and index.
  ISBN 0-85199-516-0 (pbk.)
    1. Medical helminthology. 2. Helminthiasis. I. Wakelin, Derek. II. Muller, Ralph, 1933- Worms and disease. III. Title.
  [DNLM: 1. Helminths--pathogenicity. 2. Helminthiasis. QX 200 M958w 2001]
RC119.7 .M84 2001

                                                      2001025591

ISBN 0 85199 516 0

Typeset in Melior by Columns Design Ltd, Reading.
Printed and bound in the UK by Biddles Ltd, Guildford and King's Lynn.

Contents

Acknowledgements

It is a pleasure to thank SmithKline Beecham (now GlaxoSmithKline) for a grant that has made possible the plates of colour pictures, which have greatly increased the usefulness of the whole book, and Dr John Horton of SmithKline Beecham for his advice and also for the provision of colour photographs (Plates 24 and 25). Thanks also to Dr R. Neafie for providing photographs from the Armed Forces Institute of Pathology collection (Figs 54, 62, 66, 67, 68, 75, 77 and 96 and Plate 18), to Dr L. Savioli for photographs and a booklet from the World Health Organization (WHO) and to Professor T. Polderman for a photograph of *Oesophagostum* (Plate 17). Other photographs were kindly provided by Dr J. Anderson (Fig. 100 and Plates 29 and 30), Dr Kemal Arab (Plate 23), Dr N. Ashton (Fig. 72), Prof. E.A. Bianco (Plate 27), Dr A. Bryceson (Fig. 46), Dr P. Choyce (Fig. 107), Dr D. Denham (Plate 21), Prof. D. Dennis (Plate 28), Dr F. Etges (Fig. 14), Dr R. Feachem (Plate 5), Dr D. Flavell (Plate 6), Dr H. Fuglsang (Fig. 106), Dr L.M. Gibbons (Figs 34, 57, 61 and 85), Prof. D.B. Holliman (Figs 64 and 71 and Plates 11, 12, 13, and 16), Prof. S. Lucas (Plate 19), Dr D. McLaren (Figs 5 and 80), Prof. C. Macpherson (Plate 10), Prof. Y. Matsukado (Fig. 20), Prof. M. Murray (Plate 7), Dr Nagano (Plate 21), Prof. G.S. Nelson (Fig. 44), Dr M.J. Taylor (Fig. 95), Dr A.C. Templeton (Fig. 40), Dr S. Townson (Plate 31), Dr S. Vajrasthira (Fig. 18), Dr E. Watty (Plate 17), Prof. G. Webbe (Plate 3) and the WHO (Plates 26 and 32). Thanks to Edward Arnold and Professor D. Crompton for permission to reproduce Fig. 65, to CAB *International*, and Dr P. Jordan and Dr R. Sturrock for permission to reproduce Fig. 17 and to Dr J. Baker and Harcourt for permission to publish Fig. 132.

My daughter Harriet kindly helped with maps and drawings and I would also like to acknowledge the help and information provided by many colleagues.

Professor Derek Wakelin has, in addition to writing the sections on immunology for various groups of parasites as well as the general chapter on the subject, provided useful criticism and advice on statements on immunology and immunodiagnosis included in the treatments of many of the individual parasites (possible errors in these parts are, of course, not his responsibility).

Introduction

While this book is the second edition of *Worms and Disease: a Manual of Medical Helminthology* (1975), because of the long time that has elapsed since the publication of the earlier book, it has been so extensively revised and brought up to date that virtually every chapter has had to be almost completely rewritten. In the intervening years the importance to humans of some new helminths has emerged, such as *Oesophagostomum bifurcum* and *Parastrongylus costaricensis*, but principally the changes have been necessitated by the great strides that have been made in knowledge of the diagnosis, treatment, immunology and molecular biology of parasites. The chapter on the immunology of helminths (now written by Derek Wakelin) has been greatly amplified, with the addition of more detailed paragraphs in the appropriate sections, together with the latest information on the prospects for specific vaccines. There has also been exciting progress in the field of global control of various helminths, such as the schistosomes, soil-transmitted nematodes, filariae (both those causing lymphatic filariasis and those causing onchocerciasis) and the guinea worm. Most of these campaigns have been possible because of recent advances in chemotherapy and, in some cases, of diagnosis; many have been linked with efforts to improve sanitation and general health.

The book is intended principally as a practical guide in human helminthology for physicians and medical technologists concerned with tropical and exotic diseases and for students taking postgraduate degrees and diplomas in aspects of tropical and infectious diseases. It should also prove useful as an accessory text and reference source for undergraduate medical, zoological and tropical health engineering students, and for medical technologists, microbiologists and physicians in temperate climates. With increase in air travel, most hospitals and medical practitioners in developed countries are meeting cases of parasitic infections that may have been very rare occurrences in the past, and it is becoming increasingly necessary to ask of almost all patients 'Unde venis?'. Also, if global warming increases, it is likely that the endemicity of some helminth infections will extend to higher latitudes.

The format of this book is fairly conventional, with parasites considered in order of their zoological relationships rather than their location in the body. The latter approach may be useful for diagnosis but is not practical for other aspects of the subject, as some parasites can occupy a wide range of sites in the body, so that there would be a great deal of repetition, and also because the relationships between many similar parasites that occupy different organs would be obscured. However, the various possible locations in the body of all the important helminths are shown in Fig. 132 and alternative diagnoses are discussed in the appropriate individual sections. An attempt has also been made to have the best of both worlds, e.g. all the intestinal nematodes are considered in the same section so that the new global measures being advocated for all the geohelminths can be considered together, even though they are not all closely related.

Most of the figures for infection rates have been obtained from the CD-ROM PARASITE database produced by CAB *International* or from MEDLINE. Maps have concentrated principally on helminth infections that have a focal distribution.

The term helminth (Greek ελμνξ) means worm, although it is usually restricted to the parasitic worms. The term does not refer to any one zoological taxon but those members parasitic in humans belong almost entirely to two main groups; the phylum Platyhelminthes, which includes the trematodes (flukes) and the cestodes (tapeworms), and the phylum Nematoda, comprising the nematodes (roundworms). This book provides a comprehensive account of all important helminths found in humans, with a mention of all others reported, however occasionally (a total of 267 species), and includes a brief consideration of other metazoan parasites sometimes found in humans, such as the pentastomids, dipteran fly larvae and leeches, which may be confused with the true helminths.

While the title is *Worms and Human Disease*, it must not be assumed that helminth infection invariably results in disease; most of the helminths that are predominantly human parasites are pathogenic only when worm burdens are high and, as there is no multiplication within the body, light infections become clinically important only following reinfection. The majority of helminth infections are light and cause little morbidity (although in some cases more than was previously thought), but many are so widespread that the low percentage of patients who suffer severe clinical disease represents a problem of great medical and economic importance.

1

The Trematodes

Adult trematodes, or flukes, may be found in the intestinal tract, bile-ducts, lungs or blood of humans. Some details concerning the medically most important species are shown in Table 1. All the trematodes mentioned in the table are normal human parasites, except some species of *Paragonimus* and *Fasciola* and some heterophyids and echinostomes, which are accidental parasites with humans not being involved in their transmission cycles. However, almost all trematodes are very catholic in their choice of definitive hosts (a notable exception is *Schistosoma haematobium*) and have a wide range of animal reservoirs; 144 species that have been found in humans are mentioned in the text, most of which are natural animal parasites. Not shown in the table are various aberrant forms, such as the cercarial larvae of animal and bird schistosomes, which can penetrate the skin of humans but are not able to mature.

Pre-eminent in medical and economic importance are the schistosomes, or blood flukes, which are the cause of one of the major human diseases, schistosomiasis. This is a source of suffering in many warm countries and is a major cause of morbidity. No other trematode is the cause of such widespread morbidity, but liver flukes (*Clonorchis* and the closely related *Opisthorchis*) and lung flukes (*Paragonimus*) are important parasites in areas of Asia and their presence may result in severe disease and possibly death.

It needs to be stressed that the presence of trematode parasites in the body is by no means synonymous with the presence of disease. In contrast to viruses, bacteria or protozoans, trematodes do not multiply within the human body and the few organisms present in the great majority of infected persons are tolerated with the minimum of inconvenience and are often not diagnosed. It is the small percentage of patients with large worm burdens (so-called 'wormy people') or in whom the parasites or their eggs are in ectopic sites in the body who give cause for alarm.

The digenetic trematodes are members of the phylum Platyhelminthes, which also includes the cestodes (tapeworms), monogeneans (ectoparasites of fishes and amphibians) and free-living turbellarians (planarians, etc.). Platyhelminthes, or flatworms, are acoelomate bilateria (bilaterally symmetrical and lacking a coelom). The excretory system is based on the flame cell, or protonephridium, and often the pattern of flame cells can be of importance in classification. Trematodes are characteristically flat and leaflike, or occasionally globular, hermaphroditic organisms (except for the schistosomes, which have a male folded about its long axis and a cylindrical female (Figs 3 and 4)). All have complicated life cycles with alternating sexual and asexual development in different hosts. Asexual multiplication takes place in a snail, and for parasites of medical importance this is always a gastropod snail. It is believed that the trematodes were originally parasites of molluscs and they are still always very specific in their choice of snail host;

Table 1. Trematodes of medical importance.

Habitat	Species	Situation of adult	Eggs recovered from	Snail intermediate host	Other intermediate or transport hosts	Geographical distribution
Blood	*Schistosoma mansoni*	Mesenteric veins	Faeces	*Biomphalaria* spp.	None (active penetration by cercariae)	Africa, South America
	S. japonicum	Mesenteric veins	Faeces	*Oncomelania* spp.	None (active penetration by cercariae)	China, South-East Asia
	S. mekongi	Mesenteric veins	Faeces	*Neotricula*	None (active penetration by cercariae)	Cambodia, Laos
	S. intercalatum	Mesenteric veins	Faeces	*Bulinus* spp.	None (active penetration by cercariae)	Central Africa
	S. haematobium	Vesicular veins	Urine	*Bulinus* spp.	None (active penetration by cercariae)	Africa, Middle East
Lungs	*Paragonimus westermani*	Cysts in lungs	Sputum and faeces	*Semisulcospirura Thiara Oncomelania*	Edible crustaceans containing metacercariae	South-East Asia, China, Japan
	Paragonimus spp.	Cysts in lungs	Sputum and faeces	Various	Edible crustaceans containing metacercariae	South-East Asia, West Africa, South and Central America
Liver	*Clonorchis sinensis*	Bile and pancreatic ducts	Faeces	*Bulimus Parafossarulus*	Freshwater food fish containing metacercariae	South-East Asia
	Opisthorchis felineus	Bile and pancreatic ducts	Faeces	*Bithynia*	Freshwater food fish containing metacercariae	Siberia, East Europe
	O. viverrini	Bile and pancreatic ducts	Faeces	*Bithynia*	Freshwater food fish containing metacercariae	Thailand, Laos
	Fasciola hepatica	Bile ducts	Faeces	*Lymnaea*	Metacercariae encysted on plants	Cosmopolitan (mainly temperate areas)
Intestine	*Fasciolopsis buski*	Small intestine	Faeces	*Segmentina*	Metacercariae on water plants	South-East Asia, India
	Heterophyes heterophyes	Small intestine	Faeces	*Pirenella Cerithidea*	Freshwater food fish containing metacercariae	South-East Asia, Middle East, Egypt, southern Europe
	Metagonimus yokogawai	Small intestine	Faeces	*Semisulcospira*	Freshwater food fish containing metacercariae	South-East Asia, Russia (Siberia), southern Europe
	Other heterophyids	Small intestine	Faeces	Various	Freshwater food fish containing metacercariae	Worldwide in warm countries
	Echinostomes	Small intestine	Faeces	Various	Freshwater fish or snails containing metacercariae	Mostly South-East Asia, India
	Gastrodiscoides hominis	Caecum and colon	Faeces	*Helicorbis*	Metacercariae on water plants	South-East Asia

identification and study of the biology of the particular snails involved in transmission form an important aspect of the epidemiology of trematode diseases, known as medical malacology.

Detailed consideration of snail intermediate hosts is outside the scope of this book. For the practical field worker it is necessary to consult a specialized monograph (e.g. Malek, 1963; Brown, 1980) or send specimens to an expert, as in most habitats there are species of snails present which do not transmit human helminth infections but closely resemble those that do. Some of the important snail intermediate hosts involved in the dissemination of trematodes of medical importance are shown in Fig. 1.

Morphology

The outer surface or tegument is a non-cellular syncytial extension of the sunken tegumental cells, and may have spines embedded in it. During the last few years a great deal of interest has been shown in the physiology and fine structure of the tegument of both trematodes and cestodes, because of its importance in nutrition and in antigenic stimulation (it is considered in more detail on p. 63 in the section on cestodes).

Two suckers are present in all trematodes found in humans, an anterior oral sucker into which the alimentary canal

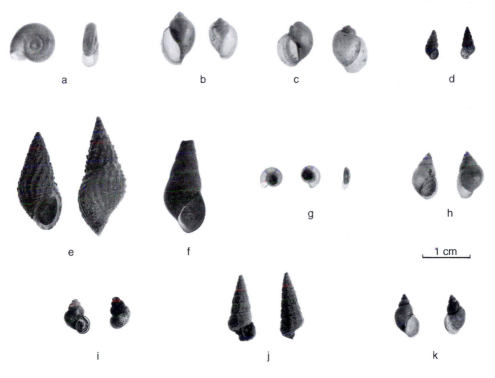

Fig. 1. Snails that act as first intermediate hosts of the trematodes of medical importance. (a) *Biomphalaria glabrata* from Brazil, host of *Schistosoma mansoni*. (b) *Bulinus* (*Physopsis*) *globosus* from Nigeria and (c) *Bulinus* (*Bulinus*) *truncatus* from Iran, hosts of *S. haematobium*. (d) *Oncomelania hupensis nosophora* from Japan, host of *S. japonicum*. (e) *Thiara granifera* from China and (f) *Semisulcospira libertina* from China, hosts of *Paragonimus westermani* and *Metagonimus yokogawai*. (g) *Polypylis hemisphaerula* from China, host of *Fasciolopsis buski*. (h) *Parafossarulus manchouricus* from China, host of *Clonorchis sinensis*. (i) *Codiella* (= *Bithynia*) *leachi* from Germany, host of *Opisthorchis felineus*. (j) *Pirenella conica* (from Egypt) host of *Heterophyes heterophyes*. (k) *Lymnaea truncatula* from England, host of *Fasciola hepatica*.

opens and a more posterior ventral sucker, or acetabulum, by which the worm attaches itself to its host. In *Heterophyes* there is also an accessory genital sucker.

The features of importance in the recognition and classification of a trematode are shown in Fig. 2 and the morphology of the flukes of medical importance in Fig. 3.

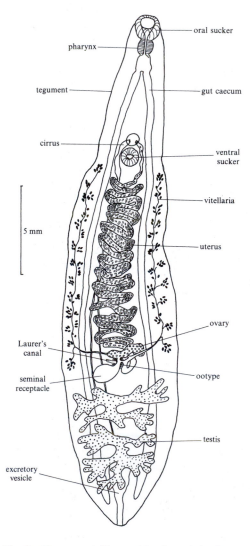

Fig. 2. Diagram of *Clonorchis sinensis* to show the features of taxonomic importance in the digenetic trematodes.

Life Cycle Stages

Adults are hermaphrodite, except for the schistosomes, which have separate sexes – the *egg* reaches water (in the schistosomes, opisthorchiids and heterophyids the egg contains a larva, termed a miracidium, when passed out; in other trematodes the larva develops inside the egg over a few weeks) – the ciliated *miracidium* larva hatches from the egg and penetrates a specific freshwater snail (except in opisthorchiids, where the egg containing a larva is ingested by the snail) – inside the snail the miracidium develops into an irregular sac-like sporocyst – germ cells inside this *primary sporocyst* form the next larval stage (these are termed *rediae* in most trematodes, where they have a rudimentary gut, but *secondary sporocysts* in schistosomes, where they are similar to the primary sporocysts), which burst out and invade new tissues of the snail (principally the digestive gland) – germ cells inside these in turn develop into the next larval stages, the tailed *cercariae*, which escape from the snail into the water (in some forms there are two redial generations). Thus one miracidium can give rise to many thousands of cercariae, the process taking several weeks or even months. The cercariae actively penetrate through the skin, as in the schistosomes, or form cysts (*metacercariae*) in a second intermediate host or on vegetation and are passively ingested in all other trematodes.

Classification

The classification given below is based principally on that of La Rue (1957), in which the life history and the larval stages are considered as well as the morphology of the adult; more conservative classifications were based entirely on the adult. The divisions at the family level are generally accepted by most authorities, but those taxa above this level are still controversial (Gibson and Bray, 1994). Recent studies utilizing computer-based cladistic analysis and molecular biology might alter the familiar groupings in the future (Brooks *et al.*, 1985; Rohde *et al.*, 1993), but changes are not generally accepted. Only a very few of the numerous families comprising the subclass Digenea are included (Yamaguti, 1971) – those which have members of medical importance.

The modes of infection of trematodes of medical importance shown in Table 2 reflect quite well the taxonomic divisions (the odd one out being *Echinostoma*, in which it might be expected that the cercariae would encyst on vegetation).

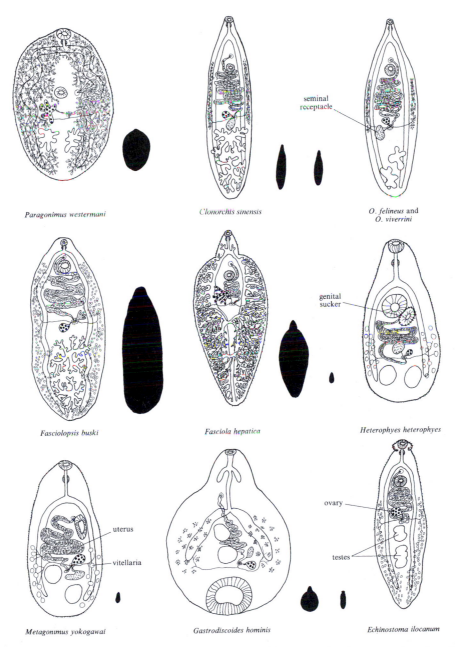

Fig. 3. Diagrams of the shape and principal organ systems of the hermaphrodite trematodes of medical importance (schistosomes are shown in Fig. 4). Comparative sizes shown in silhouette.

Table 2. Mode of infection of trematodes of medical importance.

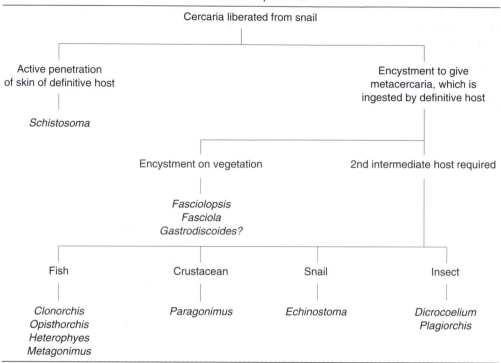

KEY: Members of the group occur in M = mammals, B = birds, R = reptiles, A = amphibians, F = fish.

PHYLUM PLATYHELMINTHES

CLASS TREMATODA

SUBCLASS DIGENEA
Endoparasites with an indirect life cycle utilizing a snail as an intermediate host. Uterus has numerous coils containing many eggs. Single excretory pore at posterior end of the body.

SUPERORDER ANEPITHELOICYSTIDA
The cercaria has a thin-walled, non-epithelial bladder.

Order Strigeida
Cercaria fork-tailed.

SUPERFAMILY SCHISTOSOMATOIDEA
Family Schistosomatidae (MB)

Dioecious
Schistosoma

SUPERFAMILY DIPLOSTOMOIDEA
Family Diplostomidae (MB)
Body usually divided into two regions. Metacercariae in fishes or amphibians.
Alaria, Neodiplostomum

SUPERFAMILY GYMNOPHALLIOIDEA
Family Gymnophallidae (MB)
Large oral sucker, small ventral sucker. Tegument with spines.
Gymnophalloides

Order Echinostomomida
Eggs operculate. Cercariae encyst on herbage or in other molluscs.

SUPERFAMILY ECHINOSTOMATOIDEA
Testes in tandem behind ovary.
Family Echinostomatidae (MBRF)
Head collar with row of spines.
Echinostoma

Family Fasciolidae (M)
Suckers close to each other. Large, spiny, lanceolate flukes, usually found in herbivores.
Fasciolopsis, Fasciola

SUPERFAMILY PARAMPHISTOMATOIDEA (MB)
Sucker at anterior and posterior extremities of body but no oral sucker.
Family Paramphistomatidae (or *Zygocotylidae*)
Body thick and fleshy. Testes in tandem in front of ovary. Metacercariae on vegetation or on snail.
Gastrodiscoides, Watsonius

SUPERORDER EPITHELIOCYSTIDA
Cercaria has an additional thick-walled epithelial bladder.

Order Plagiorchiida
Eggs operculate.

SUPERFAMILY DICROCOELIOIDEA
Cercariae encyst in arthropods and have an oral stylet.
Family Dicrocoeliidae (MBRA)
Found in intestine, liver, gall-bladder and pancreas. The oral sucker is subterminal. Testes adjacent or in tandem, anterior to ovary. Vitellaria posterior to ventral sucker.
Dicrocoelium

SUPERFAMILY OPISTHORCHIOIDEA (MBR)
Cercariae encyst in or on fish.
Family Opisthorchiidae (MB)
Suckers weak. Semi-transparent flukes found in bile-ducts and gall-bladder. Testes in tandem behind ovary.
Clonorchis, Opisthorchis, Metorchis

Family Heterophyidae (MB)
This is a large family. All members are potential parasites of humans. They are minute flukes with a spinose tegument. Testes adjacent behind ovary.
Heterophyes, Metagonimus

SUPERFAMILY PLAGIORCHIOIDEA
Family Lecinthodendriidae (MBRA)
Small spiny flukes with gonads in fore-body. Oral sucker large, ventral sucker small. Metacercariae in aquatic insects.
Phaneropsolus, Prosthodendrium

Family Paragonimidae (MB)
Many are parasites of the lungs. Vitellaria compact and dense. Cuticle spinous. Testes adjacent behind ovary. Cercariae encyst in crustaceans.
Paragonimus

Family Plagiorchiidae (MBRAF)
Cuticle spinous. Suckers well apart. Testes in tandem behind ovary. Metacercariae in insects.
Plagiorchis

Family Troglotrematidae (M)
Cercariae encyst in fish or crustaceans. Genital pore posterior to ventral sucker. Spinous body.
Nanophyetus

Family Schistosomatidae

Schistosomes

At least seven species are parasites of humans: **Schistosoma haematobium** (Bilharz, 1852); Weinland, 1858; **S. mansoni** Sambon, 1907; **S. japonicum** Katsurada, 1904; **S. intercalatum** Fischer, 1934; **S. malayensis** Greer, Ow-Yang and Yong, 1988; **S. mekongi** Voge, Bruckner and Bruce, 1978; **S. sinensium** Pao, 1959.

SYNONYMS (for *S. haematobium*)
Distoma haematobia Bilharz, 1852; *Bilharzia haematobium* Diesing, 1859.

LOCAL NAMES
Au chung (Chinese), Tsagiya (Hausa, *S. haematobium*), Katayamabayo, Suishochoman or Harapari (Japanese), Laremo (Luo, *S. haematobium* haematuria), Kadi dhig (Somali, *S. haematobium* haematuria), Kichocho (Swahili), Pa-yard bai-mai lohit (Thai), Atosi eleje (Yoruba, *S. haematobium*).

DISEASE AND POPULAR NAMES

Schistosomiasis or schistosomosis*, urinary schistosomiasis (*S. haematobium*), intestinal schistosomiasis (*S. mansoni, S. japonicum, S. intercalatum* and *S. mekongi*), schistosomiasis haematobium, intercalatum, japonicum, mansoni or mekongi; Katayama disease (early phase of *S. japonicum*); bilharziasis; bilharzia.

GEOGRAPHICAL DISTRIBUTION

It has been estimated that about 220 million people are infected in the world in 74 countries, with 600 million at risk; of those infected 20 million have severe disease, 120 million have mild symptoms and 80 million are symptomless (WHO, 1993).

S. haematobium. Africa: most of the countries of North Africa; widespread in Central and West Africa; in eastern Africa present from Somalia to the Cape and on the islands offshore, including Madagascar and Mauritius. Middle East: present in most countries. There might also be small foci in India around Bombay and in Madras State. A total of about 90 million people are infected worldwide.

S. mansoni. Africa: North Africa (Morocco, Tunisia, Egypt, southern Sudan); East Africa (from Ethiopia down to South Africa and Madagascar); most countries of Central and West Africa; Middle East (Lebanon, Oman, Saudi Arabia, Somalia, Yemen); Americas: in South America and some of the Caribbean islands.

S. intercalatum. There are limited foci in Central Africa including Cameroon, Congo, Congo Democratic Republic (Zaire), Equatorial Guinea, Gabon, São Tomé and Principe, and possibly in Central African Republic, Chad, Mali and Nigeria.

S. japonicum. China, Indonesia, Philippines, Thailand (an *S. japonicum*-like parasite which is probably distinct).

S. malayensis. Malaysia.

S. mekongi. Cambodia, Laos.

S. sinensium. China, Thailand.

MORPHOLOGY

Unlike all the other trematodes of medical importance, the sexes are separate (dioecious). In all species the male worm is characteristically boat-shaped, with a central canal (gynaecophoric canal) in which the female lives. The cuticle of the male is smooth in *S. japonicum* (the adults of *S. malayensis* and *S. mekongi* are identical) but has tuberculations in the other three important species. There are two small suckers and a varying number of testes in the different species. The female is longer than the male but much thinner and circular in cross-section. The two suckers of the female are very small and weak. The characteristics of the various species are given in Table 3 and Fig. 4.

S. haematobium. The male measures 10–20 mm × 0.9 mm and the cuticle has fine tuberculations. There are 4–5 testes. The female has a long uterus, with the ovary in the posterior third of the body. There are 10–100 eggs in the uterus at one time.

S. mansoni (Fig. 5). The adults are smaller than those of the other species. The male measures 6–13 mm × 0.75–1.0 mm and the cuticle has coarse tuberculations. There are 4–13 (usually 6–9) testes. The ovary of the female is situated anteriorly. There is usually only 1 egg in the uterus at one time.

---

*This is the standardized nomenclature for parasitic diseases advocated by the World Association for the Advancement of Veterinary Parasitology (WAAVP) (Kassai *et al.*, 1988. *Veterinary Parasitology* 29, 299–326) and the World Federation of Parasitologists (WFP), but has not been widely adopted in medical helminthology, particularly by the World Health Organization (WHO). For instance, of the titles of references in this book, 112 have -iasis endings and 16 -osis, most of which are mentioning cysticercosis or echinococcosis – used in both systems.

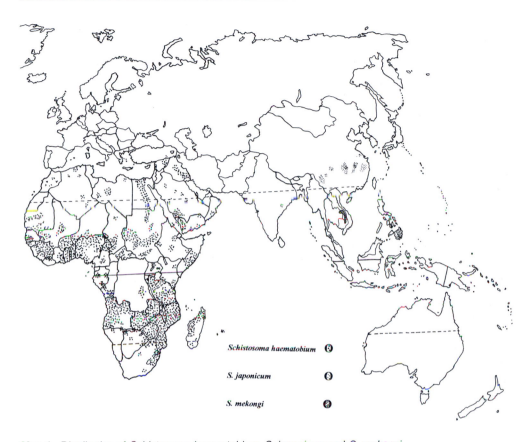

Map 1. Distribution of *Schistosoma haematobium, S. japonicum* and *S. mekongi.*

S. japonicum (S. malayensis and *S. mekongi).* The male measures 12–20 mm × 0.5–0.55 mm and has no cuticular tuberculations. There are 6–7 testes. The female has the ovary at about the middle of the body. There are 5–200 eggs in the uterus at one time.

S. intercalatum. The male measures 11–14 mm × 0.3–0.4 mm. There are 2–7 testes. The female has 5–60 eggs in the uterus at one time.

Of the complete 270 Mb genome of *Schistosoma*, 18–24% has so far been deposited in a database (Williams and Johnston, 1999).

LIFE CYCLE

The eggs are passed in urine in *S. haematobium* and in the faeces in all the other species and contain a fully formed miracid-

ium. Eggs of each species can be recognized by differences in size and morphology (Table 3 and Fig. 6). On immersion in fresh water, particularly under conditions of warmth and light, they hatch almost immediately. The miracidium larvae (Fig. 7) swim actively by means of the cilia with which they are covered and attempt to penetrate any freshwater snail they come into contact with. The miracidia die in 16–32 h if they do not succeed in reaching a suitable snail intermediate host. Like all trematodes they are extremely host-specific in regard to the snails in which they will develop, often far more so than in the definitive host. The species of snail parasitized depends on the geographical region, but *S. haematobium* and *S. intercalatum* develop in snails of the genus *Bulinus*, *S. mansoni* in *Biomphalaria* and *S. japonicum* in *Oncomelania*. *Oncomelania* differs from the other two

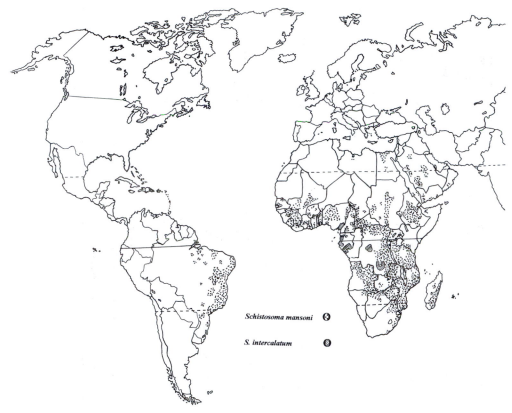

Map 2. Distribution of *Schistosoma mansoni* and *S. intercalatum*.

genera of snails in that it is amphibious, rather than aquatic, and dioecious (with separate sexes) and has an operculum on the bottom surface of the foot (to prevent drying up). Once in a susceptible snail, the miracidium loses its outer ciliated epidermal layer and develops into a mother sporocyst. This becomes filled with germ balls, which burst out after about 8 days, and most of these migrate to the digestive gland, where each develops into a thin-walled daughter sporocyst. A further process of asexual multiplication takes place and each daughter sporocyst becomes filled with the final larval stages, the cercariae. Thus one miracidium can give rise to thousands of cercariae, all of the same sex. At about 26°C, the cercariae of *S. intercalatum* begin to emerge 3 weeks after infection, those of *S. mansoni* after 4–5 weeks, those of *S. haematobium* after 5–6

weeks and those of *S. japonicum* after 7 weeks. The principal stimulus for emergence is light and different species emerge at various times in the day. The cercariae measure 300–400 μm × 50–70 μm and have forked tails (furcocercus type) (Fig. 8). They swim around in the water, usually tail first, and often hang from the surface film. They are infective for only a day or so in water. Not all the cercariae mature at the same time and usually a proportion continue to emerge throughout the life of the snail, which may be many months. When humans enter the water the cercariae penetrate the skin, often between the hair follicles, by means of the anterior spines and the cytolytic secretions of the cephalic glands. The tail is shed in the penetration process, which takes 3–5 min, and the immature schistosomes (known as schistosomula) enter peripheral lymphatics or

Table 3. Differential features of schistosomes of humans.

	Schistosoma japonicum	Schistosoma mansoni	Schistosoma haematobium	Schistosoma intercalatum	Schistosoma mekongi
Situation in human	Mesenteric veins	Mesenteric veins	Vesical veins	Mesenteric veins	Mesenteric veins
Male					
Length (mm)	10–20	6–12	10–14	11–14	15
Width (mm)	0.5	1.1	0.9	0.3–0.4	0.4
No. of testes	6–7	4–13 (usually 6–9)	4–5	2–7 (usually 4–5)	6–9
Tuberculations	None	Coarse	Fine	Fine	None
Caecal junction	Posterior third of body	Anterior third of body	Middle	Middle	Posterior third of body
Female					
Length (mm)	20–30	10–20	16–20	10–14	12
Width (mm)	0.3	0.16	0.25	0.15–0.18	0.23
Uterus	Anterior half of body	Anterior half of body	Anterior two-thirds of body	Anterior two-thirds of body	Anterior half of body
Number of eggs in uterus	50–200	1–2	10–50	5–60	10+
Position of ovary	Middle	Anterior third of body	Posterior third of body	Posterior half of body	Posterior half of body
Mature egg shape and mean size	Round with small knob 85 μm × 60 μm	Lateral spined 140 μm × 61 μm	Terminal spined 150 μm × 62 μm	Terminal spined 176 μm × 61 μm	Round, small knob 57 μm × 66 μm
Mode of voiding eggs	Faeces	Faeces	Urine	Faeces	Faeces
Egg production per female per day (in experimental animals)	3500	100–300	20–300	150–400	?
Reaction of egg to Ziehl–Neelsen stain	Positive	Positive	Negative	Positive	Positive?
Intermediate host snail	Oncomelania	Biomphalaria	Bulinus	Bulinus	Tricula
Distribution overlap	None	Over most of Africa	Throughout range	None	

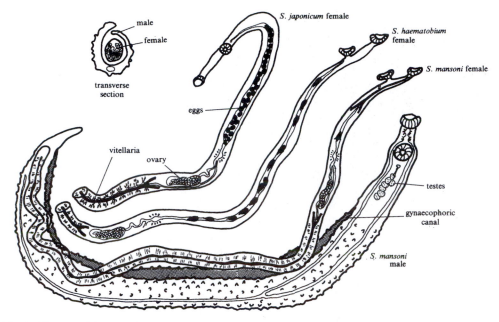

Fig. 4. Diagram of the structures of the three major schistosome species. Only the male of *S. mansoni* is shown. The males of the other species differ principally in the number of testes, while that of *S. japonicum* has a smooth tegument.

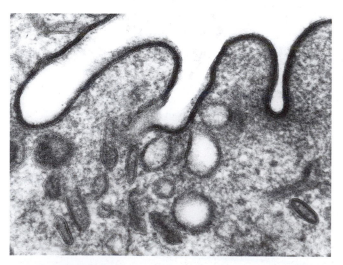

Fig. 5. Integument and double outer membrane of *S. mansoni*. Electron micrograph. Original magnification × 83,500.

venous vessels and are carried to the lungs 4–7 days after penetration (Figs 9 and 10). The schistosomula move from the lungs to the portal vessels and there grow into adult schistosomes, which mate and remain in pairs. The schistosomula are usually assumed to travel to the liver via the blood system (against the blood flow) but, at least for those of *S. japonicum,* some penetrate directly through the diaphragm. The adult

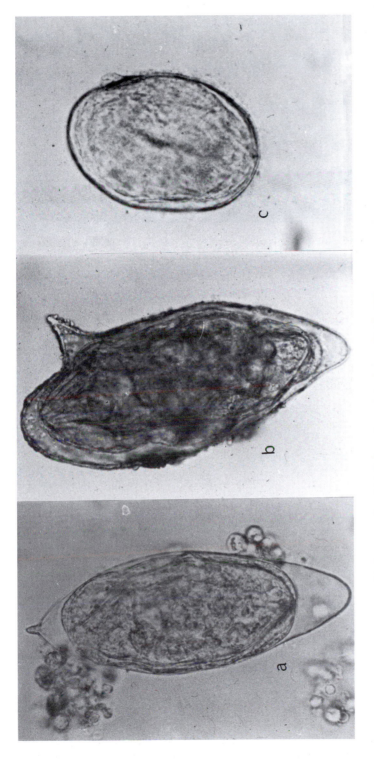

Fig. 6. Eggs of (a) *S. haematobium*, (b) *S. mansoni* and (c) *S. japonicum*. Actual size of (a) is 125 μm.

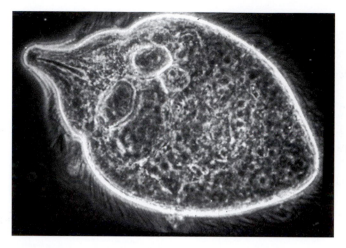

Fig. 7. Ciliated miracidium of *S. mansoni*. Note anterior penetration glands. Dark field. Actual size 80 µm.

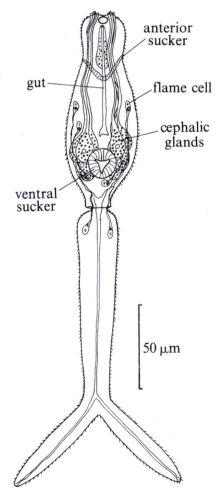

Fig. 8. Diagram of the cercaria of *S. japonicum*.

worm pairs migrate to the mesenteric veins (*S. intercalatum, S. japonicum, S. mansoni* and *S. mekongi*) or the veins of the vesical plexus surrounding the bladder, migrating through the anastomoses between the portal and systemic veins in the pelvis (*S. haematobium*).

Eggs of *S. japonicum* and *S. mansoni* first appear in the stools 25–28 days after cercarial penetration, those of *S. intercalatum* after 50–60 days and those of *S. haematobium* in the urine after 54–84 days. Adult worms of each species can live for as long as 25 years in people who have moved from a non-endemic area, but it is probable that longevity is usually considerably less in endemic areas (3–10 years) and in children is about 2–5 years. Large numbers of worms may be present, up to 400 having been found at autopsy, but in most cases there are fewer than ten worm pairs present. Each female of *S. japonicum* produces about 3500 eggs per 24 h, of *S. mansoni* 100–300, of *S. haematobium* 20–30 and of *S. intercalatum* 150–400. The number of eggs produced by *S. haematobium* decreases with age (Agnew *et al.*, 1996).

It has been reported that *S. japonicum* can undergo vertical transmission (cf. *Alaria*; p. 59), but this appears to be coincidental (Shoop, 1994).

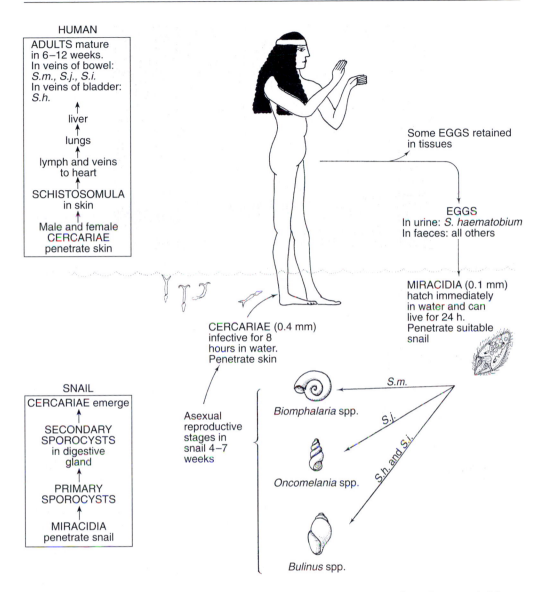

HUMAN

ADULTS mature
in 6–12 weeks.
In veins of bowel:
S.m., S.j., S.i.
In veins of bladder:
S.h.

↑

liver

↑

lungs

↑

lymph and veins
to heart

↑

SCHISTOSOMULA
in skin

↑

Male and female
CERCARIAE
penetrate skin

Some EGGS retained
in tissues

EGGS
In urine: *S. haematobium*
In faeces: all others

MIRACIDIA (0.1 mm)
hatch immediately
in water and can
live for 24 h.
Penetrate suitable
snail

CERCARIAE (0.4 mm)
infective for 8
hours in water.
Penetrate skin

SNAIL

CERCARIAE emerge

↑

SECONDARY
SPOROCYSTS
in digestive
gland

↑

PRIMARY
SPOROCYSTS

↑

MIRACIDIA
penetrate snail

Asexual
reproductive
stages in
snail 4–7
weeks

Biomphalaria spp.

S.m.

S.j.

S.h. and S.i.

Oncomelania spp.

Bulinus spp.

Fig. 9. The life cycle of schistosomes. Figure from Book of the Dead papyrus. *S.m., S. mansoni; S.j., S. japonicum; S.h., S. haematobium; S.i., S. intercalatum.*

CLINICAL MANIFESTATIONS AND PATHOGENESIS

The clinical manifestations and pathogenesis of *S. haematobium* infection differ from those caused by the other species and will therefore be considered separately. Briefly, this is because with *S. haematobium* the eggs accumulate progressively in the bladder and ureters and the reaction to them leads to cystitis, hydronephrosis, ureteric obstruction and occasionally cancer of the bladder, while with *S. japonicum, S. mansoni, S. mekongi* and, to a lesser extent, *S. intercalatum,* the granulomas surrounding the eggs cause colitis, and eggs reaching the liver cause presinusoidal block to the hepatic portal flow, leading to portal hypertension. However, with all species, the pathology depends on the target organs, intensity and duration of infection, host human leucocyte antigen (HLA) type and

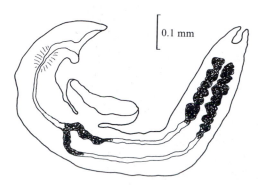

Fig. 10. Diagram of a 12-day-old schistosomulum of *S. mansoni* recovered from the lungs.

race, host immunological responses and concomitant infections such as hepatitis.

S. haematobium

Invasive stage. A cercarial dermatitis ('swimmer's itch') may appear 24 h after first infection but seldom lasts more than 48 h. It is rarely met with in people indigenous to an endemic region and is more common after penetration by cercariae of non-human species of schistosomes.

Acute phase. There are usually no symptoms until 5–10 weeks after infection, when there may be mild allergic manifestations in visitors but these are rare in indigenous populations.

Chronic phase. Maximum egg production begins 10–12 weeks after infection. In schistosomiasis it is the egg that is the important pathogenic agent. The majority of eggs pass through the bladder but an unknown proportion are trapped in the bladder wall and ureters and eventually die and calcify. The earliest bladder lesion is the pseudotubercle, but in long-standing infections nests of calcified ova ('sandy patches') (Fig. 11) are surrounded by fibrous tissue in the submucosa and make the bladder wall visible on X-ray or by ultrasonography (Hatz, 2000).

Haematuria (found in about 50% of cases), dysuria and increased frequency of

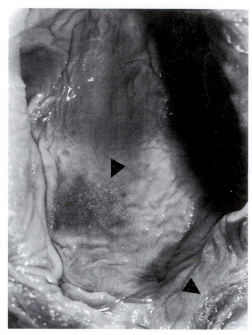

Fig. 11. Inner surface of the bladder showing nests of calcified ova ('sandy patches') (arrowed) of *S. haematobium*.

micturition are typical clinical signs and may persist intermittently for years. Cystitis is caused by hyperplasia of the epithelium (which occasionally becomes 2–3 cm thick), sometimes with papilloma formation, and a markedly reduced bladder capacity often results. This, together with the ureteritis, can lead to hydroureter, hydronephrosis (Fig. 12) and uraemia. Hydronephrosis is not necessarily only a late sequel of infection, as it has been observed in over 8% of preadolescent children in both East and West Africa. It may be reversible after antischistosomal treatment (Subramanian *et al.*, 1999) and is probably caused by oedema, congestion, inflammation and possibly proliferative lesions (although granulomas of the kidneys are very rare).

Fibrosis of the ureteral wall usually leads to dilatation, while strictures occur in less than 1% of patients. Cancer of the bladder is particularly common in Egypt and Mozambique and is clearly predisposed to by urinary schistosomiasis (IARC Working Group, 1994) but some other precipitating

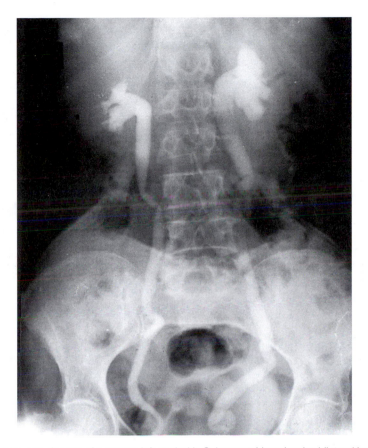

Fig. 12. Intravenous pyelogram of a woman infected with *S. haematobium* showing bilateral hydronephrosis with deformity of both ureters.

factors, such as the presence of nitrosamines in the urine, are probably involved (Mostafa *et al.*, 1995). Squamous carcinoma is more common than transitional carcinoma (Fig. 13). It has been estimated that schistosomiasis is responsible for about 16% of cases of bladder cancer in Egypt. In the Nile Delta region, men do most of the agricultural work and thus become infected, resulting in a 12:1 male-to-female bladder cancer ratio. Pulmonary arteritis progressing to irreversible and lethal cor pulmonale because of capillary damage by eggs sometimes occurs when eggs are swept back into the lungs. The presence of adult worms in the lungs following drug treatment is also a possible cause of pulmonary damage. In women, eggs may cause lesions in the ovaries, Fallopian tubes and uterus or in the lower parts of the genital tract, including the cervix, vagina and vulva, and about 6–27% of such cases result in sterility.

S. japonicum, S. mekongi, S. mansoni and S. intercalatum

Invasive phase. As for *S. haematobium*.

Acute phase. Allergic manifestations, such as pyrexia, headache, oedema, cough, dysenteric symptoms, pruritus and urticaria, occur 3–8 weeks after infection with *S. japonicum*. This is known as the Katayama syndrome and may be accompanied by tenderness in the liver region, mild abdominal pain, lymphadenopathy and splenomegaly, with an accompanying

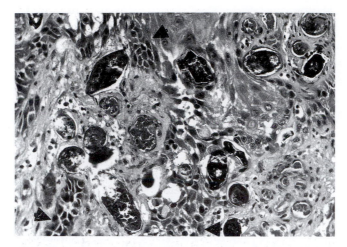

Fig. 13. Section of bladder. Eggs of *S. haematobium* (many are calcified or 'black' eggs) can be seen with epithelial squamous cell metaplasia (arrowed).

eosinophilia. This is possibly caused by a form of 'serum sickness' (acute immune complex disease) resulting from an excess of antigen when eggs are first produced. The acute phase of *S. mansoni* and *S. intercalatum* infection is rarely recognized in an indigenous population.

Chronic phase. In the majority of individuals, infection is light and symptoms are entirely absent, but in heavy infections about 50% of the eggs are trapped in the mucosa and submucosa of the colon, resulting in the formation of pseudotubercles, which coalesce and form larger granulomatous reactions and pseudopapillomas. Eggs of *S. japonicum*, in particular, are inclined to die and eventually to calcify in the colon and many thousands of calcified eggs may be found in the thickened mucosa (Plate 1). Intestinal damage, however, is usually accompanied by few symptoms except a vague feeling of ill health, with perhaps headache, abdominal pain and diarrhoea. Papillomas and inflammatory polyps often develop, and in severe cases, can lead to obstruction of the lumen of the colon. The ulceration of the colon caused by the eggs of *S. mansoni* can result in a blood loss of up to 12.5 ml day^{-1} by patients in Egypt, where papillomas are particularly common. Carcinomas of the large intestine are also

associated with chronic lesions of *S. japonicum* in a small proportion of cases (IARC Working Group, 1994). The increasing fibrosis of the colon wall means that eggs are repeatedly carried to the liver in the portal veins and become lodged in the portal tracts or, less frequently, in the lobules or sinusoids. The eggs become the centre of a pseudotubercle, in which they are engulfed by multinucleate giant cells and surrounded by inflammatory cells (eosinophils, macrophages and polymorphonuclear leucocytes). In the early stages there is a microabscess surrounding each egg, resembling miliary tuberculosis (Fig. 14). However, the cell types differ from a typical tubercle. As the lesion heals, some degree of fibrosis is usually left. Finally the miracidium in the egg dies and the mononuclear cells form Langhans-type giant cells. Experiments in mice have demonstrated that CD4+ T lymphocytes are necessary for the formation of granulomas. While the formation of granulomas is usually taken to be a host response to sequester the eggs, it is possible that mobile granulomas can aid in 'transporting' the eggs across tissues to reach the faeces or urine (Doenhoff *et al.*, 1986; Damian, 1987). Pigment, chemically but not structurally indistinguishable from malarial pigment, becomes deposited in the Kupffer cells, portal tracts and

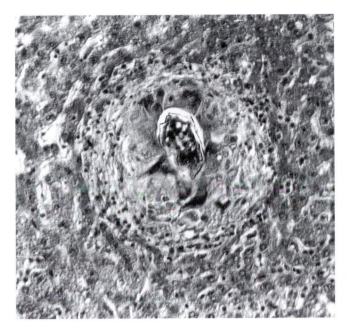

Fig. 14. Egg granuloma of *S. mansoni* in liver with surrounding epitheloid cells and some leucocytic infiltration (see Plate 1 for more advanced stage).

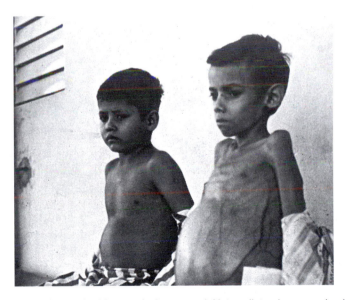

Fig. 15. Two boys with advanced schistosomiasis mansoni. Note collateral venous circulation in nearest patient.

lobules. Liver enlargement is common and splenomegaly often follows the portal hypertension (Fig. 15). Hepatosplenic schistosomiasis mansoni is more common in Brazil and Egypt than in Africa south of the Sahara and signs of portal hypertension are always present in such cases. Anaemia may be found when there is splenomegaly and is more severe after repeated haematemesis. The reaction to the eggs in the liver may

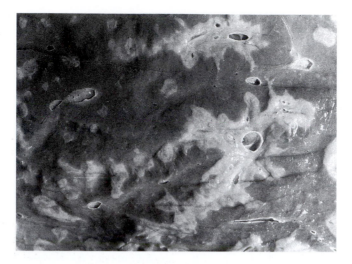

Fig. 16. 'Symmer's clay pipestem' fibrosis caused by eggs of *S. japonicum* surrounding portal veins in liver.

eventually cause the periportal fibrotic reaction termed 'Symmer's clay pipestem' fibrosis (Fig. 16). Liver function tests, however, are not altered in schistosome fibrosis, as they are in true cirrhosis, and, although there may be severe pathological lesions, there is no liver failure. Severe disease, with hepatosplenomegaly, occurs in about 10% of cases of schistosomiasis mansoni, but takes 5–15 years to develop, and in children infection can have effects on nutrition (Stephenson, 1993).

As the portal pressure increases, a collateral venous circulation becomes established and severe or even fatal episodes of bleeding can result from the oesophageal varices. The portal systemic shunt results in the eggs bypassing the liver and being deposited in the lungs. An obstructive and destructive arteritis may follow, which can lead to systematic arterial hypertension and eventually to hypertrophy of the right ventricle.

The adult worms in the blood-vessels do little damage when living but their death can lead to focal necrosis of the liver cells and to granulomas. The more severe pathology thought to be produced by infection with *S. japonicum* is usually explained by the greater egg production, the spherical shape of the egg lacking a large spine resulting in more eggs being

distributed throughout the body, and the greater longevity of the adult worms.

Brain involvement is most common in *S. japonicum* infections and two types of brain lesions have been reported. In the first type there is diffuse involvement with scattered lesions, probably caused by eggs being carried to the brain in the bloodstream, and this type usually results in no symptoms. In the second type a localized granulomatous mass is present, containing large numbers of eggs deposited by ectopic adult worms in the blood-vessels of the brain. These granulomas can cause a wide range of symptoms, depending on the anatomical location of the lesion in the brain.

A transverse myelitis can result from the presence of eggs in the spinal cord and is most commonly found in infections with *S. mansoni* and *S. haematobium*.

In order for the eggs to make their way through the tissues into the gut, the miracidia release proteolytic enzymes and other material, which diffuses through pores in the eggshell. This material (soluble egg antigen (SEA)) is highly immunogenic, and the immune response made against it leads to the formation of the large granulomas that are responsible for most of the pathology in this phase. Evidence for this and analysis of the mechanisms involved have come largely from experiments in mice. Granulomas can be induced in the lungs of mice by intravenous injection of eggs, and this process is prevented by immunosuppressive treatments that interfere with cellular responses. The degree of response to eggs and the pathology that results, following infection in mice, are strongly influenced by genetic factors, and this also reflects different degrees of immune responsiveness. It has recently been shown in humans that at least some of the variation in pathology seen in infected populations is due to the activity of particular major genes, which are associated with T-cell function (e.g. a codominant major gene, SM1, on chromosome 5). The immunology of granuloma formation is complex and involves the activity of both major subsets of CD4+ T-helper (Th) cells. SEA is a powerful inducer of Th2 responses, but Th1 cells also play a role. The cellular response is initiated and controlled by the cytokines released and in mice the phenomenon of immunomodulation occurs – i.e. early granulomas tend to be much larger than those formed later in infection.

Antigen–antibody complexes have been shown by fluorescent antibody studies to be the cause of the Splendore–Hoeppli phenomenon that occurs in sensitized hosts. Glomerulonephritis has been reported as an immune-complex disease in schistosomiasis mansoni.

IMMUNOLOGY OF SCHISTOSOMES

Although it has been established for many years that laboratory animals, including primates, develop immunologically mediated resistance to experimental infections, definite proof that acquired immunity to schistosome infections occurs in humans has been very difficult to demonstrate. It is clear that intensity of infection and prevalence with *S. haematobium* and *S. mansoni* is greatest in 10–14-year-olds and declines in older age-groups, but this could be explained by a decrease in water contact. However, longitudinal studies and detailed monitoring of reinfection after elimination of an existing infection by chemotherapy have demonstrated that age-dependent resistance does

occur against these species (Wilkins *et al.*, 1984, 1987; Butterworth, 1998; Kabatereine *et al.*, 1999), and studies in Brazil link resistance to particular genetic characteristics (Abel and Dessein, 1997). Infections with *S. japonicum* do not show this picture, although there appears to be an age-related reduction in pathology (Ross *et al.*, 2000). The slow acquisition of immunity against *S. haematobium* and *S. mansoni* correlates with a change in the balance between antiparasite immunoglobulin E (IgE) and IgG4, the former promoting protective responses against incoming larvae, perhaps by antibody-dependent cellular cytotoxic (ADCC) mechanisms directed against antigens expressed on the surface tegument. As shown by work carried out in the 1960s, adult schistosomes are largely unaffected by immunity and continue to survive in hosts immune to larval stages (concomitant immunity). One way in which this is achieved is by the adult schistosomes masking the foreign nature of their surface antigens by incorporating host-derived molecules into the tegument and by rapid replacement of the tegument (antigenic disguise). Schistosomes, like many other helminths, exert profound effects on the host's immune response. Not only do these parasites tend to polarize the T-cell response selectively towards Th2 activity, but they may also modulate other components in ways that result in a more general suppression of immune and inflammatory responses.

Immunomodulation can influence the ability of the host to respond successfully to other infections, and there is recent evidence that schistosomes and soil-transmitted nematodes may increase susceptibility to both AIDS and tuberculosis (Bundy *et al.*, 2000).

DIAGNOSIS

Parasitological. The presence of eggs in the faeces or urine is still the most widely used method of diagnosis. This usually poses no problems in heavy infections but diagnosis may not be so easy in light infections, as occur in the majority of cases, particularly in tourists, who have probably been infected only once. In general, it is only the presence of eggs containing live miracidia that indicates an active infection requiring treatment.

The eggs of *S. haematobium,* which occur in the urine, can be detected by sedimentation of a 10 ml sample (best collected around midday) in a urinalysis flask, the deposit being examined under the microscope for eggs. Alternatively, a 10 ml sample can be passed through a polycarbonate or polyamide membrane, washed, removed and stained in 1% trypan blue (or 2.5% ninhydrin, 5% iodine, eosin or methylene blue) for a few minutes. After washing again (and drying at 37°C if wished), the filter is examined in a few drops of saline on a microscopic slide. It is probably not wise to reuse filters. In about 5% of patients, eggs may also be found in the faeces.

Cytoscopy may be performed as a final diagnostic measure when no eggs can be found in the urine, but the danger of secondary infection makes this a possibly hazardous procedure.

The eggs of the other species occur in the faeces and concentration techniques, such as the formol–ether or Kato–Katz thick-smear methods (p. 258), are necessary. A modification of the thick-smear method can be used for quantitative determinations and, in some studies, has given a good indication of the number of adult worms, as can filtration staining techniques. In the latter, eggs from faeces are stained with ninhydrin on filter-paper and counted.

Rectal biopsy is often effective (even in about 50% of cases of *S. haematobium*), an unstained squash being examined under the microscope.

Clinical. In the field, haematuria can provide a quick and inexpensive indicator of urinary schistosomiasis; microhaematuria (measured by means of a reagent strip) or proteinuria correlates well with the intensity of infection. Even self-reporting by children can provide a useful epidemiological record of community prevalence, although this is likely to give an overestimate, depending on the species of worm and level of infection (Ansell and Guyatt, 1999); using models for each species more accurate estimates are possible (Guyatt *et al.*, 1999).

Portable ultrasound can be used for diagnosis of the degree of pathology, particularly in the liver or bladder, and can screen populations at the community level; it can also be used for determining the effect of chemotherapy (Hatz, 2000).

Immunological. There are numerous immunological tests for diagnosis but those involving various ELISA and immunoblotting techniques are the most convenient. A dipstick ELISA for urine samples, using an SEA can effectively diagnose schistosomiasis and correlates well with quantitative egg counts. Circulating cathodic antigen (CCA) is the dominant antigen in the urine of *S. mansoni* patients and can be detected by a monoclonal antibody (mAb) of 41/42 kDa. There are also circulating soluble adult-derived antigens (Sm31/32 and Sj31/32) in serum, which can be detected by dot ELISA, and an IgG ELISA can be used to detect antibodies against them.

TREATMENT

Chemotherapy. *Praziquantel* (usually in a single oral dose of 40 mg kg^{-1}) is the drug of choice for all species of schistosome and has virtually superseded almost all the agents previously used. It has few side-effects (except sometimes in patients with very heavy worm loads), although it is probably better not to give it during early pregnancy. Praziquantel is a heterocyclic pyrazine-isoquinoline unrelated to other anthelminthics – chemical formula 2-(cyclohexylcarbonyl)-1,2,3,6,7,11-*b*-hexahydro-4*H*-pyrazino[2,1a]isoquinolin-4-one. It is quickly metabolized, crosses the blood–brain barrier and appears to act by causing spastic paralysis and vacuolization of the tegument of the worm, possibly from interference with inorganic ion transport and an increase in membrane permeability; it may also destroy lysosomes. Two target antigens are also affected (a surface tubercle glycoprotein of 200 kDa and an esterase of 27 kDa) and maybe epitopes become exposed so that the drug evokes an effective immune response (Brindley, 1994; Dupre *et al.*, 1999).

Metrifonate is cheap and safe to use against *S. haematobium* infection. Its main disadvantage is that repeated treatment is necessary (usually 7.5–10 mg kg^{-1} given orally in each of three doses at fortnightly intervals). As an organophosphate compound, it inactivates the enzyme, destroying acetylcholinesterase, but its mode of action against the worms is obscure. Atropine sulphate can be used if symptoms of cholinergic activity occur.

Oxamniquine is a tetrahydroquinoline derivative that has activity only against *S. mansoni* (given at a single oral dose of 15 mg kg^{-1}) and can be used for advanced cases of the disease. It should be avoided in early pregnancy and in cases of epilepsy, and can cause drowsiness. Resistance to the drug has also been reported, and it is in limited supply. The mode of action is unknown.

The antimalarial compound *artemether* or *artesunate* (oil and water soluble forms of an artemisinin derivative) is being tested as a prophylactic against *S. japonicum* in China and in one trial was shown to reduce egg production of *S. mansoni* and *S. haematobium* by 15% after 12 weeks when given in the usual dose for malaria. It also acts principally against developing worms, unlike the two compounds at present in use; cyclosporin has similar modes of action but would be too expensive for general use. Caution needs to be exercised in relation to malaria resistance.

Surgery. In advanced cases with liver fibrosis, portocaval shunt and occasionally splenectomy have been used to relieve the portal hypertension, but the results have been disappointing.

EPIDEMIOLOGY
Schistosomiasis, particularly when due to *S. haematobium*, is very much a focal disease and many prevalence figures are based on limited surveys, which are not always typical of the country as a whole. However, estimates in millions of overall prevalence in each endemic country have been made

recently (Chitsulo *et al.*, 2000).

S. japonicum. China 1.06 (0.09% of total population), Philippines 0.43 (0.6%), Indonesia (Sulawesi) 0.0002 (0.0001%), Thailand very rare ('*S. japonicum*-like').

S. mansoni. Antigua fewer than 0.0001*, Brazil 7.01 (4%), with a mortality rate of 0.44 per 100,000, Burundi 0.84 (13%), Dominican Republic 0.23 (3%), Eritrea 0.26 (7%), Guadeloupe 0.033 (8%)*, Martinique 0.005 (1.3%)*, Puerto Rico 0.015 (0.4%)*, St Lucia 0.0019 (1.2%)*, Rwanda 0.38 (6%), Surinam 0.0037 (0.9%) and rising in children, Venezuela 0.0338 (0.2%).

S. haematobium. Algeria 2.1 (7.5%), India (Bombay area) very rare, Iran 0.042 (0.07%), Iraq 0.042 (0.2%), Jordan 0.0001 (0.002%), Lebanon very rare*, Libya 0.27 (5%), Mauritius 0.016 (1.5%)*, Syria 0.003 (0.02%)*, Turkey 0.0006 (0.001%)*.

S. mansoni and *S. haematobium.* Angola 4.8 (44%), Benin 1.95 (35%), Botswana 0.15 (10%), Burkina Faso 6.24 (60%), Cameroon 3.02 (23%), Central African Republic 0.33 (10%), Chad 2.78 (43%), Congo 0.89 (34%), Congo Republic (Zaire) 13.84 (28%), Côte d'Ivoire 5.6 (40%), Egypt 10.06 (17%), Equatorial Guinea 0.008 (2%), Ethiopia 4.0 (7%), Gabon 0.5 (45%), Gambia 0.33 (30%), Ghana 12.4 (73%), Guinea 1.7 (26%), Guinea Bissau 0.33 (30%), Kenya 6.14 (23%), Liberia 0.648 (24%), Madagascar 7.54 (55%), Malawi 4.2 (43%), Mali 5.88 (60%), Mauritania 0.63 (27%), Mozambique 11.3 (70%), Namibia 0.009 (0.6%), Niger 2.4 (27%), Nigeria 25.83 (23%), Senegal 1.3 (15%), Sierra Leone 2.5 (60%), South Africa 4.5 (11%), Swaziland 0.23 (26%), Togo 1.03 (25%), Uganda 6.14 (32%), Tanzania 15.24 (51%), Yemen 2.23, Zambia 2.39 (27%), Zimbabwe 4.4 (40%).

S. intercalatum. Cameroon locally in forest areas, Congo (16% in children in one area), Congo Republic (Zaire) sporadic, Equatorial Guinea (13% in Bata city),

*It is probable that in these countries transmission has now ceased and these are residual cases.

Gabon (29% in one area), São Tomé and Principe 0.005 (4%). Confirmation needed for presence in Central African Republic, Chad, Mali and Nigeria.

S. mekongi. Cambodia 0.07 (0.7%), Laos 0.12 (2%) and recent cases in refugee camps in Thailand.

S. malayensis. Malaysia very rare (Shekar, 1991).

In most areas endemic for *S. haematobium* there is a very high prevalence rate, with almost everyone in the community lightly infected before the age of 10 years. Studies in Brazil, St Lucia, Tanzania and Uganda demonstrated a relationship between egg output and prevalence of *S. mansoni* in children (Fig. 17). Above 50–60% prevalence, a small extra rise is accompanied by a considerable increase in egg output and thus in the severity of disease. Post-mortem studies and blood-filtration studies after chemotherapy for counting adults have shown a good relationship between the last two parameters so that intensity of infection can be expressed in terms of eggs per gram of faeces or per 10 ml of urine. To determine the intensity of infection of different age-groups, the frequency of occurrence of the different levels of egg output can be conveniently plotted and provides a good indicator of the proportion of the com-

munity that has levels of egg output likely to cause morbidity (Jordan *et al.*, 1993). This demonstrates the importance of quantitative determinations of egg output in schistosomiasis (p. 260). The ecological factors associated with the transmission of schistosomiasis vary markedly with the species of schistosome, owing to the differing habitats of the snails involved. The amphibious snail hosts of *S. japonicum* live mainly in rice paddies and muddy habitats beside rivers; the aquatic snail hosts of *S. mansoni* live principally in gently flowing running water (less than 0.3 m s^{-1}) such as irrigation channels, streams, lakes and ponds (Plate 2); those transmitting *S. haematobium* live almost entirely in still water, such as ponds, pools, lakes and marshy areas. Snail populations usually show marked seasonal fluctuations, the most important factors influencing numbers being rainfall and temperature. The effect of rainfall varies, depending on the yearly rainfall figures. In drier regions of Africa rainfall stimulates the production of young bulinid and planorbid snails, while in equatorial regions with a higher rainfall, snails are washed away during the rainy season and breeding takes place principally in the months following. Temperature is another factor limiting population densities, the temperature range for optimal expansion of snail numbers being 20–28°C.

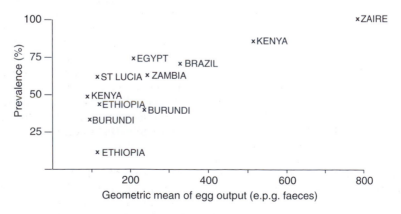

Fig. 17. Relationship between overall prevalence and intensity of *S. mansoni* infection as determined by egg output (measured by Kato–Katz technique) in various endemic areas. Each determination is based on studies by different workers. e.p.g., eggs per gram. (From Jordan *et al.*, 1993.)

Seasonal variations in the cercarial transmission rates in snails are most marked with the bulinid hosts of *S. haematobium* living in temporary bodies of water. In hyperendemic habitats, such as canals, there may be large numbers of snails producing cercariae of *S. mansoni* throughout the year.

Diurnal fluctuations in the production of cercariae occur; cercariae of *S. japonicum* (which is adapted for transmission among the nocturnal animal reservoir hosts) are mostly produced in the evening, while those of *S. mansoni* and *S. haematobium* are produced in the middle of the day. This factor is not usually of practical importance except where *S. mansoni* transmission occurs in running water, in which case washing and bathing are likely to be much safer in the morning and evening, when cercariae are less abundant.

SNAIL HOSTS OF SCHISTOSOMES

S. japonicum. *Oncomelania* is a conical, amphibious, prosobranch snail measuring 3–10 mm and having 4–8 whorls, a dextral opening and an operculum covering the foot. Species involved are *O. hupensis* from mainland China, *O. nosophora* from south-west China (and Japan), *O. formosana* from Taiwan, *O. quadrasi* from the Philippines and *O. lindoensis* from Sulawesi.

S. mekongi. *Neotricula aperta* is an aquatic snail found in the Mekong River and it probably also transmits *S. sinensium.* *Robertsiella* spp. are found in Malaysia and transmit *S. malayensis.*

S. mansoni. *Biomphalaria* is a flattened pulmonate, planorbid snail with 3.5–7 whorls, measuring 7–22 mm. Four main groups are found in Africa: (i) the *pfeifferi* group (four species), which include the most important hosts in Africa and the Middle East; (ii) the *sudanica* group (three species), which occur in both East and West Africa; (iii) the *choanomphala* group (three species), which live in the great lakes and act as hosts in Lake Victoria; and (iv) the *alexandria* group (two species), which occur sporadically in North, East and South Africa. In the western hemisphere *B. glabrata* is the most important snail host, with seven other species locally involved.

S. haematobium. *Bulinus* is a turreted pulmonate snail with a left-handed opening when looked at with the spire upwards (Fig. 1). The height varies from 4 to 23 mm. The subgenus *B. (Physopsis)* is differentiated from *B. (Bulinus)* by having a truncate columella and a pointed end to the foot in living specimens. Two main groups of bulinid snails are important as hosts: (i) the *africanus* group (ten species) of the subgenus *Physopsis* is the more important group in eastern and southern Africa and in most parts south of the Sahara; and (ii) the *truncatus, forskali* and *reticulatus* groups (27 species) of the *Bulinus* subgenus of snails act as hosts in the Near East (Iran, Egypt and Sudan), in Madagascar and in parts of both East and West Africa.

S. intercalatum. *B. (Physopsis) africanus* acts as snail intermediate host in Congo Republic and *B. (Bulinus) camerunensis* in Cameroon.

It must be borne in mind when attempting to identify a snail that there are usually many other types of snail present in the same body of water as the ones transmitting schistosomiasis, and they may be difficult to differentiate. Specialized monographs need to be consulted (Brown, 1980) or expert advice sought. It is also important to distinguish clearly the cercarial species emerging, because of the large number of animal and bird schistosomes that use the same snail hosts and produce cercariae similar to the human schistosomes. In detailed epidemiological studies, it may be necessary to expose laboratory animals to the cercariae and to identifiy any adult schistosomes that develop.

PREVENTION AND CONTROL

Personal prevention is by avoidance of water sources containing cercariae, impossible for fishermen to carry out and extremely difficult for children to be convinced of the necessity thereof. The most common source of infection in tourists to Africa appears to be swimming in Lake Malawi. Thorough and speedy towelling after swimming or wading in marshes may prevent cercariae from penetrating.

Before attempting any control measure, it is essential to define its objectives – i.e. whether it is intended to prevent apread of the disease, to reduce morbidity or transmission or to permanently interrupt transmission (elimination in an area or eradication in a country or worldwide). Until the aims of a project have been clearly defined, it is difficult to work out techniques and costings, or even to evaluate its eventual success. While eradication must be the ultimate objective, it is not yet a feasible proposition in many areas.

There are five principal methods of control: mass chemotherapy, destruction of snails, environmental sanitation, prevention of water contact and the possible use of mass vaccination. Which method or methods are to be employed will depend very much on the conditions where they are to be applied but it is usually essential to provide alternatives or to use two or more methods simultaneously (e.g. chemotherapy, snail control and health education). It is also important to determine at the beginning how the success of the campaign is to be measured, and various indices can be used. The most common assessment is that of prevalence, but incidence (measurement of the rate at which people become infected) is more sensitive and is particularly useful in mass chemotherapy campaigns. Other measures of assessment that can be used are the effect on egg output (i.e. on intensity of infection) or on severity of clinical disease (morbidity), immunological methods and various indirect biological methods. The most common biological method of assessing the success of measures against the intermediate host is a periodic snail count but determinations of the infection rates in snails have been used.

Mass (universal) chemotherapy. The primary objective should be the reduction and prevention of morbidity, although a decrease in the intensity of transmission is also important. Campaigns have been carried out in many countries, often with great success, and at the outset are vertical, involving specialized control units that have identified and mapped transmission sites, assessed the level of morbidity and educated health workers and the community about the control programme (WHO, 1993; Savioli *et al.*, 1997). Later, community-based control programmes can be instigated, utilizing trained community health workers. If transmission is intense (over 50% in children), then the whole population can be treated; otherwise, 7- to 14-year-old schoolchildren can be targeted, since they can be easily tested, treated and followed up and are likely to be the most heavily infected section of the population. A small number of heavily infected individuals produce a large percentage of the eggs reaching the environment (in one classic study with *S. mansoni*, 51% of patients had fewer than ten worm pairs while only 7% had more than 80 – although one girl who died had 1600 worm pairs). In all campaigns periodic re-treatment is essential in order to have a lasting effect. After campaigns with praziquantel in China, Indonesia and the Philippines, reduction in the size of the liver and spleen was reported (WHO, 1993), while in patients with schistosomiasis mansoni, hepatomegaly and periportal fibrosis have regressed after treatment as measured by ultrasound (Boisier *et al.*, 1998; Frenzel *et al.*, 1999).

CONTROL OF SNAILS

Chemical control. The relationship between the population dynamics of snail intermediate hosts and disease transmission to humans is poorly understood and complete eradication of snails from large areas is not feasible. Mollusciciding is likely to be most effective in targeted focal sites, say where children habitually bathe. Infection vanished from Tunisia in 1983 after treatment of oases.

Niclosamide (Bayluscide) can be used at a concentration of 8 p.p.m. hours (e.g. 0.33 p.p.m. for 24 h) for aquatic snails (Plate 3) or 0.2 g m^{-2} on moist soil for amphibious hosts of *S. japonicum*.

Biological control. Carnivorous snails, such as *Marisa cornuarietis*, or competitors, such as *Melanoides tuberculata* and *Tarebia granifera,* have been added to habitats in Guadeloupe, Martinique, Puerto Rico and St Lucia, with the result that *Biomphalaria* has vanished from all or almost all areas (Giboda *et al.*, 1997; Pointier and Jourdane, 2000).

Ecological methods of control. Habitats can be made unsuitable for snails by alternate flooding and drying of water channels or covering and lining of canal systems, as in Egypt and Sudan, and filling in of marshy areas. In many areas such measures are likely to be permanently successful, but they require close cooperation between irrigation engineers and public health workers. In rice-growing areas of mainland China and in Leyte Island (Philippines) widespread cleaning of irrigation ditches and filling in of ponds have resulted in a great reduction in schistosomiasis japonicum infection in recent years.

Prevention of water contact. The provision of piped water supplies and alternative bathing and clothes-washing places can be effective in preventing human contact with infested water and, while expensive, does have wide-ranging health benefits.

For visitors and tourists, prevention can be achieved by avoidance of contact with water in ponds, canals, slow-flowing streams and the shallow edge of lakes in endemic areas (although in Lake Victoria in East Africa the snail *Biomphalaria choanomphala* transmits *S. mansoni* in water 2 m deep). For tourists, swimming in Lake Malawi or Lake Kariba is often followed by infection. Dibutyl phthalate or hexachlorophene spread over the skin will protect for about 4 h.

Health education. Knowledge of the role of indiscriminate defecation and urination in spreading the disease to members of a community and the personal importance of avoiding contaminated water needs to be effectively communicated, particularly to children and adolescents. While it is probably impossible in Africa to prevent children swimming in the water, they could be taught to urinate (and perhaps defecate) before entry.

Present position and future outlook for control. Present control methods are capable of substantially reducing transmission and particularly morbidity in most areas provided that they are properly designed and carried out and if adequate funds are available. However, new irrigation and hydroelectric schemes in many endemic countries have increased the number of snail habitats. New human-made lakes have followed the building of dams in many countries: Côte d'Ivoire (Lakes Kossou and Taasbo), Egypt and Sudan (Lake Nasser); Ghana (Volta Lake); Nigeria (Kainji Lake); Zambia and Zimbabwe (Lake Kariba); Senegal (Lake Guiers below the Diama dam and Manantali dam in Mali). The incidence of schistosomiasis in the populations bordering these lakes or the irrigation channels coming from them (as in Egypt and the Gezira scheme in Sudan) almost always rises. In Côte d'Ivoire around Lake Kossou there used to be an infection rate of 14% with *S. haematobium*, which has now risen to 53%, and around Lake Taabo the rate has risen from 0% to 73% (although the 2% infection rate with *S. mansoni* has not changed so far); around Lake Kainji the infection rate with *S. haematobium* is now 14% in children (from nothing); around Lake Kariba there is now a 70% infection rate in children with *S. haematobium*; infection has spread greatly in the Senegal River basin since the building of the dams and there is now a prevalence of 91% with *S. mansoni* (from 1%) and of 28% with *S. haematobium* (Southgate, 1997). One trend in Africa caused by changes in ecology following the building of dams in Africa (e.g. in delta areas of Cameroon, Ghana and Egypt) is the replacement of *S. haematobium* by *S. mansoni*. The new opportunities for agriculture are also attracting possibly infected migrants and this is particularly apparent in the Gezira and in Ethiopia (although the building of the Koka dam initially reduced transmission).

Infection has been eliminated from Japan, Tunisia and Montserrat recently and campaigns against *S. haematobium* are being mounted in Mauritius (1.3% in adults only), Morocco (2.3% overall) and Tanzania (45% in Zanzibar), against *S. mansoni* in Brazil, Burundi, St Lucia and Venezuela (risen from 0.1% to 0.9% in under-10-year-olds in the last few years) and against both species in Egypt, Ghana, Madagascar, Malawi, Mali, Nigeria, Saudi Arabia, Sudan and Zimbabwe; against *S. japonicum* in China, Indonesia (1% overall infection rate) and the Philippines (3.6%); and against *S. mekongi* in Laos (72%) (WHO, 1993).

China has had control campaigns involving mass treatment of people and cattle with anthelminthics (nowadays praziquantel), snail control and environmental engineering for the last 50 years but there were still estimated to be 1.06 million cases in humans and 0.25 million cases in cattle in 1997. However, *S. japonicum* has been eliminated from 150 of the formerly 378 endemic counties in 12 provinces south of the Yangtze River (Ross *et al.*, 1997), while in 1955 there were estimated to be over 11 million cases. Unfortunately, recent flooding has increased the extent of snail habitats. The Three Gorges dam under construction on the Yangtze River will, within the next 10 years, create the largest lake in the world in a highly populous region where schistosomiasis japonicum already occurs and where there will have to be about 2 million extra migrants from highly endemic areas, which will be flooded. The building of the dam should reduce the overall density of snails along the river banks but will provide many more suitable, contaminated, marshland habitats and an increased contact with water.

Towards a vaccine. The need for a vaccine against schistosomiasis is underscored by the fact that, although chemotherapy with praziquantel is very effective, in the absence of an effective immune response reinfection tends to occur quite quickly.

Progress to date indicates that a vaccine is feasible, since protection against sheep schistosomiasis (a problem in Sudan) using irradiated cercariae has been successfully achieved. However, any human vaccine will have to consist of defined components, as cercariae might introduce viruses.

Various types of vaccine are being investigated (Capron, 1998). These include the following.

1. Peptide components of protective antigens. These can be used to generate differential responses, e.g. one elicits eosinophil-dependent ADCC, another stimulates delayed-type hypersensitivity (DTH) reactions with macrophage activation. Recently a multiple antigen peptide (MAP) vaccine has shown very promising results, inducing both T-cell and B-cell responses in mice and in monkeys, reducing parasite fecundity and egg viability and decreasing liver pathology by over 70%.
2. Excretory/secretory (ES) antigens. ES material obtained from postcercarial schistosomula kept *in vitro* is effective in immunizing rats to subsequent infection. The secretions contained proteins in the range 22–26 kDa (amplified by PCR) and induce an IgE-dependent ADCC.
3. Membrane antigens. Molecules with a molecular weight of 23 kDa (e.g. Sm23 and Sj23) occur in the tegument of all stages of the parasite but are often species-specific.
4. Paramyosin. This 97 kDa internal antigen (e.g. Sm97), obtained from schistosomula or adults, induces responses that affect the muscles and tegument of adults (Gobert, 1998).
5. DNA vaccines. Direct injection of the coding sequence for known antigens is being investigated. Such a vaccine can be used alone or combined with chemotherapy, e.g. immunization with DNA for Sm28 glutathione-*S*-transferase (GST) together with praziquantel prevented the formation of pathological lesions in mice (Dupre *et al.*, 1999).
6. Irradiated live cercarial vaccines. Although these are not directly suitable for human use, they might provide useful pointers to promising leads (Coulson, 1997).

The most promising six antigens were recently selected by the World Health Organization (WHO) for testing as vaccines but at best gave only a maximum of 60% protection (Katz, 1999).

A general problem facing the development of vaccines against any infectious disease is the generation of an appropriate T-cell response (e.g. CD4+ or CD8) and, if CD4+, then the appropriate Th subset, Th1 or Th2. In addition, where the disease associated with infection is immune-mediated, as in schistosomiasis, vaccination must not induce pathological responses. There is controversy about whether Th1 or Th2 responses are most important and appropriate for vaccine-induced resistance to schistosome infection, but it is probable that a balanced response would be best (Wynn and Hoffmann, 2000).

The route of administration of any vaccine is also very important, as is the choice of a suitable adjuvant. Presentation of antigens via an engineered vector organism can overcome both problems. For example, Bacillus Calmette–Guérin (BCG) has been engineered to produce an intracellular schistosome GST and this has induced a strong and long-lasting response in mice when given by the intranasal route (a mixed response of GST-specific immunoglobulin – IgG2a, IgG2b and IgA in serum and IgA in bronchial lavage fluids). A vaccine against schistosomiasis haematobium (Sh28GST – Bilhvax) together with praziquantel treatment is undergoing field trials in Senegal.

ZOONOTIC ASPECTS

Animal hosts are extremely important in the transmission of *S. japonicum* and *S. mekongi* and in some countries can maintain the parasite in the absence of humans. In mainland China infection occurs in 40 species of domestic and wild animals (Jordan *et al.*, 1993) and is important as a serious cause of morbidity and mortality in cattle and goats. In the Dongting Lake area of Hunan, 60% of cattle and buffaloes, 24% of pigs, 9% of dogs and 7% of people were found to be infected. Dogs and pigs play an important part in maintaining transmission

on the island of Leyte in the Philippines, although many other species of animals are infected, as they are on Sulawesi (Indonesia) and used to be in Japan. Molecular studies indicate that *S. japonicum* is a species complex of many sibling species, and in Taiwan the local form of *S. japonicum* occurs only in animals and is not infective to humans. The dog appears to be the only reservoir host of *S. mekongi* in Laos. *S. sinensium* is a little known species with a laterally spined egg found a few times in humans and rodents in China and Thailand (Greer *et al.*, 1989), while the 'Tonle Sap schistosome' has been newly discovered in humans living around Lake Tonle Sap in Cambodia (Pecoulas *et al.*, 1995).

S. mansoni has been reported frequently from animals (of 38 species) but in many cases they do not appear to have any epidemiological significance. However, baboons and green monkeys are apparently maintaining infections among themselves in areas of East Africa and rodents may act as reservoir hosts in East Africa, Senegal and Guadeloupe and particularly in Brazil, where up to 15 species appear to be of increasing importance in maintaining infection in urban and periurban areas of the north-east (Mott *et al.*, 1995).

Animals appear to be of little or no importance in the transmission of *S. haematobium*, although various primates have been found infected, nor are they for *S. intercalatum*.

The schistosomes found in humans and animals in Africa can be divided into two groups of sibling species. Hybridization can occur experimentally within members of each group but is not common in nature. In the *S. haematobium/S. intercalatum* group, *S. mattheei* Veglia and Le Roux, 1929, is a parasite of sheep, cattle, wild animals and occasionally humans in southern Africa. The eggs in the faeces or urine have a terminal spine and measure 120–180 μm in length (Fig. 124). Curiously, in all human cases, the eggs have occurred together with those of *S. haematobium* or *S. mansoni*; the females of *S. mattheei* are known to be capable of producing eggs parthenogenetically and are perhaps carried by excess males of the other species. *S. bovis* (Sonsino, 1876) Blanchard, 1895, is similar to *S. haematobium* and is found in cattle in southern Europe, in Iraq and over much of Africa, but there have been very few genuine infections in humans (Mouchet *et al.*, 1988). *S. margrebowiei* Le Roux, 1933, is a common parasite of antelopes in Africa but the few human cases reported might be spurious. *S. rodhaini* Brumpt, 1931, is closely related to *S. mansoni* and is found in rodents and carnivores in Central Africa; it has been reported once from a human. *S. curassoni*, Brumpt 1931, is a parasite of domestic ruminants in West Africa and has been doubtfully reported from humans.

The cercariae of various mammal and bird schistosomes penetrate the skin of humans in many areas of the world but do not develop further. In a sensitized host they cause dermatitis at the site of entry, with irritation, pruritus, macules and papules ('swimmers' itch' or 'schistosome dermatitis'). Examples are the cercariae of the bird parasites *Austrobilharzia terrigalensis* (Australia), *Bilharziella polonica* (Europe), *Gigantobilharzia sturniae* (Japan), *G. huttoni* (Florida, USA), *Microbilharzia variglandis* (Delaware, USA), *Trichobilharzia brevis* (Japan), *T. maegraithi* (Thailand), *T. ocellata* (worldwide) and *T. stagnicolae* (USA) and cercariae of mammalian species of schistosomes, such as *Heterobilharzia americana* (Louisiana, USA), *Orientobilharzia turkestanica* (China and Iran), *Ornithobilharzia turkestanicum* (Iran), *Schistosoma bovis* (Africa), *S. spindale* (Asia) and *Schistosomatium douthitti* (North America).

Schistosome dermatitis is more of a nuisance than a serious medical problem when it occurs in bathers or water-sports enthusiasts using lakes frequented by waterfowl, but is of real economic importance among rice planters in China, Malaysia and Vietnam.

Family Paragonimidae

Paragonimus westermani
(Kerbert, 1878) Braun, 1899

SYNONYMS
Distoma westermani (*D. westermanii*) Kerbert, 1878; *D. ringeri* Cobbold, 1880.

DISEASE AND COMMON NAMES
Paragonimiasis or paragonimosis; pulmonary distomiasis, Oriental lung fluke infection.

LOCAL NAMES
Pa-yard bai-mai nai pod (Thai).

GEOGRAPHICAL DISTRIBUTION
Paragonimus westermani is widely distributed in the Chekiang Province of China, Korea, Laos, the Philippines, Taiwan and Thailand and also occurs in smaller areas of India, Indonesia, Japan, Malaysia and Vietnam, with one or two cases in Russia and Poland. Although there are at least 14 other species that have been reported from humans, most of the estimated 21 million cases in 39 countries worldwide are due to *P. westermani*, with 195 million people at risk.

LOCATION IN HOST
The adults are typically found in pulmonary cysts, usually in pairs.

MORPHOLOGY
A living *Paragonimus* is a thick fleshy fluke measuring 8–16 × 4–8 mm and is reddish-brown in colour, with a tegument covered in simple or toothed spines. The ventral sucker lies just anterior to the middle of the body and is about the same size as the oral sucker. The testes are almost side by side in the posterior part of the body. The large excretory bladder is usually apparent in sections of the worm (Fig. 18 and Plate 4). The yellowish-brown egg is ovoid and thick-shelled. It measures 80–110 µm × 50–60 µm, with a rather flattened operculum, which gives the impression of being too small, and is unembryonated when laid (Fig. 123).

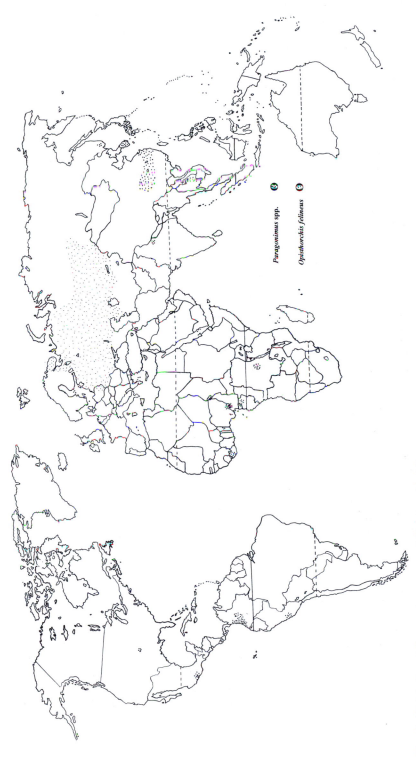

Paragonimus spp.

Opisthorchis felineus

Map 3. Distribution of *Paragonimus* spp. and *Opisthorchis felineus*.

LIFE CYCLE

The eggs are usually swallowed and pass out in the faeces but may also escape in sputum. For further development they have to reach water. The miracidia hatch after 3 weeks in water (at an optimum temperature of 27°C) and penetrate freshwater snails. These are operculate genera, of which the most important is *Semisulcospira* (*S. libertina* is an intermediate host species in China, Japan, Taiwan and Korea). Other important snails are *S. amurensis, Thiara granifera* and *Oncomelania nosophora* (see Fig. 1).

In the snail the miracidia develop into sporocysts followed by two generations of rediae, and finally, in about 3 months, give rise to very short-tailed cercariae. The cercariae emerge from the snail and swim in the water, where they can survive for only 24–48 h.

If cercariae find freshwater crabs, principally *Eriocheir*, the mitten crab in Asia and also *Potamon* (Fig. 19) and *Sesarma*, or freshwater crayfish (*Astacus*), they penetrate and encyst in the gills or muscles as metacercariae (measuring 250–500 μm). Freshwater crustaceans can probably also become infected by ingesting unencysted cercariae in the water or even inside an infected snail.

The crustacean intermediate hosts are eaten by humans as food. If they are eaten raw, the metacercariae hatch in the duodenum and young worms penetrate through the intestinal wall and pass across to the abdominal wall in about 6 h. The immature flukes burrow through the diaphragm to the

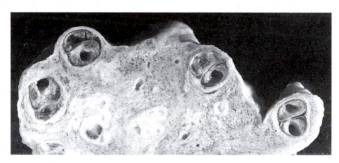

Fig. 18. Cut portion of lung (of a tiger) with cysts containing pairs of adult *Paragonimus.* Note large excretory bladder in each fluke.

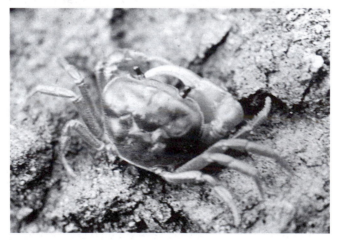

Fig. 19. *Potamon*, a crab second intermediate host of *Paragonimus* in Asia.

pleural cavity in 6–10 days and enter the lung capsule in 15–20 days. The first eggs are passed 60–70 days after infection. Although *Paragonimus* is hermaphrodite, two worms are necessary for fertilization to take place (Fig. 19 and Plate 4). This is true for the usual diploid form of *P. westermani*, but there is also a triploid form, in which parthenogenesis can occur; the adults of the latter are larger and more pathogenic and the eggs differ in size and shape (see Blair *et al.*, 1999). The adult worms can live for 20 years but usually die after about 6 years.

CLINICAL MANIFESTATIONS

There are no recognizable symptoms accompanying the migratory phases.

The first signs are usually fever with a dry cough, sometimes accompanied by bloodstained sputum containing eggs after rupture of the cysts. Chest pain can be severe and, if the infection is heavy, there is sometimes increasing dyspnoea and bronchitis. Many patients with haemoptysis are diagnosed as suffering from pulmonary tuberculosis.

Cerebral paragonimiasis may result in epileptic seizures, as well as headaches, visual disturbances and symptoms of meningitis.

PATHOGENESIS

Pulmonary. As flukes grow in the lungs they cause an inflammatory reaction and become surrounded by a cyst, possibly caused by softening followed by fibrosis (Plate 4). However, as the cyst wall is usually lined with columnar epithelium, it is probable that, in most cases, it represents the expanded wall of a bronchus. The capsule is collagenous and oedematous, with plasma cells, eosinophils, neutrophils, macrophages and fibroblasts. The cyst measures about 1 cm in diameter after 90 days and is filled with a thick brownish fluid containing eggs. Bronchopneumonia may result when a cyst bursts or retains an opening into a bronchus. Eggs are often present in the lung tissues and cause pseudotubercles similar to those caused by schistosome eggs, with infiltration by eosinophils and lymphocytes, followed by giant cells and fibroblasts.

Extrapulmonary. Adults are sometimes found in many parts of the body, particularly in the organs of the abdominal cavity or subcutaneous tissues. In these sites the worms are rarely fertilized and presumably have developed from larvae that lost their way. This occurs more frequently with species of *Paragonimus* which are less adapted to humans than *P. westermani*. Most serious complications follow the presence of flukes in the brain (Fig. 20). This may be common in areas of high endemicity (e.g. over 5000 cases per annum in South Korea). Adults found in

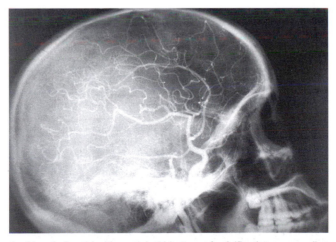

Fig. 20. Radiograph of head of a girl with soap-bubble type of calcification surrounding cysts containing adult *Paragonimus* in occipital lobes.

the brain usually have eggs, unlike those recovered from other extrapulmonary sites; it is believed that they migrate from ruptured lung cysts along the soft tissues surrounding the veins into the cranium. The flukes cause necrosis of the surrounding brain substance and are eventually encapsulated, with granulomas surrounding released eggs lying along the fibrous wall of the cyst. When a fluke dies, the cavity of the lesion becomes filled with purulent material. Lesions may occur in the cerebral cortex, cerebellum, basal ganglia and medulla oblongata. Cerebral paragonimiasis can easily be confused with brain disease caused by other helminths, such as *Schistosoma japonicum, Gnathostoma spinigerum* and *Parastrongylus cantonensis* or larvae of *Echinococcus granulosus* and *Taenia solium*, as well as with viral or bacterial infections and with brain tumours.

Levels of non-specific IgE are elevated in infection and IgG4 levels are also very high, possibly to obstruct IgE-mediated immunopathogenicity. Immune evasion mechanisms are probably employed by the parasites, with periodic sloughing of the outer calyx layer on the tegument.

DIAGNOSIS

Clinical. A cough with brown sputum but otherwise good health is often indicative of a light infection in a patient from an endemic area. Characteristic nodular or ring shadows apparent on X-ray or computer-assisted tomography (CT) scan can be recognized by an expert, but the disease is often mistaken for tuberculosis.

Parasitological. A certain method of diagnosis is to find the characteristic eggs in sputum or faeces, which need to be differentiated from those of *Achillurbainia* (see below). Various concentration techniques may be necessary for detection of eggs in faeces (see p. 258) as, in chronic infections, very few eggs may be passed; centrifugation with 2% NaOH is a method that can be used.

Immunological. The intradermal (ID) test has been widely used for many years and is useful in differentiating paragonimiasis from tuberculosis, but it is very non-specific and the test lasts for many years after cure or the death of parasites. There have been numerous trials of ELISA tests in the last 20 years, some using crude antigens, but recently more specific ES antigens (probably cysteine proteases) and tests for parasite antigen using mAbs have increased sensitivity and specificity (Ikeda, 1998; Blair *et al.*, 1999). Dot ELISAs using dried antigens dotted on nitrocellulose plates are also being used. Immunological techniques can differentiate between species of *Paragonimus*, particularly between *P. heterotremus* and *P. westermani* (Dekumyoy *et al.*, 1998).

TREATMENT

The drug praziquantel has revolutionized treatment in the last few years when given at 25 mg kg^{-1}, three times a day after meals for 3 days. Side-effects are usually minor and short-lived. Triclabendazole at 5 mg kg^{-1} daily for 3 days has also proved to be effective in cases in Africa and South America, one of which was resistant to praziquantel.

Surgery, which used to be necessary for cerebral cases, is now rarely used since the advent of effective drug therapy, except for some cases of cutaneous infection where flukes can be easily removed.

EPIDEMIOLOGY

Paragonimiasis can be contracted from both raw and pickled crabs and crayfish. In the Philippines a dish called kinagang is made from crab juice and in the Chekiang province of China 'drunken crabs' (*Potamon* sp.) are eaten alive after steeping in rice wine. In Japan crabs (usually *Eriocheir* sp.) are usually eaten well-cooked but the metacercariae contaminate knives, hands and chopping-boards during preparation in the kitchen and are then accidentally transferred to salad vegetables. Crushed crayfish juice is used as a treatment of measles in Korea and in this way young children become infected. In Japan, wild boar, hens and ducks appear to act as paratenic hosts. Paratenic hosts (including rodents) are likely to be important in transmission to large carnivores.

Metacercarial cysts accumulate during the life of the crab and in large specimens there may be as many as 1000 cysts g^{-1} of tissue.

PREVENTION AND CONTROL

Metacercarial cysts in the crustaceans are killed by heating in water at 55°C for 5 min and even light cooking renders them safe. However, cysts can live for up to 48 h when frozen at -20°C, although they die in minutes when dried.

Where zoonotic infections are rare, sanitary improvements to prevent eggs reaching snail habitats in water can be used. In Korea there has been a reduction in prevalence caused by increasing industrialization and pollution of habitats.

National campaigns need to involve public awareness and community participation, food control, sanitary waste disposal and adequate monitoring and surveillance (WHO, 1995).

ZOONOTIC ASPECTS

Paragonimus westermani is a natural parasite of carnivores; in fact, the specific name honours a director of Amsterdam zoo, where the first specimens were found in the lungs of a tiger. It is found especially in the members of the cat family, such as the tiger, leopard and domestic cat, in most parts of its range but has also been reported from dogs, pigs and monkeys. In China, Japan and Korea, animal hosts are probably not of importance in transmission to humans, while in Indonesia, Malaysia and Sri Lanka infection is confined entirely to animals and human cases do not occur.

Over 30 probably valid species of *Paragonimus* have been described (Blair *et al.*, 1999) differing (often slightly) in morphology and life cycle. Many cause zoonotic infections in humans in various parts of the world (WHO, 1995), as outlined below.

Africa. *P. africanus* Voelker and Vogel, 1965, and *P. uterobilateralis* Voelker and Vogel, 1965, are parasites of the mongoose, civet cat and humans in Cameroon and eastern Nigeria and occasionally also in 12 other countries of West and Central Africa (WHO, 1995).

Americas. *P. caliensis* Little, 1968, is a natural parasite of opossums in Central and South America. *P. kellicotti* Ward, 1908, is found in many carnivores, pigs and opossums in North America, with a few cases in humans in Canada and two in the USA. *P. mexicanus* Miyazaki and Ishii, 1968, is found in many carnivores and opossums and occasionally humans in North, Central and South America; most cases are in Ecuador and cerebral infections are not infrequent.

Asia. *P. bangkokensis* Miyazaki and Vajrasthira, 1967, is found in cats and other carnivores in China, Russia and Thailand. *P. heterotremus* Chen and Hsia, 1964, is found in carnivores and rodents in China, Laos, Thailand and Vietnam. *P. miyazaki* Kamo *et al.*, 1961, is a parasite of carnivores in Japan, and adults do not mature in humans. *P. ohirai* Miyazaki, 1939, is a parasite of rats and mice in Japan. *P. philippinensis* Ito *et al.*, 1978, is primarily a parasite of dogs in the Philippines. *P. pulmonalis* (Baelz, 1883) Miyazaki, 1978, is found in cats and dogs in Japan, Korea and Taiwan. *P. sadoensis* Miyazaki *et al.*, 1968, has been found only in humans in Japan. *P. (= Pagumogonimus) skrjabini* Chen, 1960 (= *P. hueitungensis* Chung *et al.*, 1975) is a parasite of cats, dogs and palm civets in China: in human infections worms do not mature and the young migratory worms are often subcutaneous or cerebral.

Family Achillurbainiidae

Achillurbainia nouveli Dolfuss, 1939, was first found in a palpebro-orbital abscess from a Malayan leopard in a zoo in France. An adult was subsequently found in a 10-year-old Chinese girl. The adults are common in the lungs of rats (*Rattus muelleri*) in West Malaysia and freshwater crabs probably act as second intermediate hosts. *A. recondita* Travassos, 1942, developmental stages have been found in humans in Brazil, Honduras and Louisiana, USA; adults are usually in opossums.

Poikilorchis (or probably *Achillurbainia*) **congolensis** Fain and Vandepitte, 1957, is a similar parasite and was first found in a retroauricular cyst in Congo Republic. Similar eggs have been found in cysts in two boys in Sarawak and in Cameroon and Nigeria. The eggs are similar to those of *Paragonimus* but are smaller (63 μm × 40 μm).

Family Opisthorchidae

Clonorchis sinensis
(Cobbold, 1875) Looss, 1907

SYNONYMS
Distoma sinense Cobbold, 1875; *Opisthorchis sinensis* Blanchard, 1895.

Clonorchis was erected as a genus on the basis of the shape of the testes, but it is doubtful that this is sufficient to warrant separation from the very closely related genus *Opisthorchis*. However, it still persists in the literature and, unless there is a formal decision by the International Commisssion on Zoological Nomenclature, it is reluctantly retained here.

DISEASE AND POPULAR NAMES
Clonorchiasis or clonorchiosis, opisthorchiasis sinense; Chinese liver fluke disease.

LOCAL NAMES
Oogyubyo, Hareyamai or Suishobyo (Japanese).

GEOGRAPHICAL DISTRIBUTION
About 7 million cases in nine countries in the world (with 290 million people at risk); in China (4.7 million cases), Hong Kong (0.3 million), India (rare in Assam), North Korea (0.95 million), Russia (Siberia), Taiwan and Vietnam (1 million).

LOCATION IN HOST
Adults inhabit the bile-ducts just under the liver capsule, but in massive infections may be found in the gall-bladder, pancreatic ducts and all bile-ducts as well.

MORPHOLOGY
Adult flukes measure 11–20 mm × 3–4.5 mm and are elongated and extremely flat, tapering anteriorly and rounded posteriorly; when living they are almost transparent. There can be a wide variation in the size of adults, depending upon the intensity of infection and on the diameter of the bile-ducts in which they are living. The tegument has no spines. The ventral sucker is smaller than the oral and is situated about a quarter of the length from the anterior end. The two deeply lobed testes lie one behind the other at the posterior end. They provide an important identification feature, particularly in stained specimens (Fig. 2).

LIFE CYCLE (Fig. 21)
In most infections there are usually only a few adults present but there can be up to 6000 and a daily egg production of 1000 eggs ml^{-1} bile or 600 g^{-1} faeces may be recorded.

The small yellowish-brown eggs (Fig. 123) measure 23–35 μm × 10–20 μm and have an operculum at one end and a small knob at the other. The eggs contain a fully formed miracidium when laid and pass from the bile-ducts into the intestine and out with the faeces. They have to reach water, where they do not hatch but are ingested by various species of snails (*Alocinma longicornis* in southern China, *Bulimus fuchsiana* in northern China and *Parafossarulus manchouricus* in most endemic areas are commonly infected species). The miracidia hatch in the rectum of the snail and develop into sporocysts in the hepatopancreas, where they give rise to numerous rediae.

Cercariae are produced 21–30 days after infection. These have an unforked keeled tail, and emerge into water, where they live for only 1–2 days, unless they can penetrate beneath the scales of freshwater fish and form a metacercarial cyst in the subcutaneous connective tissues, usually those near the caudal fin.

Over 100 species of fish have been implicated as secondary intermediate hosts of *C. sinensis* and up to 3000 cysts

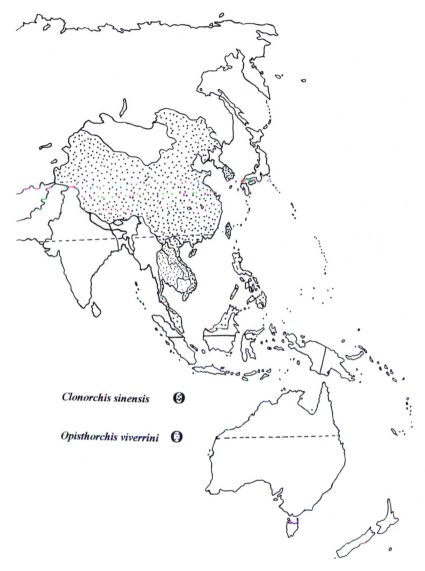

Map 4. Distribution of *Clonorchis sinensis* and *Opisthorchis viverrini*.

have been found in a single fish. Metacercarial cysts measure 140 µm × 120 µm and are infective in about 23 days. When fish are eaten raw or undercooked, the metacercarial cysts hatch out in the human duodenum and the young flukes migrate up the bile-ducts, maturing in 3–4 weeks. The adult flukes can live for up to 26 years but on average survive for 10 years (Chen *et al.*, 1994).

CLINICAL MANIFESTATIONS

The majority of infections (about 70%) are symptomless and the presence of worms is only diagnosed at autopsy, when up to 100 flukes may be found in the bile-ducts. Moderate infections, due to the presence of 100–1000 flukes, result in diarrhoea, abdominal discomfort and some splenomegaly. When a heavy infection, which may consist of many thousands of worms (the maximum recorded being 21,000), is contracted at one time, there

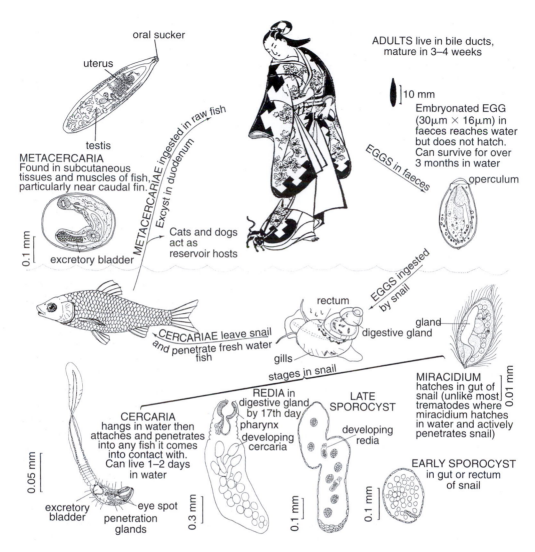

Fig. 21. Life cycle of *Clonorchis sinensis*. Figure of courtesan and cat by Kaigetsudo.

are additional symptoms, such as a sudden onset of fever, acute pain in the upper right quadrant, liver enlargement and tenderness, oedema, an increased erythrocyte sedimentation rate and up to 40% eosinophilia; symptoms of cholecystitis and hepatitis follow a few weeks later, and there may also be bouts of recurrent gall-bladder colic. There is usually loss of weight, with slight jaundice, and later there may be tachycardia, with palpitations and vertigo. However, in an endemic area, parasites are often acquired progressively over a period of months or years, and the onset of symptoms is more insidious.

Portal hypertension may occur with splenomegaly (this is found in 20–40% of autopsies) and ascites is almost always present in fatal cases, although not usually diagnosed during life.

Prognosis depends largely on the number of parasites present and, as the great majority of cases have only light infections, no ill health ensues. However, the prevalence can be so high in endemic regions that even the low proportion of heavily infected individuals can provide an important source of morbidity.

Death is only likely to occur where there is an intercurrent bacterial infection (apart from the possibility of cholangiocarcinoma); salmonellae in particular flourish in bile-ducts attacked by *Clonorchis*. A similar relationship has been reported with urinary schistosomiasis, where it has been shown that *Salmonella typhi* may live on the inside and outside of the body of the schistosomes.

PATHOGENESIS

At operation the presence of severe infection is obvious from gross examination of the liver because the thickened bile-ducts appear as pale patches on the surface. If the liver is cut, the slimy, brownish flukes often emerge from the ducts.

The adult worms presumably feed mainly on the biliary epithelium but, unlike *Fasciola hepatica*, have no spines on the tegument to cause mechanical damage. In the early stages there is an inflammatory reaction in the biliary epithelium and in heavy infections there is cellular infiltration, consisting mainly of lymphocytes and leucocytes, particularly in the outer part of the fibrous wall. This is followed by hyperplasia and metaplasia of the epithelium, with much mucus, and there may be the formation of new biliary ductules (Fig. 22). Because immature *Clonorchis* migrate up the bile-ducts, there is not the pathology associated with early *Fasciola* infections, which burrow through the liver parenchyma (see p. 47). In the chronic stage there is an encapsulating fibrosis of the ducts and destruction of the adjacent liver parenchyma. A fibrotic reaction surrounds eggs that reach the liver parenchyma, but there is not the granuloma formation around intact eggs which occurs in schistosomiasis (Fig. 14).

Stones are common in the bile-ducts and gall-bladder in cases of *C. sinensis* infection and were found in 70% of autopsies in a study in Hong Kong. The remains of adult worms are sometimes found inside the stones. Recurrent pyogenic cholangitis is one of the most important complications of clonorchiasis, as well as of ascariasis (p. 151). The cholangitis often follows a long relapsing course, eventually leading to widespread fibrosis. Cirrhosis of the liver is found in about 10% of autopsies, but there is no evidence that it is directly related to the presence of the parasite and it may be coincidental or accentuated by an accompanying bacterial infection. *Clonorchis* often enters the pancreatic ducts and causes pancreatitis, with adenomatous hyperplasia; occasionally there may be acute inflammation.

Carcinoma of the bile-ducts is found in association with clonorchiasis in Canton and Hong Kong and is far more common than in non-endemic regions (IARC Working Group, 1994); it has also been reported from experimental infections in dogs and cats.

IMMUNOLOGY OF LIVER FLUKES

Immunological aspects of infection with *Fasciola hepatica* (see p. 46) have been extensively studied in domestic ruminants and in laboratory rodents. Infections are associated with blood eosinophilia, strong antibody responses and immune-mediated inflammation in the liver and bile-ducts. Evidence sluggests that infection elicits strongly polarized Th2 responses but also that flukes are capable of down-regulating host immunity in various ways. Infections with *Clonorchis sinensis* similarly induce eosinophils and profound inflammatory responses in the liver (in some cases resulting in cholangiocarcinoma) as well as parasite-specific IgA, IgE and IgG; it can be assumed therefore that a similar polarization of the immune response occurs. Evidence for immunity to reinfection in humans is not strong, there being no decline in prevalence or intensity of infection in chronically exposed populations. Experimental studies using *Opisthorchis viverrini* in hamsters have clarified some aspects of the immune response and suggested the operation of a degree of immune protection. This has also been proposed in human infections with this species. In an endemic area individuals who were egg-negative had higher levels of IgA, IgG and IgM than those who were egg-positive and they showed recognition of specific antibodies not detected by antigens of infected individuals. Studies in hamsters have also

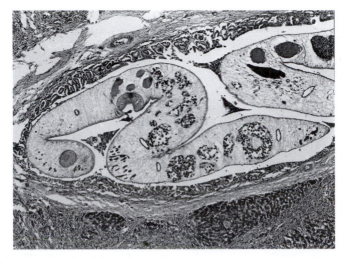

Fig. 22. Section of liver with two adult *Clonorchis* in bile-duct. There is marked epithelial proliferation, oedema of the mucosa and some fibrosis (see also Plate 6). The ventral sucker, uterus filled with many eggs and testes (in fluke on left) are apparent.

shown that parasite antigen accumulates in the tissues around the worms and is associatated with marked inflammatory responses.

DIAGNOSIS

Parasitological. The most important method of diagnosis is examination of the faeces for eggs (p. 254). When eggs are scanty, concentration methods (Kato–Katz or sedimentation techniques) can be used or a duodenal aspirate taken. In symptomless infections large numbers of eggs are usually produced. Any eggs found need to be distinguished from those of *Heterophyes, Metagonimus, Metorchis* or rarely *Dicrocoelium,* which are similar.

Immunodiagnosis. Intradermal and complement fixation tests have been in use for many years but remain positive for many years after cure and they also cross-react with *Paragonimus* and *Schistosoma.*

An ELISA using a purified recombinant antigen of adult worms (mol. weight 28 kDa) looks promising (Yong *et al.*, 1998), as does application of a dot-immunogold–silver stain (Liu *et al.*, 1995).

TREATMENT

Praziquantel at three times 25 mg kg^{-1} daily for 1–3 days or at a single dose of 40 mg kg^{-1} (given in Korea to reduce side-effects) is stated to be effective for adults or children over the age of 4. However, *Clonorchis* is not nearly as sensitive to the paralytic action of the drug as are the schistosomes.

EPIDEMIOLOGY

Infection is widespread in some endemic areas: 40% in adults in the Red River delta region of North Korea, 24% in some villages of the Amur River area of Siberia, 23% in Hong Kong, 15% in Guangdong (China).

Infection is usually contracted from eating raw or undercooked fish and fish dishes (usually cyprinids, such as *Carassius carassius, Cyprio carpus* and *Pseudorasbora parva,* but about 110 species have been incriminated (see WHO, 1995)). However, the metacercarial cysts are very sticky and can stick to the hands and to knives and boards, which are subsequently used for chopping salad vegetables, so that the parasite can sometimes be transmitted even when fishes are cooked before eating.

In South Fukien province in China, fish is not commonly eaten raw, but decoctions of raw crushed fish are used as a cure for asthma and freshwater shrimps (which can act as a secondary intermediate host in this area) are eaten as a cure for nosebleeds. Human cases in this province are mostly in children; the parasite being maintained in dogs. In South Korea, infection formerly occurred in men, who traditionally eat raw fish to increase their thirst at rice wine drinking parties.

In rural areas of China, human faeces ('night-soil') was commonly used to enrich ponds containing food fish and, as these ponds also often contain suitable snails, maximum opportunities for continuation of the life cycle were provided (Plate 5). Nowadays, however, untreated faeces are not commonly used in mainland China.

There is a recent tendency in many people in Europe and North America to eat more raw and lightly cooked fish and there is a danger of cases of food-borne helminths increasing in tourists and from imported foodstuffs.

CONTROL AND PREVENTION

The most obvious method of prevention is thorough cooking of fish, but this is not always feasible as raw fish is a traditional item of diet in endemic regions. Deep-freezing of fish at $-30°C$ for 32 h is recommended for killing cysts.

Control is possible by sanitary disposal of faeces to prevent eggs reaching ponds or slow-flowing streams and canals. Even storage of faeces for a few days or addition of ammonium salts as fertilizer before adding to ponds is an effective measure. The use of molluscicides is difficult because of toxicity to fish.

National campaigns should follow the same guidelines as for *Paragonimus* and other food-borne trematodes (see WHO, 1995).

ZOONOTIC ASPECTS

Dogs are the most important reservoir hosts but infections occur in most fish-eating carnivores. Pigs and rats can also be naturally infected.

In the South Fukien province of China, about 30% of dogs are infected and these are almost entirely responsible for perpetuating infection.

Opisthorchis viverrini
(Poirer, 1886) Stiles and Hassall, 1896

SYNONYM
Distoma viverrini Poirer, 1886. The name should more correctly have been *O. viverrinae*.

DISEASE AND LOCAL NAME
Opisthorchiasis or opisthorchiosis viverrini; Pa-yard bai-mai nai tub (Thai).

GEOGRAPHICAL DISTRIBUTION
Thailand, Cambodia and Laos, with about 9 million cases (and 50 million at risk), of which 7.3 million are in Thailand (see Map 4, p. 39).

LOCATION IN HOST
Adults inhabit the bile-ducts.

MORPHOLOGY
The adults are very similar to those of *C. sinensis* but the testes are lobed rather than dendritic, and there are differences in the flame-cell pattern.

LIFE CYCLE
Very similar to that of *C. sinensis*. Snails involved in Thailand are subspecies of *Bithynia siamensis*, with 15 species of fish belonging to seven genera acting as second intermediate hosts (WHO, 1995), such as *Puntius orphoides* ('pla pok' in Thai) and *Hampala dispar* ('pla suud'), which are eaten either raw ('koi pla') or semi-fermented ('pla ra').

CLINICAL MANIFESTATIONS AND PATHOGENESIS
The majority of infected individuals (about 80%) show no symptoms or signs attributable to the parasite apart from eosinophilia and there are likely to be less than 1000 eggs g^{-1} faeces. Although there may be local damage to the bile-duct epithelium, there is

no noticeable damage to liver function. With heavier infections (10,000–30,000 eggs g^{-1} faeces), diarrhoea, epigastric and upper right-quadrant pain, anorexia, lassitude, jaundice and mild fever may slowly develop. In long-standing infections there may be oedema of the legs, accompanied by ascites, mild periportal fibrosis, hepatomegaly, inflammation and biliary epithelium hyperplasia.

In heavy infections the gall-bladder becomes enlarged and non-functional, with cholecystitis, cholangitis, liver abscess and gallstones. Cholangiocarcinoma is strongly correlated with *O. viverrini* infection (Plate 6) and few patients live longer than 6 months after diagnosis (Elkins *et al.*, 1990; IARC Working Group, 1994).

The immunology of liver-fluke infections is discussed on p. 41.

DIAGNOSIS AND TREATMENT

Diagnosis is by finding eggs in the faeces. They are similar to those of *C. sinensis* but are slightly narrower (30 μm × 12 μm) and more regularly ovoid, without such a clear shoulder at the operculum (Fig. 123). The eggs of an intestinal fluke, *Phaneropsolus bonnei* (see p. 59), which has been reported from humans in north-east Thailand, are similar in size but are smoothly ovoid and contain an undifferentiated ovum when passed in the faeces.

Immunodiagnosis is not widely used but a mAb ELISA using mAbs that can detect an 89 kDa metabolic antigen from *O. viverrini* in faeces is stated to be both sensitive and specific (Sirisinha *et al.*, 1995).

Praziquantel can be given as for *Clonorchis* and is equally effective.

EPIDEMIOLOGY

There are prevalence rates of over 70% in ethnically similar rural communities of north-eastern Thailand (35% overall) and Laos, and it has been estimated that infection costs $120 million annually in lost wages and medical care. Infection in humans occurs principally at the end of the rainy season and the beginning of the dry season (September to February), as fish contain more metacercariae and are more easily caught before

ponds dry in March. Infection is very uncommon in children under the age of 5.

The metacercarial cysts are slightly less resistant to pickling than those of *C. sinensis,* but thorough cooking or deep-freezing of fish is the only sure method of personal prevention.

ZOONOTIC ASPECTS

O. viverrini is a natural parasite of the civet cat but is common in domestic cats and dogs, which play a role in maintaining transmission, although human-to-human transmission is common.

Opisthorchis felineus
(Rivolta, 1884) Blanchard, 1895

SYNONYMS

Distoma felineum Rivolta, 1884; *D. sibiricum* Winogradoff, 1892 (first report from humans).

DISEASE AND POPULAR NAME

Opisthorchiasis or opisthorchiosis felineus; cat liver-fluke disease.

GEOGRAPHICAL DISTRIBUTION

About 1.5 million cases (with 14 million at risk): Russia (Siberia with 1.2 million cases), Belarus, Kazakhstan, Ukraine (0.3 million) (see Map 3, p. 33).

LOCATION IN HOST

Adults are found in the distal bile-ducts and sometimes proximal ducts also.

MORPHOLOGY

Adults are identical to those of *O. viverrini*. Differentiation is based on differences in the flame-cell patterns of the cercariae and in the life cycle.

LIFE CYCLE

Very similar to the previous two species. The snail intermediate hosts are species of *Codiella* (= *Bithynia*), particularly *C. leachi*. Twenty-two species of fish belonging to 17 genera transmit infection (see WHO, 1995).

CLINICAL MANIFESTATIONS

Similar to the other two species, except that symptoms are more likely to occur in the acute phase (2–4 weeks after infection), such as high fever, abdominal pain and hepatitis-like symptoms, accompanied by eosinophilia (possibly because more infections are in adult immigrants).

The connection with cholangiocarcinoma is not as clear as with *O. viverrini* or *C. sinensis* (IARC Working Group, 1994), although the ratio of hepatic cell carcinoma to bile-duct carcinoma in uninfected individuals from an endemic area of Siberia was found to be 8:1, while in infected people the ratio was reversed. In a fatal case in Russia, a total of 7400 worms were recovered.

DIAGNOSIS AND TREATMENT

Eggs, which are identical to those of *O. viverrini*, can be recognized in the faeces. They are likely to be scanty in clinically important infections and concentration techniques may be necessary. Immunodiagnostic tests are being investigated.

Treatment as for *C. sinensis*.

EPIDEMIOLOGY

In the central area of western Siberia there are prevalence rates of 40–95% and the highest infection rates in Russia in general are found in river basin areas. In endemic areas of Ukraine rates vary from 5% to 40%. There may be very heavy infections of metacercariae in food fish.

A popular raw fish dish, 'stroganina', is responsible for many infections.

ZOONOTIC ASPECTS

Cats provide an important reservoir host and may have high infection rates. Infection in a range of animals, such as foxes, dogs, cats and pigs, is found over a wide area of eastern Europe. *O. guayaquilensis* is a parasite of cats and dogs with a human focus in an area of Ecuador and *O. noverca* is a common parasite of pigs and dogs with two human cases in India.

Metorchis albidus (Braun, 1893) Looss, 1899, and **M. conjunctus** (Cobbold, 1864) Looss, 1899, are two liver flukes found in North American fish-eating carnivores. The latter species was responsible for infection in 19 people in Canada who ate sashimi in a restaurant. They suffered from upper abdominal pain, low-grade fever and eosinophilia, lasting for up to 4 weeks; praziquantel was very effective in treatment (MacLean *et al.*, 1996).

Pseudamphistomum truncatum (Rudolphi, 1819), Luhe, 1909 is a liver parasite of wild carnivores, cats and dogs and has occasionally been found in humans in Russia (Siberia) from eating raw fish. *P. aethiopicum* Pierantoni, 1942, was reported once from a human in Ethiopia.

Family Dicrocoeliidae

Dicrocoelium dendriticum
(Rudolphi, 1818) Looss, 1899

SYNONYMS

Fasciola lanceolata, F. dendritica, D. lanceolatum.

DISEASE AND POPULAR NAME

Dicrocoeliasis or dicrocoeliosis; lancet-fluke infection.

GEOGRAPHICAL DISTRIBUTION

Dicrocoelium is a cosmopolitan parasite of the bile-ducts of sheep and other herbivores. True human infections are rare, but spurious infections from ingestion of eggs in liver are not uncommon. Real or spurious infection was found in 0.2% of about 27,000 patients in a hospital in Riyadh, Saudi Arabia, and in 0.2% of a rural population in Turkey, and occasional human cases are reported worldwide.

LOCATION IN HOST

Adults live in the bile-ducts.

MORPHOLOGY

Adult worms are flat and lancet-shaped, measuring 5–15 mm × 1.5–2.5 mm. The testes are in tandem just behind the ventral sucker. The vitellaria are restricted and the uterus takes up most of the posterior part of the body.

LIFE CYCLE
This is of great interest zoologically, as *Dicrocoelium* is one of the few trematodes that utilize terrestrial snails as intermediate hosts (*Zebrina* or *Helicella* in Germany). The snail ingests the eggs containing miracidia and eventually the cercariae leave the snail in slime balls, each containing 200–400 cercariae. These are then ingested by ants, and the ants infected with metacercariae are eaten by sheep (or rarely humans) on vegetation. *Dicrocoelium* was present in the livers of 37 autopsy cases in Uzbekistan and infected ants were found on local mulberry trees (Azizova *et al.*, 1988).

CLINICAL MANIFESTATIONS AND PATHOGENESIS
In the few proven cases detected in life, symptoms have been of mild hepatitis.
　　Pathology in animals is similar to that of *Fasciola* but less severe.

DIAGNOSIS AND TREATMENT
Characteristic eggs, measuring 38–45 µm $\times$ 22–30 µm, may be found in the faeces (Fig. 124). It is essential that patients are kept on a liver-free diet for a few days in order to rule out spurious infections. Treatment of one case with triclabendazole was not successful.

Dicrocoelium hospes Looss, 1907, is found in domesticated and wild herbivores in Africa and human cases have been reported from Ethiopia, Ghana, Kenya, Mali and Sierra Leone.

Eurytrema pancreaticum (Janson, 1889) Looss, 1907, is a parasite of the pancreatic ducts of domestic herbivores in Asia and South America. Grasshoppers act as second intermediate hosts. Three cases have been reported from humans (Ishii *et al.*, 1983), with worms in the dilated pancreatic ducts.

Family Fasciolidae

Fasciola hepatica Linnaeus, 1758

SYNONYM
Distomum hepaticum L., 1758.

DISEASE AND POPULAR NAMES
Fascioliasis or fasciolosis, distomiasis; liver-fluke infection, liver-rot (in sheep).

GEOGRAPHICAL DISTRIBUTION
About 2.4 million human cases in 61 countries worldwide (with 180 million at risk). *Fasciola* is primarily an animal parasite of great veterinary importance and is found in sheep and cattle kept on damp and muddy pastures in all the sheep- and cattle-raising areas of the world. Human infections have been reported most frequently from Bolivia, Cuba, Ecuador, Egypt, France, Iran, Peru, Portugal and North Africa and are much more common than previously thought.

LOCATION IN HOST
Adult worms inhabit the bile-ducts.

MORPHOLOGY
The hermaphroditic adult flukes measure 20–30 mm $\times$ 13 mm wide (specimens are usually smaller in heavy infections) and are flat and leaflike, with a spiny tegument (Plate 7).
　　The oral sucker measures 1.0 mm in diameter and the ventral sucker, which lies close behind it, about 1.6 mm. The male and female reproductive systems are both very dendritic, as in *Fasciolopsis buski*, but in *Fasciola* the two gut caeca are also highly branched.
　　The dendritic testes lie one behind the other in the middle portion of the body. The small, highly branched, ovary is in front of the anterior testis. The dendritic vitellaria lie in the lateral fields and have vitelline ducts leading to the ootype. The uterus, filled with eggs, is confined to the anterior third of the body.

LIFE CYCLE
In sheep the eggs are laid in the biliary tracts, reach the intestine and are passed out in the faeces. The undifferentiated ovum develops into a miracidium under moist conditions in 9–15 days at 22–25°C. The miracidium that hatches out of the egg lives for only about 8 h and can move in a film of moisture on damp pastures. For further

development the free-living miracidium must penetrate an amphibious snail, usually a species of *Lymnaea* (mainly *L. truncatula* in Europe, *L. tomentosa* in north-west Africa and *L. viatrix* in South America).

Once inside the snail, there is a sporocyst, followed by two redia stages; the cercariae, which emerge 30–40 days after penetration at 24°C, encyst as metacercariae on vegetation (Fig. 23). This is usually wet grass, but watercress, water mint (in Iran) or other salad vegetables are of most importance in human infections (or perhaps sometimes in drinking water). When cysts are ingested, the larvae excyst in the duodenum, migrate through the intestinal wall and reach the bile-ducts by eating their way through the hepatic parenchyma from the surface of the liver. The adult worms mature in 3–4 months and live for 5–12 years.

CLINICAL MANIFESTATIONS

There is an acute phase corresponding to the period when the young flukes are migrating through the liver tissues (4–8 weeks). Symptoms of dyspepsia, nausea and vomiting, abdominal pain localized to the right hypochondrium or epigastrium and high fever (up to 40°C) ensue, often with sudden onset. Allergic symptoms, such as pruritus and urticaria, can also occur. Anaemia is found in a proportion of cases and the erythrocyte sedimentation rate is often raised. There is a leucocytosis in 50–100% of cases, with high eosinophilia (up to 60%).

The chronic phase ensues when the flukes reach the bile-ducts. There is often painful liver enlargement and occasionally an obstructive jaundice develops later; there may also be pains in the lower chest, with loss of weight. Symptoms are due to inflammation of the epithelial lining of the duct or to obstruction of its lumen and they closely resemble those of biliary disease, with obstructive jaundice and centrilobular cholestasis. Cholelithiasis can also occur as a complication. Many chronic cases are probably asymptomatic and undiagnosed, so the proportion of such cases is unknown. Sometimes parasites in humans develop in ectopic sites in other organs or in the wall of the peritoneal cavity, and cause granulomas.

The parasite is responsible for few deaths but in one case 40 flukes were found to be blocking the bile-ducts at autopsy.

PATHOGENESIS

Most of the knowledge on pathology is based on studies in animals. In sheep, the tracts of the migrating flukes show a coagulation necrosis of the liver cords, with numerous neutrophils, lymphocytes and erythrocytes. The traumatic damage caused is roughly proportional to the number of parasites present and, in sheep, death is usually caused by the presence of over 600 worms. The mature flukes in the bile-ducts cause a secondary adenomatous hyperplasia and desquamation of the lining epithelium of the bile-ducts (which becomes over 2.0 mm thick) with exaggerated Aschoff–Rokitansky crypts. The plasma cells, lymphocytes and eosinophils in the periductal tissues are replaced by a fibrotic reaction leading to great thickening of the walls and a much reduced lumen (Plate 7). Bile-duct hyperplasia and fibrosis of portal tracts has been seen in biopsy specimens in human infections.

The immunology of liver-fluke infections in general is discussed on p. 41.

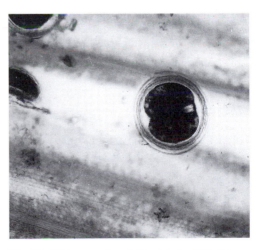

Fig. 23. Metacercariae of *Fasciola hepatica* on blades of grass (actual size 0.3 mm).

DIAGNOSIS

Clinical. Clinical signs are often variable but a triad of fever, liver enlargement and high eosinophilia is very suggestive, particularly if combined with a history of having eaten home-grown watercress a few weeks before.

CT and ultrasound can be of use in visualizing worms in the bile-ducts.

Parasitological. Eggs in the faeces are often scanty and duodenal or bile-duct aspirates can be used. Eggs are large, measuring 130–150 μm × 60–85 μm, and ovoid, with an inconspicuous operculum (Fig. 123). Faeces concentration techniques can be employed, but in about 30% of human cases no eggs can be found in faeces or bile. Spurious infections from ingestion of infected liver can be ruled out by keeping the patient on a liver-free diet for a week.

Immunological. An intradermal test has been used for many years but is not very specific and only becomes positive after a few weeks. Passive haemagglutination is another test that is well established. In the last few years there have been many studies utilizing ELISAs. For instance an IgG4 ELISA, using either recombinant or native protein (cathepsin L1 cysteine proteinase) as antigen, gives very sensitive results with finger-prick blood (O'Neill et al., 1999). An antigen-detection test using sandwich ELISA detected infection by 1 week, with an optimum at 3 weeks. Western immunoblots are useful for confirmation of infection. Tests for detection of Fasciola coproantigens also show great promise. These recent immunological tests can be used for detecting early infections and also for assessing the success of a cure.

TREATMENT

Praziquantel, which has been so effective against almost all other trematode infections, has little effect in fascioliasis. The standard treatment for many years was with bithionol (30–50 mg kg^{-1} given orally on alternate days for 10–15 days or as a single dose of 45 g for an adult and half this for a child) and this is still used. Recently triclabendazole at 10 mg kg^{-1} for 1 or 2 days has given cure rates of 80–90% and is now the drug of choice.

EPIDEMIOLOGY AND ZOONOTIC ASPECTS

There are occasional human cases reported from many countries (61 in total) following ingestion of infected watercress or lettuce and epidemics may occur locally in particularly wet years (e.g. in France a total of 10,000 cases were recorded between 1956 and 1982, principally in two wet and warm periods). Infection is spreading in many parts of the world and it is clear that there are some human endemic regions where human-to-human transmission takes place (Mas Coma et al., 1999). In the Andean altiplano areas of Bolivia there are prevalences of 15–100% and in children in central Peru of 10–34% and probably many cases also at high altitudes in Ecuador. There are also much higher infection rates in the Nile delta, in the Tadzhik Republic (Samarkand) and in the Caspian region of Iran than previously thought. In these areas of high intensity, infections are more common in children (Dalton, 1998).

Infection occurs in up to 50% of sheep and 70% of cattle in many parts of the world and is a major veterinary problem in many countries, but flukes may also be found in goats, donkeys, pigs, camels, horses, rabbits and deer.

The eggs of Fasciola do not usually develop below 10°C (or over 30°C) and in many temperate countries they rest over the winter on pastures, the miracidia hatching out in the spring. However, eggs can develop at lower temperatures in the high Andes foci. Studies of the temperature, of developmental factors in the intermediate and definitive hosts and of rainfall have enabled accurate forecasts of the likely build-up of infection in domestic stock in countries in Europe (Fig. 24).

PREVENTION AND CONTROL

In commercial watercress beds there must be precautions to prevent pollution by faeces of domestic stock.

A vaccine for infections in cattle and sheep is being investigated (Dalton, 1998).

Fasciola gigantica Cobbold, 1856, is a common parasite of cattle, camels and other herbivores in Africa, in Asia and on some Pacific islands. The eggs are larger than those of *F. hepatica* (160–190 µm × 70–90 µm) and the adults are longer (25–75 mm × 12 mm), with more anterior testes, a larger ventral sucker and not so pronounced 'shoulders'. Sporadic cases have been reported from humans in tropical Africa, China, Egypt, Hawaii, Iran, Thailand, Turkey and Uzbekistan. The life cycle and clinical effects are similar to those of *F. hepatica* except that the snail hosts, such as *Lymnaea natalensis* in Africa, are often aquatic, not amphibious.

Immunodiagnostic tests, such as SDS-PAGE using an ES antigen of 27 kDa or a somatic antigen of 38 kDa, or IgM or IgG ELISA, appear to be as effective as for *F. hepatica* and do not cross-react with schistosomiasis.

Fasciola indica Varma, 1953, is found in buffaloes and other herbivorous mammals in Asia, with a very few human cases reported from India and Korea. In Russia *Lymnaea truncatula* acts as first intermediate host for all three species.

Fasciolopsis buski
(Lankester, 1857) Odhner, 1902

SYNONYMS
Distoma buski Lankester, 1857, *Distoma crassum* Busk, 1859.

DISEASE, POPULAR AND LOCAL NAMES
Fasciolopsiasis or fasciolopsiosis; Busk's fluke infection; Pa-yard bai-mai nai lumsi (Thai).

GEOGRAPHICAL DISTRIBUTION
The largest endemic foci of infection are in the Yangtze basin provinces of China but infection also occurs in Bangladesh, Cambodia, India (particularly Assam, but also in Bihar, Madras and Orissa), Indonesia, Laos, Taiwan and central Thailand.

LOCATION IN HOST
Adult flukes are found in the small intestine, attached by the ventral sucker. In heavy infections they may also be present in the stomach and colon.

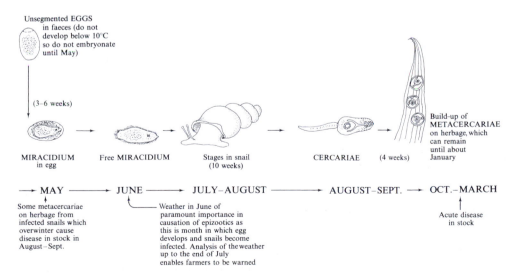

Fig. 24. Effect of weather on the life cycle of *F. hepatica* in western Europe.

MORPHOLOGY

Fasciolopsis is the largest human trematode, measuring on average 30 (20–70) mm × 12 (8–20) mm (Fig. 3). It is a thick, ovoid worm without a cephalic cone and, when living, is pinkish in colour. The tegument is covered with transverse rows of small spines, which are most numerous around the ventral sucker. The ventral sucker is a short distance behind the oral sucker and is about four times as large. The testes are highly branched and lie one behind the other in the posterior part of the body. The organs of the female reproductive system are also branched, as is typical of members of the family Fasciolidae but, unlike the liver fluke *Fasciola,* the two gut caeca are unbranched. The egg is large, 130–140 μm × 80–85 μm (Fig. 123); the yellowish-brown shell is clear and thick and has a small operculum. The egg is unembryonated when laid and is almost identical to that of *Fasciola hepatica*; they can sometimes be differentiated with difficulty when living by the distribution of the lipid granules in the yolk cells, which are uniformly arranged in *Fasciolopsis* and concentrated around the nucleus in *Fasciola,* by differences in the number of yolk cells and by the size of the germinal area. Daily egg production is about 25,000 per fluke.

LIFE CYCLE

Eggs passed in the faeces need to reach water for further development and they take 3–7 weeks at 27–32°C to embryonate fully (they can survive for 3–4 months at 4°C but do not develop). The miracidium that hatches out enters a freshwater planorbid snail, such as *Gyraulis chinensis, Hippeutis cantori* or *Polypylis* (= *Segmentina*) *hemisphaerula,* in which a sporocyst and two redial stages are found. The xiphidocercous cercariae, which emerge from the second-generation rediae, leave the snail and swim in the water. They encyst on the roots or fruits of various freshwater plants, such as the water caltrop (*Trapa bicornis* and *T. natans*) or water chestnut (*Eliocharis tuberosa*), to give an encysted metacercarial stage.

When ingested on edible plants, the metacercariae excyst in the duodenum and the young flukes take 3–4 months to mature in the ileum. The adult worms can produce up to 28,000 eggs 24 h^{-1} but live for only about 6–12 months in humans.

CLINICAL MANIFESTATIONS

In the majority of cases infection is light (fewer than 20 worms or 5000 eggs g^{-1} faeces) and there are no symptoms. With a heavy worm burden there is nausea and diarrhoea, accompanied by intense griping pains in the morning which are relieved by food. Oedema, including a characteristic facial swelling more prominent in the periorbital region, is often found. In children with more than 100 worms the abdomen is usually distended and there may be stunting of growth. The presence of more than 400 worms usually proves fatal to young children.

In about 40% of cases there is an eosinophilia of up to 30%.

PATHOGENESIS

The adult worms cause traumatic inflammatory damage to the mucosa at the site of attachment, often leading to ulceration and haemorrhage, and make the mucosa hyperaemic. They also provoke an excessive secretion of mucus. Toxic by-products produced by the adults are said to cause the facial oedema that is sometimes found and can result in a toxic diarrhoea, but this may be due to a protein-losing enteropathy. When many worms are present, there is also the possibility of obstruction of the bowel, with resultant stasis.

DIAGNOSIS

Recovery of eggs in faeces is the only method used in practice and various concentration methods can be employed if necessary. The eggs can be easily differentiated from those of *Gastrodiscoides* and are larger than those of echinostomes but cannot usually be distinguished from those of *Fasciola*.

TREATMENT

Praziquantel (15–60 mg kg^{-1}) and albendazole have both been used successfully, although the latter had some failures with children.

EPIDEMIOLOGY

There are often high prevalence rates in endemic areas: 39% in Dacca, Bangladesh, 70% in Jiangxi, China, 70% in Maharashtra and 29% in Bombay, India, 27% in South Kalimantan, Indonesia (57% in children), 3.8% in Vientiane, Laos, and 17% in Supanburi, Thailand (Yu and Mott, 1994).

The seed pods of water caltrop (also known as water ling) are probably the most important source of human infection, because this plant is grown in ponds fertilized with night-soil, while the other plants involved are usually grown in running streams. Before the nuts of the water caltrop or the bulbs of water chestnut are eaten, the outer covering is removed with the teeth and this provides the principal mode of infection. This habit is particularly common in children, who are usually more heavily infected than adults. In markets caltrop nuts are kept fresh by sprinkling with water and thus the cysts are prevented from drying.

In Vietnam the roots of the water bamboo (*Zizania aquatica*, *Salvinia natans* and *Lemna polyrhiza*) and water hyacinth (*Eichornia crassipes*) are also eaten, and in Thailand lotus (*Nymphoea lotus*), a watercress (*Neptunia cleracea*) and water morning glory (*Ipomea aquatica*).

In Taiwan and Thailand water plants are collected and fed to pigs, which helps to maintain a reservoir of infection. In Thailand infection is confined to regions growing water caltrops although the nuts are grown in many other non-endemic areas also; this is probably because cysts dry up during transport or because the nuts are only eaten cooked in these other regions.

PREVENTION AND CONTROL

Water vegetables need to be carefully peeled and washed. Boiling for 1–2 min is sufficient to kill the metacercarial cysts. In some areas free metacercarial cysts have been found floating on the water surface and may be ingested in drinking water.

Night-soil, as once commonly used in China, should be stored before being added as fertilizer to submerged fields. Sanitary disposal of faeces would probably be effective, although there is still the possibility of zoonotic infections. Molluscicides could possibly be used for snail control but their efficacy has not been tested.

ZOONOTIC ASPECTS

Pigs act as important reservoir hosts. The endemic region in central Thailand is a perennial flood basin where rice is grown and houses are built on stilts. Pigs are also kept in pens on stilts and fed on water plants; the faeces of the pigs passes into the water below, in which snails live and food plants are grown.

There are high prevalence rates in pigs in areas of Bangladesh, Burma (Myanmar), Cambodia and India but few human infections, as the appropriate plants are not eaten raw.

Family Heterophyidae

Heterophyes heterophyes
(von Siebold, 1852) Stiles and Hassall, 1900

SYNONYMS
Distoma heterophyes von Siebold, 1852; *Heterophyes aegyptiaca* Cobbold, 1866; *Heterophyes nocens* Onji and Nishio, 1915.

DISEASE AND POPULAR NAMES
Heterophyiasis, heterophyosis; von Siebold's fluke infection, dwarf-fluke infection.

GEOGRAPHICAL DISTRIBUTION
Asia (southern China, Japan, Indonesia, Korea, the Philippines, Taiwan), North Africa and Middle East (Egypt, Iran, Sudan, Tunisia, Turkey) and southern Europe (Greece and Romania).

LOCATION IN HOST
Adults are attached to the wall of the jejunum and upper ileum, often in the crypts of Lieberkühn (Fig. 25).

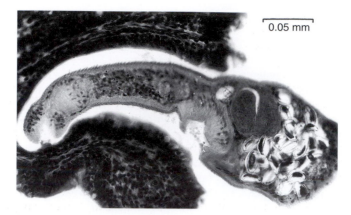

0.05 mm

Fig. 25. Section of the intestinal mucosa (of cat) with adult *Heterophyes* attached by the oral sucker. The ventral sucker and uterus filled with eggs can also be seen.

MORPHOLOGY

Heterophyes is a small hermaphroditic fluke, measuring 1.0–1.7 mm × 0.3–0.7 mm (Fig. 3). It has an elongate ovoid shape and is greyish when living. The tegument is covered by fine scale-like spines, most numerous at the anterior end. The oral sucker is much smaller (90 µm) than the ventral (230 µm), which lies in the middle third of the body. A genital sucker (150 µm in diameter), capable of protrusion but not adherence, lies near the left posterior margin of the ventral sucker; it bears a number of radiating rows of small spines and is interrupted at the end part nearest the ventral sucker. The alimentary tract consists of a narrow prepharynx, a small bulbous pharynx, a narrow oesophagus and two gut caeca, which arise towards the middle of the body and extend to the posterior end of the fluke. The tubular excretory bladder lies in the posterior fifth of the body.

The two ovoid testes lie side by side, near the posterior end of the body. The male duct has a large seminal vesicle, which opens into the genital atrium in the genital sucker by a muscular ejaculatory duct. The rounded ovary is situated in the midline about one-third of the way from the posterior end of the body and there is a seminal receptacle and Laurer's canal. The closely coiled uterus opens into the genital sucker. The vitelline glands consist of about 14 large follicles in a limited posterior area of the body.

LIFE CYCLE

The brown eggs are about the same size as those of *Clonorchis* (30 µm × 15 µm) and have a very slight shoulder to take the operculum (Fig. 123) and there may be a small knob at the opposite end. The egg contains a fully developed miracidium when discharged in the faeces, which hatches out only when the egg is ingested by a suitable water snail (these are of the operculate type, with a cap on the base of the foot to close the shell). Important species are *Pirenella conica* in the Nile Delta (Fig. 1) and *Cerithidea cingulata microptera* in China and Japan.

Asexual multiplication in the snail consists of a sporocyst and one or two redial generations before the cercarial stage is reached. The lophocercous cercariae emerge 3–4 weeks after ingestion of the egg and encyst in a folded position under the scales, on the fins, tail and gills and in the superficial muscles of various freshwater fishes. The metacercariae measure about 160 µm and are infective in 15–21 days.

Species of fish involved include *Mugil cephalus* (brackish water mullet), *Aphasia fasciatus* and *Tilapia nilotica* in Egypt and Greece and *Mugil* spp. and *Acanthogobius* spp. in Japan. When the fish is eaten uncooked the metacercariae escape and develop in the small intestine. The flukes mature in 15–20 days and the adults live for about 2 months.

CLINICAL MANIFESTATIONS

In light infections there are usually no symptoms. In heavy infections, nausea and intermittent chronic diarrhoea, sometimes with the passage of blood and abdominal discomfort with colicky pains and tenderness, have been reported beginning 9 days after ingestion of cysts. Symptoms resemble those of amoebiasis or heartburn and there may be vomiting, simulating a peptic ulcer. Slight eosinophilia is sometimes found.

PATHOGENESIS

A mild inflammation of the mucosa at the site of attachment and sometimes a superficial necrosis occur if there are thousands of worms present; up to 4000 have been reported.

Eggs of many species of heterophyids have been found at necropsy from various sites in the body, either because the eggs themselves have succeeded in filtering through the intestinal wall to the mesenteric lymphatics or venules or because the adults have penetrated the gut wall and laid eggs in the peritoneal cavity. This phenomenon appears to be a reaction to humans as abnormal hosts, and embolization of the eggs may occur. Cardiac lesions caused by *Heterophyes* or other members of the same family include fibrosis surrounding eggs in the mitral valve and myocardium, with consequent heart failure. Eggs have been found in the brain on a few occasions, as have encapsulated adults.

DIAGNOSIS

This is by recovery of eggs following suggestive clinical findings, either by direct faecal smears or by concentration methods. The eggs can be differentiated from those of opisthorchids by the less well-developed shoulders at the operculum giving a more oval outline and by the smaller posterior

knob. The contained miracidium also has bilaterally symmetrical penetration glands (Fig. 123).

TREATMENT

Niclosamide (2 g day^{-1} for 2 days for an adult) has been used for many years but more recently praziquantel (a single dose of 20 mg kg^{-1}) has become the drug of choice.

EPIDEMIOLOGY

Transmission is by eating fresh or salted uncooked fish. There may be heavy infections in both rural and urban communities in the Nile Delta region of Egypt, who traditionally eat pickled mullet ('fessik') at the feast of Sham-el Nessim. An infection rate of 10% has been reported from schoolchildren in the area. However, most infections are in 20–40-year-olds, who eat freshly salted mullet; metacercariae can live for up to 7 days in these.

PREVENTION AND CONTROL

Personal prevention is by thorough cooking of fish. Partial cooking (mostly of *Tilapia nilotica*) carried out around Lakes Manzala, Borollos and Edco in the Nile Delta destroys only about 70% of cysts. Preventing pollution of the water with faeces, which in Egypt is mainly by fishermen, is a possible long-term objective.

ZOONOTIC ASPECTS

Dogs, cats, foxes and other fish-eating mammals act as reservoir hosts and can maintain the infection in the absence of humans.

Metagonimus yokogawai
Katsurada, 1912

SYNONYM

Heterophyes yokogawai Katsurada, 1912.

DISEASE AND POPULAR NAME

Metagonimiasis or metagonimosis; Yokogawa's fluke infection.

GEOGRAPHICAL DISTRIBUTION

This is probably the most common human intestinal fluke in the Far East and is endemic in China, Indonesia, southern Japan, Korea, Manchuria, Taiwan and Siberia. It has also been reported from Israel, Serbia and Spain.

LOCATION IN HOST

Adults are found in the upper and middle parts of the jejunum, rarely in the duodenum, ileum and caecum. The flukes are embedded in the crypts of Lieberkühn in the early stages or in the mucus found on the surface.

MORPHOLOGY

This genus is closely related to *Heterophyes*, the adults being similar in size and structure. The principal differences are that in *Metagonimus* the ventral sucker is situated to the right of the midline and there is no accessory sucker (Fig. 3).

LIFE CYCLE

The eggs measure 27 μm × 16 μm and are very similar to those of *Heterophyes* (Fig. 123). The life cycle is also similar. In China, Japan and Korea the snail species involved is *Semisulcospira libertina*. The second intermediate fish hosts are *Plecoglossus altivelis* (a trout, the 'ayu' or sweetfish), *Leuciscus hakuensis*, *Mugil cephalus*, *Odontobutis obscurus* and *Salmo perryi* in Japan and Siberia and also *Pseudorasbora parva* and *Carrasius carrasius* (silver carp) in Korea. Each adult fluke produces about 1500 eggs 24 h^{-1}.

CLINICAL MANIFESTATIONS AND PATHOGENESIS

Similar to *Heterophyes*, with abdominal pain, diarrhoea and lethargy. A heavy infection in Japan caused intractable diarrhoea and weight loss and from the faecal egg count it was estimated that 50,000–70,000 adult worms were present (63,587 have been recovered from one patient who had only slight symptoms (Chai and Lee, 1990)). Headache, abdominal and muscular pains, fever and urticaria have also been reported.

Pathological changes are characterized by villous atrophy and hyperplasia of the crypts, with inflammatory cell infiltration. Eggs may be carried by intestinal capillaries and lymphatics to the myocardium, brain, spinal cord and other tissues, where granulomatous changes or embolisms can be provoked by their presence.

DIAGNOSIS AND TREATMENT

As for *Heterophyes*. The eggs can, with difficulty, be differentiated from those of *Heterophyes*, as the latter have a thinner shell and are light brown in colour.

EPIDEMIOLOGY

Since the eggs of this species are so similar to those of many other parasites in this family that can infect humans, it is difficult to know the true prevalence. In ethnic minorities in Khabarovsk Territory of Siberia, there are high rates of 20–70% and, in endemic areas of coastal Korea, there appear to be 10–20% of villagers infected.

In Japan the cercariae do not emerge from the snail intermediate hosts below 18–20°C and infection does not occur in areas where summer temperatures are below this figure.

ZOONOTIC ASPECTS

Dogs, cats, rats and pigs (and perhaps pelicans and other fish-eating birds) act as reservoir hosts and infection in animals is common worldwide. Potentially all species of the family Heterophyidae could become human intestinal parasites where raw fish is eaten and it is likely that many others will be recorded as occasional human parasites (particularly in the Far East) when expelled adult worms are examined. The following species have been recorded from humans and, in some, eggs or occasionally adults have been found in the heart, brain or spinal cord: *Apophallus donicus* (eastern Europe, Canada and USA), *Centrocestus armatus* (Korea), *C. caninus* (Taiwan), *C. cuspidatus* (Egypt and Taiwan), *C. formosanus* (China and Japan), *C. kurokawai* (Japan), *C. longus* (Taiwan), *Cryptocotyle lingua* (Greenland),

Diorchitrema amplicaecale (Taiwan), *D. formosanum* (Taiwan), *D. pseudocirratum* (Hawaii and Philippines), *Haplorchis microrchis* (Japan), *H. pleurolophocerca* (Egypt), *H. pumilio* (Egypt, Iran and Far East), *H. taichui* (Bangladesh, Egypt, Iran and Far East), *H. vanissimus* (Philippines) and *H. yokogawai* (Far East and Egypt), *Heterophyes dispar* (Korea and Thailand), *H. equalis* (Egypt), *H. heterophyes nocens* (Korea and Japan), *H. katsuradai* (Japan), *Heterophyopsis continua* (Far East), *Metagonimus minutis* (China and Taiwan), *M. takahashi* (Japan and Korea), *Phagicola longa* (Brazil and Mexico), *P. ornamenta, P. ornata* and *Pharyngostomum flapi* (Egypt), *Procerovum calderoni* (China, Philippines and Egypt), *P. varium* (Japan), *Pygidiopsis summa* (Japan and Korea), *Stellantchasmus amplicaecalis* (Egypt), *S. falcatus* (Korea, Laos, Thailand and Hawaii), *Stictodora fuscata* and *S. manilensis* (Korea). See Coombs and Crompton (1991), Yu and Mott (1994), WHO (1995), Ashford and Crewe (1998) and Muller (2001), and for details of intermediate hosts, rarity and original references.

Family Paramphistomidae

Gastrodiscoides hominis
(Lewis and McConnell, 1876) Leiper, 1913.

SYNONYMS AND DISEASE
Gastrodiscoidiasis or gastrodiscoidosis; *Amphistomum hominis* Lewis and McConnell, 1876, *Gastrodiscus hominis* Fischoeder, 1902.

GEOGRAPHICAL DISTRIBUTION
Infection is most common in India, particularly Assam, Bihar and Orissa, but also occurs in Burma (Myanmar), China, Kazakhstan, the Philippines, Thailand and Vietnam.

LOCATION IN HOST
Adults attach to the wall of the caecum and ascending colon by their suckers.

MORPHOLOGY
Gastrodiscoides is the only human-parasitic member of the paramphistomes, which are important parasites of domestic herbivores. It is a dorsally convex fluke measuring 5–8 mm $\times$ 3–5 mm and, when living, is reddish in colour. The body is disc-shaped with an anterior conical projection bearing the oral sucker (Fig. 3). Like all other members of the family, the ventral sucker is close to the posterior end. The tegument is smooth. The alimentary tract consists of a pair of lateral pouches arising from the oral sucker and a slightly tortuous pharyngeal tube, which bifurcates into two gut caeca that extend only to the middle of the discoid region. The large excretory bladder is in the midline behind the ventral sucker. The two lobate testes lie in tandem just behind the bifurcation of the caeca. The common genital opening is on a cone just anterior to the bifurcation. The ovoid ovary lies just posterior to the testes near the midline. The vitelline glands are scattered and surround the caeca behind the testes. The loosely coiled uterus opens on the genital cone.

LIFE CYCLE
The eggs measure 146 (127–160) µm $\times$ 66 (62–75) µm. They are rhomboidal in shape, have a small well-fitting operculum and are transparently greenish in colour (Fig. 123). They contain about 24 vitelline cells and a central unembryonated ovum. After the eggs are expelled in the faeces and reach water, a miracidium develops in 9–14 days at 24°C. The miracidium that emerges from the egg can develop experimentally in the snail *Helicorbis coenosus* found in Uttar Pradesh and cercariae emerge 28–152 days after infection. The cercariae form metacercarial cysts on water plants; probably the water caltrop is involved in human infection but the life cycle has not been elucidated in nature.

ZOONOTIC ASPECTS
Pigs, monkeys (rhesus), apes (orang-utan), field rats and the Napu mouse deer are natural hosts, but it is not known what the

relationship is between human and animal hosts.

Watsonius watsoni (Conyngham, 1904) Stiles and Goldberg, 1910 (synonym *Amphistomum watsoni*, Conyngham, 1904), has been reported once from northern Nigeria in a patient who died of severe diarrhoea. Many worms were seen in the stools and after autopsy many more were found attached to the wall of the duodenum and jejunum and a few in the colon. Presumably infection was contracted from ingestion of metacercarial cysts on vegetation. *Watsonius* is a natural parasite of monkeys in West Africa and Singapore.

Fischoederius elongatus (Poirer, 1883) Stiles and Goldberger, 1910, is a parasite of ruminants in Asia, contracted from ingesting cysts on vegetation. Human infection has been reported from China.

Family Echinostomidae

Most of the members of this large and rather heterogeneous group are parasites of the gut of birds and lower vertebrates, but a few are found in mammals and at least 24 species are occasional parasites of humans. Typically, members have a collar of spines behind the oral sucker.

Echinostoma ilocanum
(Garrison, 1908) Odhner, 1911

SYNONYMS
Fascioletta ilocanum Garrison, 1908; *Euparyphium ilocanum* Tubangui and Pasco, 1933.

DISEASE AND POPULAR NAME
Echinostomiasis or echinostomosis; Garrison's fluke infection.

GEOGRAPHICAL DISTRIBUTION
Five human cases were found by Garrison in prisoners in Manila jail in 1907 and

occasional cases have been reported since from China (Yunnan), Indonesia, the Philippines (11–44% in northern Luzon), Thailand (8.2% in one area) and recently India (Grover *et al.*, 1998).

LOCATION IN HOST
Adults live in the jejunum; they attach by insertion of the oral end into the mucosa.

LIFE CYCLE
This is a natural parasite of dogs and cats, and eggs (measuring 100 µm × 65–70 µm) in the faeces are undifferentiated. If they reach water, the contained miracidia develop in about 8–14 days at 26°C. They emerge and penetrate into suitable freshwater snails (particularly *Hippeutis*) and multiply asexually. Cercariae that emerge then enter a wide range of other snails (such as *Pila*) and encyst as metacercariae. When these snails are eaten raw by dogs, cats or humans, they excyst and develop into adult worms. Other echinostomes utilize fish and amphibians (usually frogs) as second intermediate hosts, which are also eaten raw. It appears that cercariae can also be swallowed while swimming and cause infection.

Other Echinostomids

E. echinatum (= *lindoense*) (Zeder, 1803) formerly had a high infection rate (24–96%) around Lake Lindu in central Sulawesi but has been very uncommon since the 1970s because of changes in eating habits consequent on the introduction of tilapia into the lake. The first intermediate host is a planorbid snail or a type of mussel (*Corbicula*) and the metacercariae encyst in edible pulmonate and bivalve snails, which used to be eaten raw and are now rare (partly because they are eaten by the fish).

E. hortense Asada, 1926, has an infection rate of up to 22.4% in southern Korea and is not uncommon in north-eastern China, where loach (the usual second intermediate host) are eaten raw as a cure for jaundice; it has also been reported from Japan. The natural definitive hosts are rats and dogs.

E. malayanum Leiper, 1911, has been recovered from humans in India, Indonesia (Irian Jaya and Sumatra), the Philippines (20% in areas of Luzon) and north-east Thailand (3–8%). It is probably a natural parasite of dogs or rats and human infection is through ingestion of edible molluscs (particularly *Pila* and *Vivipara*), which act as second intermediate hosts.

E. revolutum (Froelich, 1802) Looss, 1899, is a common parasite of the caeca of duck, goose and muskrat, and most human cases come from Taiwan (2.8–6.5% infection) and north-east Thailand, with reports from China and Indonesia. Edible molluscs, such as *Corbicula,* act as second intermediate hosts.

Hypoderaeum conoideum (Bloch, 1872) Dietz, 1909, is a parasite of birds, but there can be up to 55% infection rates in norteast Thailand. Snails, such as *Planorbis* and *Lymnaea* spp., act as both first and second intermediate hosts.

There are many species of echinostomes that can act as occasional or rare parasites of humans, the numbers increasing as the use of praziquantel allows voided adult worms to be examined (for further information, see Haseeb and Eveland, 2000): *Artyfechinostomum malayanum* (Thailand), *A. mehrai* (India), *A. oraoni* (India), *A.* (= *Paryphostomum*) *sufrartyfex* (four cases in India), *Echinochasmus fujianensis* (up to 7.8% in southern Fujian, China), *E. japonicus* (China, Japan, Korea and Taiwan), *E. jiufoensis* (one fatal case in Canton, China), *E. liliputanus* (up to 23% in areas of Anhui province, China), *E. perfoliatus* (Japan, Taiwan and Europe), *Echinoparyphium paraulum* (Russia), *E. recurvatum* (Egypt, Indonesia and Taiwan), *Echinostoma* (= *Echinochasmus*) *angustitestis* (two cases in China), *E. cinetorchis* (Japan, Korea and Taiwan), *E. japonicum* (Japan and Korea), *E. macrorchis* (Indonesia, Japan, Korea and Taiwan), *Echinostoma melis* (= *Euparyphium jassyense*) (China, Romania and Taiwan), *Episthmium caninum* (Thailand) and *Himasthala muehlensi* (one case in Colombia or USA).

MORPHOLOGY

These species of echinostomes are mostly small flukes measuring 2.5–8.0 mm and all have a collar of spines behind the oral sucker (Fig. 3).

CLINICAL MANIFESTATIONS

In most infections there are no signs apart from the presence of eggs in the faeces. In heavy infections (e.g. 14,000 worms were recovered from one child at autopsy), symptoms are similar to those of *Fasciolopsis buski,* with vague abdominal manifestations, such as flatulence, intestinal colic and diarrhoea (Graczyk and Fried, 1998). Vomiting, diarrhoea, abdominal pain and swelling of the feet were reported in one case in a child (Grover *et al.*, 1998) and there may be anaemia and oedema. There have been fatalities in children from dehydration. The adult worms attach to the mucosa of the small intestine and may produce inflammatory lesions and necrosis at the site of attachment, with increased cellular infiltration in the intestinal mucosa. There may also be a generalized toxic process. In an experimental infection with 113 metacercariae of *Echinochasmus japonicus,* abdominal pain, diarrhoea and intestinal gurgling developed about 10 days after infection (Lin *et al.*, 1985).

DIAGNOSIS

Eggs found in the faeces are similar to those of *Fasciolopsis* or *Fasciola,* although somewhat smaller (most are about 100 μm × 70 μm); specific identification is almost impossible without recovery of adults after treatment.

TREATMENT

Cure is simple with a single oral dose of 10–20 mg kg^{-1} of praziquantel (or 5 mg kg^{-1} for *Echinochasmus fujianensis*).

Other Occasional and Rare Human-parasitic Trematodes

Family Diplostomidae

Alaria americana Hall and Wigdor, 1918, and *A. marcianae* (La Rue, 1917) Walton, 1950, are very similar parasites of wild carnivores and dogs and cats in North America, in which the anterior portion of the body is spoon-shaped, with an organ that secretes proteolytic enzymes. They have an unusual life cycle. When eggs from faeces reach water, the miracidia hatch out and penetrate and multiply in suitable species of snails (including *Heliosoma* spp.). The emerging cercariae develop in amphibian tadpoles into a larval stage known as a mesocercaria (midway between a cercaria and a metacercaria). Frogs and snakes ingest tadpoles and act as paratenic hosts. When these are eaten by young carnivores, metacercariae develop in the lungs, are coughed up and become adults in the small intestine in about 20 days. However, in pregnant animals the mesocercariae migrate to the mammary glands and infect the suckling young through the milk, and adults develop in these (known as 'amphiparatenesis'). They can also infect subsequent litters (Shoop, 1994). A fatal case in Canada occurred in a man who ingested frogs' legs while hiking. He was thought to be suffering from gastric flu but died 9 days later from extensive pulmonary haemorrhage and at autopsy was found to have thousands of mesocercariae in many tissues. In other cases mesocercariae have been found in the eye (Smyth, 1995). Another species in carnivores, *A. alata* (Goeze, 1782), has occasionally infected humans with mesocercariae in the Middle East. *Neodiplostomum* (= *Fibricola*) *seoulensis* (Seo, Rim and Lee, 1964) Hong and Shoop, 1994, a parasite of rats, has developed to adulthood in the human small intestine in a few cases in South Korea and is contracted from eating raw amphibians or snakes (paratenic hosts). *Diplostomum spathaceum* (Rudolphi, 1819) Olsson, 1876, is a cosmopolitan para-site of birds, with metacercariae in the eyes of fish, and there have been a few cases of swimmer's itch in the former Czecho-slovakia, but more importantly cercariae have entered the eye and caused cataracts in the lens.

Family Lecithodendriidae

Phaneropsolus bonnei Lie Kian Joe, 1951, and *Prosthodendrium molenkampi* Lie Kian Joe, 1951, were both discovered in Indonesia at autopsy and are also present in rural populations of north-east Thailand and Laos. Eggs of both species are similar to those of *Opisthorchis* and heterophyids, and insects act as second intermediate hosts. *Phaneropsolus spinicirrus, Paralecithodendrium obtusum* and *P. glandulosum* are three other poorly characterized species commonly found in Thais (Yu and Mott, 1994).

Family Plagiorchiidae

Plagiorchis harinasutai Radomyos, Bunnag and Harinasuta, 1989, *P. javensis* Sandground, 1940, *P. muris* Tanabe, 1922, and *P. philippinensis* Sandground, 1940, have insects as second intermediate hosts and have been found in humans in Thailand, Indonesia, Japan and the Philippines, respectively.

Family Troglotrematidae

Nanophyetus salmincola Chapin, 1927, is an intestinal parasite of wild carnivores, birds and domestic dogs in the Pacific north of the USA and in Siberia. Metacercariae encyst in salmonid fishes and in the USA, in dogs that eat the fish. Adults cause a haemorrhagic enteritis, with high fever, anorexia, vomiting and lymphadenopathy ('salmon poisoning'), with a high mortality 10–14 days after infection, caused by a rickettsia (*Neorickettsia helminthoeca*), which is transmitted by the trematode. Following ingestion of raw fish, some patients in both areas suffered from diarrhoea, weight loss, nausea, vomiting, fatigue, anorexia and a high eosinophilia of up to 43%; in one case there was also a high fever but the possible role of the rickettsia was not investigated (Eastburn *et al.*, 1987). Symptoms usually resolved after a few months. The parasites have been separated into two subspecies: *N. s. salmincola* in the USA and *N. s. schikhobalowi* in Siberia. Diagnosis is by finding eggs in faeces (measuring about 80 µm × 45 µm) and treatment is with praziquantel. Prevention is by not eating raw or smoked salmon in endemic areas, although there has been one case of infection through handling fish. There is a 4.2% infection rate in a focus on the lower Amur River in Siberia (and up to 60% in local ethnic minorities), and the ranges of both subspecies appear to be spreading.

Other families

Species of trematodes belonging to various other families that have occasionally been found in humans include: *Carneophallus* (= *Spelotrema*) *brevicaeca* (from shrimps and has caused fatalities in the Philippines), *Cathaemasia cabreri* (Philippines), *Clinostomum complanatum* (from fish in Japan and Middle East), *Cotylurus japonicus* (China), *Gymnophalloides seoi* (from oysters in a village in Korea), *Isoparorchis hypselobagri* (China, India), *Microphallus minus* (Japan), *Paryphostomum bangkokensis* (Thailand), *P. sufrartyfex* (India), *Philophthalmus lacrymosus* (in the eye in Serbia), *Philophthalmus* sp. (eye in Sri Lanka), *Prohemistomum vivax* (from fish in Egypt) and *Psilorchis hominis* (Japan). See Yu and Mott (1994), WHO (1995), Ashford and Crewe (1998) and Muller (2000) for further details of intermediate and definitive hosts.

References

Abel, L. and Dessein, A.J. (1997) The impact of host genetics on susceptibility to human infectious diseases. *Current Opinion in Immunology* 9, 509–516.

Agnew, A., Fulford, A.J.C., Mwanje, M.T., Gachuhi, K., Gutsam, V., Krijger, F.W., Sturrock, R.F., Vennerwald, B.J., Ouma, J.H., Butterworth, A.E. and Deelder, A.M. (1996) Age dependent reduction of schistosome fecundity in S. *haematobium* but not S. *mansoni* infections in humans. *American Journal of Tropical Medicine and Hygiene* 55, 338–343.

Ansell, J. and Guyatt, H. (1999) Self-reporting of blood in urine by schoolchildren may be the most cost-effective diagnostic test for urinary schistosomiasis. *Bulletin of Tropical Medicine and International Health* 7, 5.

Ashford, R.W. and Crewe, W. (1998) *The Parasites of* Homo sapiens. Liverpool School of Tropical Medicine, Liverpool, UK.

Azizova, O.M., Sagieva, A.T., Israilova, S., Sadykov, K.M., Shirinova, N.Sh., Mukhidinov, Sh.M., Ismatov, I., Adilova, N.B. and Saidaliev, T.S. (1988) *Dicrocoelium lanceolatum* infection in man (on autopsy data) [English summary]. *Meditsinskaya Parazitologiya i Parazitarnye Bolezni* 2, 26–28.

Blair, D., Xu, Z.-B. and Agatsuma, T. (1999) Paragonimiasis and the genus *Paragonimus*. *Advances in Parasitology* 42, 113–222.

Boisier, P., Ramarokoto, C.E., Ravaoalimalala, V.E., Rabrijaona, L., Serieye, J., Roux, J. and Esterre, P. (1998) Reversibility of *Schistosoma mansoni*-associated morbidity after yearly mass praziquantel therapy: ultrasonographic assessment. *Transactions of the Royal Society of Tropical Medicine and Hygiene* 92, 451–453.

Brindley, P.J. (1994) Relationships between chemotherapy and immunity in schistosomiasis. *Advances in Parasitology* 34, 134–161.

Brooks, D.R., O'Grady, R.T. and Glen, D.R. (1985) Phylogenetic analysis of the Digenea (Platyhelminthes: Cercomeria) with comments on their adaptive radiation. *Canadian Journal of Zoology* 63, 411–443.

Brown, D.S. (1980) *Freshwater Snails of Africa and Their Medical Importance.* Taylor and Francis, London, UK.

Bundy, D., Sher, A. and Michael, E. (2000) Helminth infections may increase susceptibility to TB and AIDS. *Parasitology Today* 16, 273–274.

Butterworth, A.E. (1998) Immunological aspects of human schistosomiasis. *British Medical Journal* 54, 357–368.

Capron, A. (1998) Schistosomiasis: 40 years' war on the worm. *Parasitology Today* 14, 379–384.

Chai, J.Y. and Lee, S.H. (1990) Intestinal trematodes of humans in Korea: *Metagonimus,* heterophyids and echinostomes. *Korean Journal of Parasitology* 28 (suppl.), 103–122.

Chen, M.G., Lu, Y., Hua, X.J. and Mott, K.E. (1994) Progress in morbidity due to *Clonorchis sinensis* infection: a review of recent literature. *Tropical Diseases Bulletin* 91, R7–R65.

Chitsulo, L., Engels, D., Montresor, A. and Savioli, L. (2000) The global status of schistosomiasis and its control. *Acta Tropica* 77, 41–51.

Coombs, I. and Crompton, D.W.T. (1991) *A Guide to Human Helminths.* Taylor and Francis, London, UK.

Coulson, P.S. (1997) The radiation-attenuated vaccine against schistosomiasis in animal models: paradigm of a human vaccine? *Advances in Parasitology* 39, 272–336.

Dalton, J.P. (ed.) (1998) *Fasciolosis.* CAB International, Wallingford, UK.

Damian, R.T. (1987) The exploitation of host immune responses by parasites. *Journal of Parasitology* 73, 1–11.

Dekumyoy, P., Waikagul, J. and Eom, K.S. (1998) Human lung fluke *Paragonimus heterotremus*: differential diagnosis between *Paragonimus heterotremus* and *Paragonimus westermani* infections by EITB. *Tropical Medicine and International Health* 3, 52–56.

Doenhoff, M.J., Hassounah, O., Murare, H., Bain, J. and Lucas, S. (1986) The schistosome egg granuloma: immunopathology in the cause of host protection or parasite survival? *Transactions of the Royal Society of Tropical Medicine and Hygiene* 80, 503–514.

Dupre, L., Herve, M., Schacht, A.M., Capron, A. and Riveau, G. (1999) Control of schistosomiasis pathology by combination of Sj28GST DNA immunization and praziquantel treatment. *Journal of Infectious Diseases* 180, 454–467.

Eastburn, R.I., Fritsche, T.R. and Terhune, C.A., Jr (1987) Human intestinal infection with *Nanophyetus salmincola* from salmonid fishes. *American Journal of Tropical Medicine and Hygiene* 36, 586–591.

Elkins, D.B., Haswell-Elkins, M.R., Mairang, E., Mairang, P., Sithithaworn, P., Kaewkes, S., Bhudhisawasdi, V. and Uttaravichien, T. (1990) A high frequency of hepatobiliary disease and suspected cholangiocarcinoma associated with heavy *Opisthorchis viverrini* infection in a small community in north-east Thailand. *Transactions of the Royal Society of Tropical Medicine and Hygiene* 84, 715–719.

Frenzel, K., Grigull, L., Odongo-Aginya, E., Ndugwa, C.M., Loroni-Lakwo, T., Schweigmann, U., Verster, U., Spannbrucker, N. and Doehring, E. (1999) Evidence for long-term effect of a single dose of praziquantel on *Schistosoma mansoni*-induced hepatosplenic lesions in northern Uganda. *American Journal of Tropical Medicine and Hygiene* 60, 927–931.

Giboda, M., Malek, E.A. and Correa, R. (1997) Human schistosomiasis in Puerto Rico: reduced prevalence rate and absence of *Biomphalaria glabrata*. *American Journal of Tropical Medicine and Hygiene* 57, 564–568.

Gibson, D.I. and Bray, R.A. (1994) The evolutionary expansion and host–parasite relationships in the Digenea. *International Journal for Parasitology* 24, 1213–1226.

Gobert, G.N. (1998) The role of microscopy in the investigation of paramyosin as a vaccine candidate against *Schistosoma japonicum. Parasitology Today* 14, 115–118.

Graczyk, T.K. and Fried, B. (1998) Echinostomiasis: a common but forgotten food-borne disease. *American Journal of Tropical Medicine and Hygiene* 58, 501–504.

Greer, G.J., Kitikoon, V. and Lohachit, C. (1989) Morphology and life cycle of *Schistosoma sinensium* Pao, 1959, from northwest Thailand. *Journal of Parasitology* 75, 98–101.

Grover, M., Dutta, R., Kumar, R., Aneja, S. and Mehta, G. (1998) *Echinostoma ilocanum* infection. *Indian Pediatrics* 35, 549–552.

Guyatt, H., Brooker, S. and Donnelly, C.A. (1999) Can prevalence of infection in school-aged children be used as an index for assessing community prevalence? *Parasitology* 118, 257–268.

Haseeb, M.A. and Eveland, L.K. (2000) Human echinostomiasis: mechanisms of pathogenesis and host resistance. In: Fried, B. and Graczyk, T.K. (eds) *Echinostomes as Experimental Models for Biological Research*. Kluwer, Dordrecht, The Netherlands, pp. 83–98.

Hatz, C.F.R. (2000) The use of ultrasound in schistosomiasis. *Advances in Parasitology* 48, 226–285.

IARC Working Group (1994) *Schistosomes, Liver Flukes and* Helicobacter pylori. IARC Monographs on the Evaluation of the Carcinogenic Risk of Chemicals to Humans, Vol. 6, World Health Organization, Geneva, Switzerland, 270 pp.

Ikeda, T. (1998) Cystatin capture enzyme-linked immunosorbent essay for immunodiagnosis of human paragonimiasis and fascioliasis. *American Journal of Tropical Medicine and Hygiene* 59, 286–290.

Ishii, Y., Koga, M., Fujino, T., Higo, H., Ishibashi, J., Oka, K. and Saito, S. (1983) Human infection with the pancreas liver fluke *Eurytrema pancreaticum*. *American Journal of Tropical Medicine and Hygiene* 32, 1019–1022.

Jordan, P., Webbe, G. and Sturrock, R. (eds) (1993) *Human Schistosomiasis*. CAB International, Wallingford, UK.

Kabatereine, N.B., Ouma, J.H., Kemijumbi, J., Butterworth, A.E., Dunne, D.W. and Fulford, A.J.C. (1999) Adult resistance to schistosomiasis mansoni: age-dependence of reinfection remains constant in communities with diverse exposure patterns. *Parasitology* 118, 101–105.

Katz, N. (1999) Schistosomiasis vaccines: the need for more research before clinical trials. *Parasitology Today* 15, 165–166.

La Rue, G.R. (1957) The classification of digenetic trematodes. *Experimental Parasitology* 6, 306–344.

Lin, J.X., Chen, Y.Z., Liang, C.Z., Yang, L.B. and Zhuang, H.J. (1985) Epidemiological investigation and experimental infection of *Echinochasmus japonicus* [in Chinese. English summary]. *Chinese Journal of Parasitology and Parasitic Diseases* 3, 89–91.

Liu, Y.S., Du W.P., Wu, Y.M., Chen, Y.G., Zhang, K.Y., Shi, J.M., Hu, X.Z., Li, G.Y., You, C.F. and Wu, Z.X. (1995) Application of dot-immunogold–silver staining in the diagnosis of clonorchiasis. *Journal of Tropical Medicine and Hygiene* 98, 151–154.

MacLean, J.D., Arthur, J.R., Ward, B.J., Gyorkos, T.W., Curtis, M.A. and Kokoskin, E. (1996) Common-source outbreak of acute infection due to the North American liver fluke *Metorchis conjunctus*. *Lancet, British Edition* 347, 154–158.

Malek, E.A. (1963) *Medical Malacology*. Burgess, Minneapolis, USA.

Mas Coma, M.S., Esteban, J.G. and Bargues, M.D. (1999) Epidemiology of human fascioliasis: a review and proposed new classification. *Bulletin of the World Health Organization* 77, 340–346.

Mostafa, M.H., Badawi, A.F. and O'Connor, P.J. (1995) Bladder cancer associated with schistosomiasis. *Parasitology Today* 11, 87–89.

Mott, K.E., Nuttall, I., Desjeux, P. and Cattond, P. (1995) Geographical approaches to control of some parasitic zoonoses. *Bulletin of the World Health Organization* 73, 247–257.

Mouchet, F., Develoux, M. and Mamadou, B.M. (1988) *Schistosoma bovis* in human stools in Republic of Niger. *Transactions of the Royal Society of Tropical Medicine and Hygiene* 82, 257.

Muller, R. (2001) Dogs and trematode zoonoses. In: Macpherson, C.N.L., Meslin, F.-X. and Wandeler, A.I. (eds) *Dogs, Zoonoses and Public Health*. CAB International, Wallingford, UK, pp. 149–176.

O'Neill, S.M., Parkinson, M., Dowd, A.J., Strauss, W., Angles, R. and Dalton, J.P. (1999) Short report: immunodiagnosis of human fascioliasis using recombinant *Fasciola hepatica* cathepsin L1 cysteine proteinase. *American Journal of Hygiene and Tropical Medicine* 60, 749–751 (also 1998, 58, 417–423).

Pecoulas, P.E., Farhati, K. and Picot, H. (1995) Les schistosomes humaines d'Asie à l'exception de *Schistosoma japonicum*. *Médecine et Maladies Infectieuses* 25, 99–106.

Pointier, J.P. and Jourdane, J. (2000) Biological control of the snail hosts of schistosomiasis in areas of low transmission: the example of the Caribbean area. *Acta Tropica* 77, 53–60.

Rohde, K., Hefford, C., Ellis, J.T., Baverstock, P.R., Johnson, A.M., Watson, N.A. and Dittman, S. (1993) Contributions to the phylogeny of the Platyhelminthes based on partial sequencing of 18s ribosomal DNA. *International Journal for Parasitology* 23, 705–724.

Ross, A.G.P., Li-TueSheng, Sleigh, A.C., McManus, D.P. and Li, Y.S. (1997) Schistosomiasis control in the People's Republic of China. *Parasitology Today* 13, 152–155.

Ross, A.G.P., Sleigh, A.C., Li, Y.S., Williams, G.M., Aligui, G.D.L. and McManus, D.P. (2000) Is there immunity to *Schistosoma japonicum*? *Parasitology Today* 16, 159–164.

Savioli L., Renganathan, E., Montresor, A., Davis, A. and Behbehani, K. (1997) Control of schisto-somiasis – a global picture. *Parasitology Today* 13, 444–448.

Shekar, K.C. (1991) *S. malayensis*: the biologic, clinical, and pathological features in man and experi-mental animals. In: Sun, T. (ed.) *Progress in Clinical Parasitology*, Vol. 2. Field and Wood, Philadelphia, USA, pp. 145–178.

Shoop, W.L. (1994) Vertical migration in the Trematoda. *Journal of the Helminthological Society of Washington* 61, 153–161.

Sirisinha, S., Chawengkirttikul, R., Haswell-Elkins, M.R., Elkins, D.B., Kaewkes, S. and Sithithaworn, P. (1995) Evaluation of a monoclonal antibody-based enzyme linked immunosorbent assay for the detection of *Opisthorchis viverrini* infection in an endemic area. *American Journal of Tropical Medicine and Hygiene* 52, 521–524.

Smyth, J.D. (1995) Rare, new and emerging helminth zoonoses. *Advances in Parasitology* 36, 1–47.

Southgate, V.R. (1997) Schistosomiasis in the Senegal River basin: before and after the construction of the dams at Diama, Senegal and Manantali, Mali and future prospects. *Journal of Helminthology* 71, 125–132.

Stephenson, L. (1993) The impact of schistosomiasis on human nutrition. *Parasitology* 107 (suppl.), S107-S123.

Subramanian, A.K., Mungai, P., Ouma, J.H., Magak, P., King, C.H., Mahmoud, A.A.F. and King, C.L. (1999) Long-term suppression of adult bladder morbidity and severe hydronephrosis following selective population chemotherapy for *Schistosoma haematobium*. *American Journal of Tropical Medicine and Hygiene* 61, 476–481.

WHO (1993) *The Control of Schistosomiasis*. Technical Report Series No. 830, World Health Organization, Geneva, Switzerland.

WHO (1995) *Control of Foodborne Trematode Infections*. World Health Organization, Geneva, Switzerland.

Wilkins, H.A., Goll, P.H., Marshall, T.F. de C. and Moore, P.J. (1984) Dynamics of *Schistosoma haematobium* infection in a Gambian community. III. Acquisition and loss of infection. *Transactions of the Royal Society of Tropical Medicine and Hygiene* 28, 227–232.

Wilkins, H.A., Blumenthal, U.J., Hagan, P., Hayes, R.J. and Tullock, S. (1987) Resistance to reinfec-tion after treatment of urinary schistosomiasis. *Transactions of the Royal Society of Tropical Medicine and Hygiene* 81, 29–35.

Williams, S.A. and Johnston, D.A. (with others) (1999) Helminth genome analysis: the current status of the filarial and schistosome genome projects. *Parasitology* 118 (suppl.), 519–538.

Wynn, T.A. and Hoffmann, K.E. (2000) Defining a schistosomiasis vaccination strategy – is it really Th1 versus Th2? *Parasitology Today* 16, 497–501.

Yamaguti, S. (1971) *Synopsis of Digenetic Trematodes of Vertebrates*. Keigaku, Tokyo, Japan.

Yong, T.S., Yang, H.J., Park, S.J., Kim, Y.K., Lee, D.H. and Lee, S.M. (1998) Immunodiagnosis of clonorchiasis using a recombinant antigen. *Korean Journal of Parasitology* 36, 183–190.

Yu, S.-H. and Mott, K.E. (1994) *Epidemiology and Morbidity of Food-borne Intestinal Trematode Infections*. WHO document: WHO/SCHISTO/94.108. World Health Organization, Geneva, Switzerland.

Further Reading

Bergquist, N.R. (1992) *Immunodiagnostic Approaches in Schistosomiasis*. John Wiley & Sons, Chichester, UK.

Jordan, P., Webbe, G. and Sturrock, R. (eds) (1993) *Human Schistosomiasis*. CAB International, Wallingford, UK.

Rollinson, D. and Simpson, A.J.G. (eds) (1986) *The Biology of Schistosomes: from Genes to Latrines*. Academic Press, London, UK.

Wellcome Trust (1998) *Schistosomiasis*. Topics in International Health CD-ROM, CAB International, Wallingford, UK.

2

The Cestodes

All adult cestodes (or tapeworms) inhabit the intestinal tract or associated tracts of vertebrates.

They are flat, ribbon-shaped worms consisting of a chain of a few or many separate proglottides, the whole chain being known as a strobila. At the anterior end is the scolex or holdfast organ, which usually attaches to the intestinal mucosa by means of suckers or sucking grooves and often has hooks. Posterior to the scolex is the narrow undifferentiated neck region, from which growth takes place to give rise to the developing proglottides.

In the order Cyclophyllidea, to which most of the adult tapeworms of humans belong, the proglottides become successively mature and then gravid, when they are filled with eggs. At the gravid stage they become detached and pass out with the faeces. All tapeworms of humans are hermaphroditic, the male organs developing first. Thus male organs alone are found in the mature proglottides nearer to the scolex; further back the organs of both sexes are present but the female organs only are functional. With large tapeworms there is often a single specimen present and cross-fertilization occurs between proglottides. The genital organs are well developed in each proglottid. The male system consists of the testes (three in number in *Hymenolepis* to over 500 in *Taenia*), the vasa efferentia, which unite to form a vas deferens, and a protrusible, muscular cirrus or penis. The cirrus opens into a common genital pore on the margin of the

proglottid just anterior to the vagina. The female organs lie ventrally in the proglottid. The ovary is usually bilobed and lies posteriorly. The ova pass into the oviduct, which joins the spermatic duct from the terminal part of the vagina or seminal receptacle. The ova then pass into the oötype, where fertilization occurs. The vitelline ducts from the vitellaria also open into the oötype and provide shell material and yolk cells. The uterus extends anteriorly from the oötype and ends blindly. The uterus fills with eggs and, when gravid, has a shape characteristic of its family (e.g. with lateral branches in taeniids and a lobate transverse sac in hymenolepids).

Members of the order Pseudophyllidea show structural and life-history differences from the Cyclophyllidea, which are mentioned in the section dealing with the only member that is an important parasite of humans, the broad fish tapeworm, *Diphyllobothrium*.

As cestodes have no gut, all nutritive and waste material must pass through the outer covering or tegument; this functions almost as an inside-out gut wall and contains specific systems of molecular and ion transport, e.g. of amino acids, hexose sugars, nucleotides, lipids, vitamins, purines and pyrimidines. The tegument consists of a syncytial distal cytoplasm with a superficial anucleate zone and an inner nucleated cytosomal zone. The external surface is covered with a row of michrotriches, similar to intestinal microvilli, which increases the surface area in a similar way (increasing the functional area by 1.7–11.8 in some cestodes investigated, compared with a 26 times increase for mouse microvilli). On the tip of each microtriche there is a glycocalyx, composed of mucopolysaccharide and glycoprotein acidic groups, which absorbs and incorporates hexose sugars and amino acids, concentrates inorganic and organic ions, binds host amylase and carries out 'contact digestion' (Smyth and McManus, 1989).

In the great majority of infections the adult tapeworms that normally occur in humans do not cause any serious pathology, although their presence can be extremely unpleasant. Accidental adult tapeworms contracted zoonotically are encountered rarely, principally in children, and are usually short-lived. However, infection with larval tapeworms is potentially very serious and in some countries cysticercosis (caused by the metacestodes of *Taenia solium*) and echinococcosis are important public health problems (56 species of adult and larval cestodes are included as having occurred in humans).

Classification

KEY: Members are parasites of M = mammals, B = birds, R = reptiles, A = amphibians, F = fish.

PHYLUM PLATYHELMINTHES

CLASS CESTODA
No digestive system. Presence of calcareous corpuscles. Usually hermaphrodite.

SUBCLASS EUCESTODA
Body typically divided into short proglottides with anterior holdfast organ, often with suckers and hooks. Egg with 6 hooks. There are many orders of no medical importance, which are not included (see Khalil *et al*., 1994).

Order Pseudophyllidea (MBRAF)
Length very variable but may be up to 30 m. Holdfast typically with dorsal and ventral sucking grooves. Genital apertures usually on ventral surface. Testes and vitellaria scattered and follicular. Eggs usually operculate. Life cycle includes procercoid and plerocercoid larvae.
Diphyllobothrium, Spirometra

Order Cyclophyllidea (MBRA)
Length variable, from 3 mm to 10 m. Holdfast typically with 4 large suckers. Apical end often with row of hooks. Proglottides usually wider than long. Genital apertures marginal. Vitellaria single, compact, postovarian. Gravid uterus without aperture and sometimes broken into capsules. Eggs non-operculate. Larva commonly a cysticercus (bladder-worm) in a vertebrate, or a cysticercoid in an arthropod.

Family Taeniidae (MB)
Rostellum of scolex non-retractable and usually with 2 circles of hammer-shaped hooks. Testes numerous. Gravid proglottides longer than broad. Gravid uterus has median stem and lateral branches. Larva a cysticercus, coenurus or hydatid in a vertebrate.
Taenia, Echinococcus

Family Hymenolepididae (MB)
Rostellum retractable, hooks thornlike. Testes rarely more than 4. Gravid uterus a transverse tube. Larva a cysticercoid in insects (except *H. nana*).
Hymenolepis

Family Dipylididae (M)
Rostellum retractable, hooks typically thorn-shaped. Genitalia single or double. Testes usually numerous. Mature proglottides longer than wide. Gravid uterus a transverse lobed sac or replaced by egg sacs. Larval stage a cysticercoid in insects.
Dipylidium

Family Anoplocephalidae (MBR)
No rostellum. Testes numerous. Gravid proglottides much wider than long. Gravid uterus often replaced by paruterine organs. Eggs often with characteristic membrane drawn out into a pair of cross-tapered processes (pyriform apparatus). Larva a cysticercoid in oribatid mites.
Bertiella, Inermicapsifer

Family Davaineidae (MB)
Rostellum retractable, hooks T-shaped. Suckers often spinose. Gravid uterus

replaced by egg pouches. Larva a cysticercoid in insects.
Raillietina

Family Mesocestoididae (MB)
No rostellum. Mature proglottides wider than long, genital apertures median. Posterior paruterine organ. First larval stage probably in oribatid mites, second tetrathyridium in vertebrates.
Mesocestoides

Order Pseudophyllidea

Diphyllobothrium latum
(Linnaeus, 1758) Lühe, 1910

SYNONYMS
Taenia lata Linnaeus, 1758; *Dibothriocephalus latus* Lühe, 1899; *Bothriocephalus latus* Bremser, 1918.

DISEASE, POPULAR AND LOCAL NAMES
Diphyllobothriasis or diphyllobothriosis; broad fish tapeworm infection; Lapamato (Finnish), Breda binnikemaskens (Swedish).

GEOGRAPHICAL DISTRIBUTION
It is estimated that there are about 20 million cases worldwide. In Europe it is found principally in countries with many lakes, such as Finland, Estonia, Russia (Don and Volga Rivers), Poland and Ukraine, with sporadic cases in Italy/Switzerland (Lake Maggiore) and Slovakia (Danube basin); in Asia, in Japan, north-eastern Russia (Amur River basin) and with a few cases in China, India (one case) and Korea; in the Americas, in the Great Lakes regions of Canada and the USA, Argentina and Chile (Valdiva River basin).

LOCATION IN HOST
The adult worm or worms inhabit the lumen of the small intestine with the scolex embedded in the mucosa.

MORPHOLOGY
Diphyllobothrium is the longest tapeworm infecting humans. It measures 3–10 m in length and may have 4000 proglottides. Each proglottid measures 2–7 mm × 10–12 mm, and contains both male and female reproductive organs (Fig. 26). *Diphyllobothrium* differs from all other human tapeworms in having a uterine pore through which eggs are discharged (this is typical of the order Pseudophyllidea and similar to the situation in trematodes). This pore and the cirrus and vagina open on the ventral surface, not at the lateral margin as in the Cyclophyllidea. The scolex measures 1–2 mm and has no suckers but attaches to the mucosa by two sucking grooves (Fig. 27).

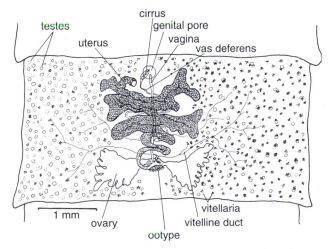

Fig. 26. Mature proglottid of *Diphyllobothrium latum*. The vitellaria are shown principally on the right-hand side, the testes on the left. Note genital uterine pore, through which eggs emerge.

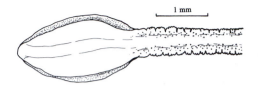

Fig. 27. Scolex with two sucking grooves.

LIFE CYCLE (Fig. 28)

Up to 1 million eggs can be produced daily and these pass out in the faeces. The ovoid eggs measure 55–80 µm × 40–60 µm and are similar in structure to those of trematodes (Fig. 123). They are yellowish-brown, operculate and with a small knob at the end opposite to the operculum. The ovum is unsegmented when laid and is surrounded by yolk cells. If the egg reaches fresh water, the ovum develops in 12 days to many weeks, depending on the temperature, into a ciliated larva (termed a coracidium) measuring 40–50 µm and with six small hooks (Fig. 29a). The coracidium larva escapes into the water through the opened operculum and swims around in an apparently aimless manner. The coracidium can survive for 1–2 days but for further development must be ingested by a suitable planktonic copepod belonging to the genus *Diaptomus* or, more rarely in Europe, *Cyclops,* living in large bodies of water (about 40 species including *D. vulgaris*, *D. gracilis, C. vicinus* and *C. strenuus*). Inside the stomach of the crustacean, the outer epithelium is lost and the enclosed larva penetrates the gut wall with the aid of the hooks. In the body cavity a procercoid larva, measuring 0.5 mm in length, develops in 14–21 days (Fig. 29b).

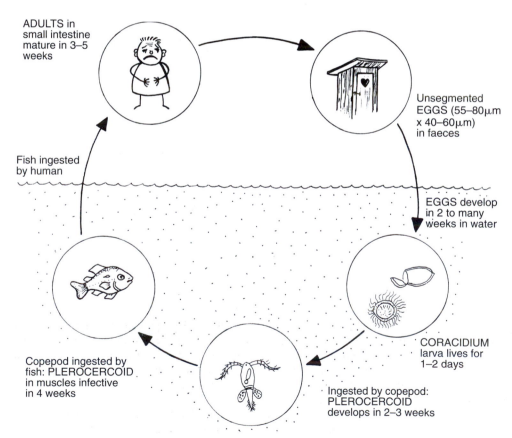

Fig. 28. Cartoon illustrating the life cycle of *Diphyllobothrium latum* (after *Tiedoksianto Information,* 1971, 12, 3–9).

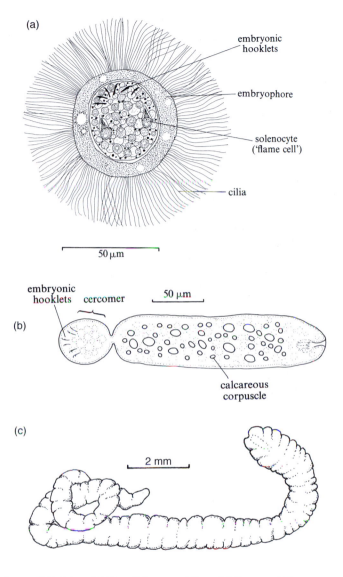

(a)

embryonic
hooklets

embryophore

solenocyte
('flame cell')

cilia

50 μm

embryonic
hooklets   cercomer   50 μm

(b)

calcareous
corpuscle

(c)

2 mm

Fig. 29. Larval stages of *D. latum*. (a) Free-living coracidium. (b) Procercoid from copepod.
(c) Plerocercoid from fish.

If the copepod is ingested by a plankton-eating freshwater fish, the procercoid larva penetrates the intestinal wall in about 4 h and develops into a plerocercoid larva in the connective tissues and muscles. The plerocercoid is an elongate wormlike larva with an inverted scolex and takes about 4 weeks to become infective (Fig. 29c). The larvae eventually become encysted but usually remain infective throughout the life of the fish. The small copepods (about 1 mm long) are often ingested by small fish and, when these are eaten by a larger fish, such as pike, perch, burbot or salmon, the released plerocercoids can penetrate the intestinal wall and remain viable. In this way the larval parasites become concentrated in the larger carnivorous food fishes, which act as paratenic hosts (e.g. the pike). Human infection occurs when fish are eaten raw or semi-cooked. The released larva attaches to the intestinal wall by the everted scolex and develops proglottides. *Diphyllobothrium* reaches maturity in 3–5 weeks and can live for up to 25 years in humans. Usually only a single worm is present. After voiding eggs, a chain of the oldest proglottides breaks off and is often passed out in the faeces (pseudoapolysis). A small form of *D. latum*, measuring about 60 cm × 2.3 mm, has been reported from Japan.

CLINICAL MANIFESTATIONS AND PATHOGENESIS
Often none. In a proportion of cases there is abdominal pain, loss of weight, anorexia and vomiting. Sometimes the worm becomes lodged in the jejunum, where it causes acute pain and vomiting of segments.

The most important pathological effect of diphyllobothriasis is anaemia, which occurs only in Finland and is of the pernicious megablastic (macrocytic) type. It used to occur in about 20% of cases but is not so common since diet has improved. The cause appears to be a competitive uptake of vitamin B_{12} by the worm, rather than any substance released by it interfering with Castle's intrinsic factor (von Bonsdorff, 1977). *Diphyllobothrium* has a vitamin B_{12} content 50 times that of *Taenia saginata* and absorbs 80–100% of radioactive B_{12} added to the diet of symptomless carriers. The North American strain of *Diphyllobothrium* takes up only 6–7%, however, and anaemia is very rare. Anaemia in Finland possibly occurs: (i) because the strain of worm is found higher up the gut, in the jejunum and nearer to the stomach; (ii) because of a reduction in intrinsic factor resulting from damage to the gastric mucosa; (iii) principally because of a low dietary intake of B_{12} (supported by the finding that pernicious anaemia has decreased greatly since the diet has improved); (iv) because of human genetic factors. There can be up to 25% eosinophilia in early infections.

Occasional cases of multiple infection have been known to cause obstruction of the small intestine.

DIAGNOSIS
This is by discovery of the characteristic eggs in the faeces but they need to be differentiated from similar trematode eggs, such as those of *Paragonimus* (Fig. 123).

Sometimes a chain of proglottides is passed in the faeces at intervals and these can be recognized by the characteristic shape of the uterus (Fig. 30), but there is no regular expulsion of gravid proglottides, as with taeniid tapeworms.

TREATMENT
Praziquantel is the drug of choice at a single oral dose of 15–30 mg kg⁻¹, but it is important to make sure that the scolex has been expelled.

Niclosamide (2,2'-dichloro-5,4'-nitrosalicylanilide) at 1 g first thing in the morning and then 1 g 1 h later (scolex is destroyed) and bithionol (50–60 mg kg⁻¹, repeated a day or so later if no scolex is recovered) have been used for many years.

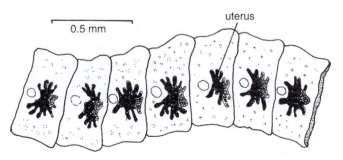

Fig. 30. Chain of proglottides as sometimes passed in the faeces. The characteristic branched uterus can be recognized by the tanned eggs.

EPIDEMIOLOGY

Raw or smoked freshwater fish is an important item of diet in many countries. In reservoirs in the Krasnoyarsk region of Siberia the tipping of untreated sewage has caused 100% infection in pike living in lakes and 5% in rivers, with 35,000 cases reported annually in Russia overall. 'Caviar' made from the roe of pike is a popular dish in that area and is the cause of a seasonal rise in the infection rate in the spring when the fish have roe. In the Archangel region (as in Finland) infection has been much reduced by improved treatment of sewage.

Around the Baltic Sea, slices of raw fish known as 'strogonina' are a popular item of diet and are important in transmission, as is 'sashimi' in Japan.

PREVENTION AND CONTROL

The plerocercoid larvae in fish are killed by freezing at −10°C for 15 min. They are also killed by complete drying or by thorough pickling.

Proper disposal and treatment of faeces are also of great importance in reducing incidence.

ZOONOTIC ASPECTS

Infection with *D. latum* has been recorded from many mammals, including dogs, cats and bears. However, with the exception of dogs, animals are probably not of importance in transmission; tapeworms in cats last only for a matter of weeks.

Numerous other species of *Diphyllobothrium* and related genera are occasionally found in humans, mostly contracted from marine fish (Ruttenber *et al.*, 1984). However, the taxonomic status of species within this genus is rather confused and it is often very difficult to differentiate them on adult characters alone, although the structure and size of eggs can be useful. *Diphyllobothrium pacificum* (Nybelin, 1931) Margolis, 1956, is a natural parasite of fur seals and sea lions with plerocercoids in marine fish (e.g. mackerel) and has been found in humans in Chile, Ecuador and Japan. Other species with a few cases in humans include: *D. cameroni*

Rausch, 1969, a natural parasite of monk seal, in Japan; *D. cordatum* Cobbold, 1879, found naturally in seals and walrus, in Alaska; *D. dalliae* Rausch, 1956, and *D. dendriticum* (Nitzsch, 1824), parasites of gulls and freshwater fish, in Alaska; *D. elegans* (Krabbe, 1865), naturally in seals and sea lion, in Japan; *D. giljacicum* (= *D. luxi*) Rutkevich, 1937, in freshwater fish and adults only known from humans in Siberia; *D. hians* (Diesing, 1850), naturally in seals, in Japan and Siberia; *D. klebanovskii* (= *D. luxi*) Muratov and Posokhov, 1988, naturally in brown bears and salmon, in Belarus and Siberia; *D. lanceolatum* (Krabbe, 1865), naturally in seals, in Alaska; *D. minus* Cholodkovsky, 1916, naturally in seagulls, in Russia; *D. nenzi* Petrov, 1938, in Russia; *D. nihonkaiense* (= *D. luxi*) Yamane *et al.*, 1986, is apparently a human parasite in Japan and Siberia contracted from salmon; *D. orcini* Hatsushika and Shirouzu,1990, naturally in killer whale, in Japan; *D. scoticum* (Rennie and Reid, 1912), naturally in seals and sea lion, in Japan; *D. skrjabini* Plotnikov, 1932, in dogs and freshwater fish, in Russia; *D. tangussicum* Podjapolskaia and Gnedina, 1932, is apparently a human parasite in Russia; *D. ursi* Rausch, 1954, naturally in bears, in Canada and Alaska; *D. yonagoense* Yamane *et al.*, 1981, natural cycle unknown, in Japan and Korea.

Diplogonoporus grandis (= *D. balanopterae*) (Blanchard, 1894) Lühe, 1899, is a parasite of whales and has been reported over 50 times from humans in Japan (causing abdominal discomfort) and Korea, with a single case in Spain. Each proglottid has a double set of reproductive organs and the eggs measure 63–68 μm × 50 μm. Other species are *D. brauni* Leon, 1907, in Romania and *D. fukuokaensis* Kamo and Miyazaki, 1970, in Japan. *Ligula intestinalis* Linnaeus (1758) Bloch, 1782, a common and widespread parasite of fish-eating birds, has been found in humans in Poland and Romania; *Schistocephalus solidus* (Mueller, 1776) Creplin, 1829, another common bird parasite, has been recorded from humans in Alaska; *Pyramicocephalus anthocephalus* (Fabricius, 1780) Monticelli,

1890, is a pseudophyllid tapeworm of seals, which has been recorded from humans in Alaska and Greenland.

Sparganosis

Sparganosis is the term used to describe infection with the plerocercoid larvae (= spargana) of diphyllobothriid tapeworms of the genus *Spirometra* (in some textbooks they are included in the genus *Diphyllobothrium,* but it is clearly a valid genus, although more correctly it should be *Luheella*).

The adult tapeworms are parasites of carnivores in tropical and subtropical regions of Africa, the Americas, Australia, Europe and Asia. The mature proglottides can be easily differentiated from those of *Diphyllobothrium* by the structure of the uterine coils, which form compact loops in the midline rather than a rosette shape (Fig. 30). The eggs can also be differentiated.

The life cycle resembles that of *Diphyllobothrium* except that the procercoids develop in cyclopoid species that inhabit small ponds rather than lakes (*Eucyclops serrulatus* and *Mesocyclops leuckarti* and probably the other species transmitting *Gnathostoma* and *Dracunculus*) (Fig. 31); also the plerocercoids do not develop in fish but, in most parts of the world, in amphibians, reptiles and small mammals and, in East Africa, in large game animals. A wide range of vertebrates, including humans, in which adult tapeworms will not develop, can also act as paratenic hosts. Human infection may occur in one of three ways:

1. By ingestion of cyclops containing procercoid larvae in drinking water from ponds or open wells; this is the most likely mode of infection in many parts of the world.
2. By application of the flesh of an infected frog to ulcers, sores and infected eyes; the procercoid is activated by warmth and enters the flesh. This form of traditional poultice is used only in areas of South-East Asia, particularly Thailand and Vietnam, and spargana in the eye can result in severe oedema and eventually nodule formation, usually of the upper eyelid; when removed the contained larva has often degenerated into a caseous mass.
3. By ingestion of raw or undercooked meat of infected frogs, snakes, mammals or birds; the contained plerocercoids burrowing through the wall of the intestine (Plate 8).

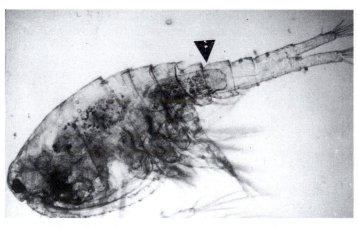

Fig. 31. *Cyclops* with procercoids of *Spirometra* sp. in the haemocoel. Calcareous bodies can be seen in the bodies of the parasites.

Spargana wander in the deep tissues and usually migrate to the subcutaneous tissues, where they eventually encyst, resulting in a fibrous nodule about 2 cm in diameter. Surgical excision of the nodule is usually possible, and the enclosed larva, which has a scolex similar to that of *Diphyllobothrium* but with a tail many centimetres in length, is sometimes mistaken for a guinea worm in Africa. The most serious effects are caused by larvae in the brain, which can cause repeated seizures (in 84% of patients), hemiparesis (59%) and headache (56%) with convulsions, and can be diagnosed by computer-assisted tomography (CT) or magnetic resonance imaging (MRI) scans (Chang *et al.*, 1992). The lesions need to be removed surgically; high dosages of praziquantel have not always been successful. Very rarely, larvae may enter the eye and cause endophthalmitis, leading to blindness (Sen *et al.*, 1989) and larvae may also enter various visceral organs. Sparganosis can be diagnosed by a chemiluminescence ELISA.

Many species of *Spirometra* have been described from various areas of the world, but most are morphologically variable and the species position is very confused. Parasites from Asia or Europe are usually termed *S. mansoni* (Cobbold, 1882), *S. houghtoni* (Kellogg, 1927) or *S. erinacei* (= *S. erinaceieuropei*) (Rudolphi, 1819), with plerocercoids in frogs and snakes and adults occurring naturally in carnivores, including cats and dogs (16% in Thailand), those from Africa *S. theileri* (Baer, 1925), with plerocercoids in wild herbivores and adults in large carnivores, and worms from the Americas *S. mansonoides* (Mueller, 1935), with plerocercoids in frogs and snakes and adults in wild carnivores and cats and dogs (the adults of this species can be differentiated morphologically from all the others and produce a growth hormone-like cysteine proteinase that causes weight gain in experimentally infected mice).

The presence of spargana is becoming more commonly identified with an increasing concern about strange growths, and there is an ELISA using crude antigens of adult or larval worms which works well.

'Sparganum proliferum' is a rare form, of unknown relationship, in which the plerocercoids become disorganized and proliferate in the tissues by lateral budding (DNA analysis shows that they are of the genus *Spirometra* but of unknown species). In human cases found at autopsy many thousands of larvae have been present in the viscera as well as in the subcutaneous tissues. It is possible that virus infection of a normal sparganum may be responsible. Three fairly recent similar cases, probably of proliferating spargana, have been described, one in an abdominal mass from an Amerindian in Paraguay (Beaver and Rolon, 1981) and two others from the lungs of a man and the spinal cord of a woman in Taiwan (Lo *et al.*, 1987).

Order Cyclophyllidea

The majority of tapeworms of medical and veterinary importance belong to this order.

Family Taeniidae

This group of taeniid tapeworms includes the most important cestode parasites of humans. The adults of two species, *Taenia saginata* and *T. solium*, are only found in humans but are usually of minor medical importance. The larval stages are always in mammals and consist of a fluid-filled cyst, which may contain a single or many protoscolices, each of which is capable of developing into an adult tapeworm in a definitive host (Fig. 32). Human infection with larval cestodes can be a very serious medical problem indeed.

Taenia saginata
Goeze, 1782

SYNONYMS
Taeniarhynchus saginatus Weinland, 1848; *Taenia africana* Linstow, 1900; *T. confusa*

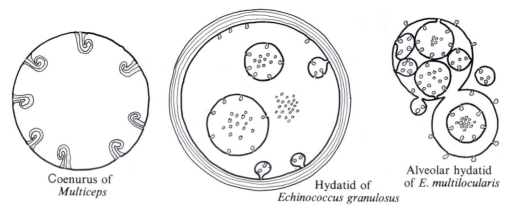

Coenurus of
Multiceps

Hydatid of
Echinococcus granulosus

Alveolar hydatid
of *E. multilocularis*

Fig. 32. The various types of taeniid larvae. They contain one or many protoscolices.

Ward, 1896; *T. hominis* Linstow, 1902. In the literature from eastern Europe this tapeworm is commonly called *Taeniarhynchus saginatus,* because some authorities believe that the lack of rostellum and hooks is sufficient to warrant a genus separate from *Taenia* (Bessenov *et al.*, 1994). However, there is evidence that there are rudimentary hooks in the cysticerci and it is likely that these have been secondarily lost.

DISEASE AND POPULAR NAME
Taeniasis or taeniosis saginata; beef tapeworm infection.

LOCAL NAMES
Dooda shareatia or dedan (Arabic), Than kaung (Burmese), San-chik (Cantonese), Sanadu mushi (Japanese), Miliny (Luo), Tegu (Swahili), Nada puchi (Tamil), Payard tua tued (Thai), Sonsono (Twi), Arán inú (Yoruba).

GEOGRAPHICAL DISTRIBUTION
Infection is cosmopolitan and occurs in almost all countries where beef is eaten raw or undercooked. In most countries it is more common than the pork tapeworm (*T. solium*), with about 60 million cases in the world.

LOCATION IN HOST
The scolex of the adult tapeworm is embedded in the mucosa of the wall of the ileum, with the rest of the tape extending throughout the lumen.

MORPHOLOGY
The scolex is pear-shaped, 1–2 mm in diameter, but with no rostellum or hooks. The adult worm is very long, sometimes exceeding 20 m. Usually, however, it is about 5 m long with 1000–2000 proglottides. Each mature proglottid measures about 12 mm wide and 10 mm long and each gravid proglottid contains about 0.8–1 $\times 10^5$ eggs.

Female organs. The ovary is in the posterior part of the proglottid and has two large lobes. The follicular vitellaria (which produce the eggshell and nutrient yolk cells) lie in a band behind the ovaries. The uterus extends forwards as a tube, slightly dilated anteriorly. In contrast to the uterus of *Diphyllobothrium*, it has no opening to the exterior. Gravid proglottides contain a characteristic taeniid type of uterus filled with eggs (Figs 33 and 34).

Male organs. The numerous follicular testes are scattered throughout the anterodorsal part of the proglottid. The vas deferens opens through the muscular cirrus at the common genital pore, which is situated irregularly on alternate lateral margins.

LIFE CYCLE
The eggs measure 43 μm × 31 μm and are identical to those of *T. solium* and many other taeniids. They are deposited in human faeces (about 0.7–1 $\times 10^6$ 24 h^{-1}), often inside the gravid proglottid, or the latter

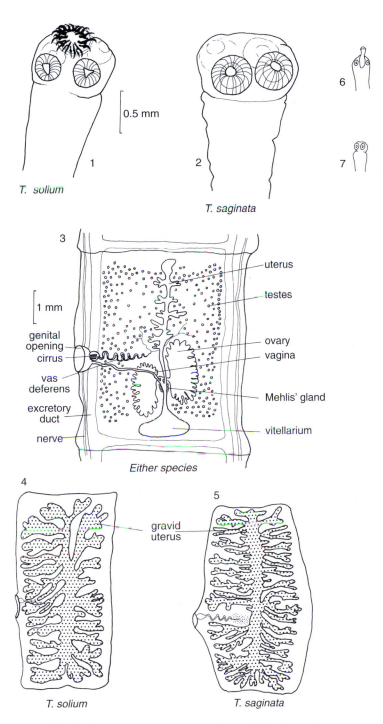

Fig. 33. Comparative morphological features of *Taenia solium* and *Taenia saginata*.
1 and 2. Scolices (6 and 7 are the scolices of *Hymenolepis nana* and *H. diminuta* at the same scale).
3. Mature proglottid of either species. 4 and 5. Gravid proglottides showing the typical numbers of branches of the uterus in each species.

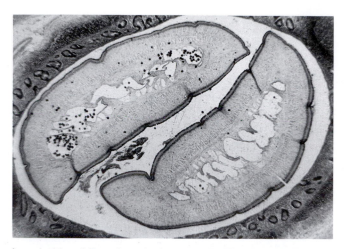

Fig. 34. Section of proglottides of *T. saginata* in the appendix. The uterus contains eggs.

may pass out through the anus and for further development need to be ingested by cattle, when the contained oncosphere larva hatches in the duodenum. The oncospheres penetrate through the intestinal wall with the aid of the six hooklets and enter the venous capillaries (or the mesenteric lymphatics) in about 30 min. The embryos are carried by the circulation until they reach the voluntary muscles, where they lose the hooks and develop into an infective cysticercus larva in 10–12 weeks, or sometimes longer. The fully formed cysticercus is ovoid and white in colour and measures about 8 mm × 5 mm (it is known to veterinarians as a 'cysticercus bovis'). The invaginated protoscolex has four suckers but no hooks. The outer wall of the fluid-filled bladder has microvilli, possibly serving a trophoblastic function.

Humans become infected from eating raw or undercooked beef. The protoscolex of the cysticercus evaginates in the duodenum, attaches to the wall of the ileum and begins to form proglottides.

CLINICAL MANIFESTATIONS
Often the first and only sign of infection is the presence of active proglottides in the faeces, perhaps preceded by the feeling of them 'crawling' out through the anus.

As the tapeworm matures, 6–8 weeks after infection, there may be epigastric or umbilical pain, nausea, weakness, loss of weight, alteration of appetite, and headache. These symptoms and signs are possibly caused by toxic products produced by the worms or are allergic reactions, and are characteristically alleviated by taking food.

Occasionally, generalized allergic manifestations, such as urticaria with pruritus ani or widespread pruritus, result. The presence of a lump in the throat is a not uncommon symptom, reported particularly by middle-aged women in Poland. Perhaps unsurprisingly, symptoms often increase in frequency and severity once patients are aware they have a tapeworm. Occasionally a worm causes obstruction due to bolus impaction in the intestine and it has been known for proglottides to be vomited and then aspirated.

A moderate eosinophilia occurs in 5–45% of patients.

PATHOGENESIS
Little pathology can be directly attributed to the physical action of the scolex on the mucosa, although inflammation of the mucosa of the ileum sometimes occurs. Over 100 cases of intestinal obstruction, perforation or appendicitis have been reported. In a recent case in Reunion island, intestinal perforation led to death from septic shock.

DIAGNOSIS

Parasitological. The presence of gravid proglottides with the characteristic taeniid branched uterus in the faeces provides the usual method of diagnosis. These are passed out in short chains of 5–8 proglottides, are very active and sometimes can be felt migrating out of the anus. When pressed between glass slides, the number of lateral branches of the uterus can be counted in order to differentiate *T. saginata* (15–32, usually 20–23, main branches) from *T. solium* (7–13, usually 9, main branches). However, in South Africa at least some degree of overlap was reported, but it is not clear how much. The two species can be clearly differentiated if the scolex is passed in the faeces after chemotherapy, because of the lack of rostellum and hooks in that of *T. saginata*. There are also small differences in the mature proglottides: those of *T. saginata* have a vaginal sphincter muscle and testes confluent posteriorly to the vitellarium, while those of *T. solium* have a third lobe to the ovary. Unfortunately, special preparation is often necessary in order to see these features.

Free eggs may be found in the faeces if the gravid proglottides have been autolysed, particularly using concentration techniques, and may also be found by taking possibly repeated anal swabs with sticky tape (p. 163) or a sticky glass spatula, as used in Russia, and examining under the microscope, although species of taeniids cannot be differentiated.

Serological. The detection of coproantigens in faeces by capture ELISA techniques has proved sensitive and also specific (Machnicka *et al.*, 1996). There are various techniques for diagnosis of cysticerci in cattle. The best probably recognize circulating excretory/secretory (ES) antigens of cysticerci by monoclonal antibody-based dot ELISA, SDS-PAGE or immunoblotting (which recognizes antigens of 65, 87 and 100 kDa).

TREATMENT

Praziquantel at a single oral dose of 5–10 mg kg^{-1} is usually completely effective.

Albendazole at a single oral dose of 800 mg has about 80% effectiveness. Niclosamide (2 g for an adult given in a divided dose over 2 days) has been in use for many years but has (usually mild) side-effects and is not always effective. With newer compounds the scolex is destroyed and so follow-up is necessary to determine that the complete worm has been expelled (if the scolex should remain embedded, a new worm can develop within weeks).

EPIDEMIOLOGY

The prevalence of *T. saginata* infection has remained high in areas of Europe; various recent regional estimates are 0.4–9.5% in Belgium, 1.3–1.7% in northern Italy, 4.0% in northern Germany, 20,000 cases annually in Russia, 0.9% in Slovakia and 2.5% in Turkey. It is rare in the UK (627 cases in England and Wales between 1990 and 1998). In other parts of the world estimates are 1.3% in Afghanistan, 0.5% in Brazil, 0.4–1.0% in Egypt, 1.0% in Ethiopia, 0.3% in Honduras, 7.7% in Iran and 2.3% in eastern and 11.5% in northern Nigeria. Estimates of cysts in cattle are 1.9% in Brazil, 8.3–28.8% in Botswana, 0.1% in Chile, 1.3% in Bulgaria, 0.72% overall in Egypt, 3.5–6.0% in northern Germany, 0.43–15.9% in Kenya, 3.2% in Poland, 1.7% in Sudan, 29% in Swaziland, 4.5% in Switzerland, 0.6–16% in Tanzania, 6.8–59% in Togo, 0.5–88% in Texas, USA, 1.6% in Vietnam and 3.2% in Zimbabwe. Raw minced beef or very rare steaks are popular items of diet in many countries.

The eggs can survive on pastures for 60–180 days, in sewage for 16 days at 18°C. and in river water for many weeks and they can survive for up to 1 h at 50°C. (Muller, 1983). In Russia eggs withstand the winter better than summer (at the optimal temperature of −4°C, they survive for 62–64 days). Moisture is a very important factor governing their survival and they die rapidly when desiccated (Muller, 1983).

Infection of cattle occurs mainly when they are young calves, sometimes from the hands of stockmen, but more usually from faecal matter spread on pastures. Proglottides can also migrate out through the anus and may contaminate pastures when an infected person walks over them. In developed countries transmission is primarily due to inadequate treatment of sewage. Eggs are very resistant and can survive the activated sludge process; thorough drying or sand filtration is necessary to remove them. In some parts of the world improperly treated effluent finds its way back to the fields.

The role of birds, particularly seagulls, in the dissemination of *T. saginata* eggs from sewage beds to fields has not been clearly established but they have been implicated in Denmark and England. Flies have also been implicated in Russia and in one survey 4.8% of all flies, particularly sarcophagid flies, were found to be infected.

Cysts in calves survive for longer (for up to 2 years) than those in mature cattle (maybe as little as 3 weeks). Cysticerci in cattle are economically very important and are estimated to cost $1000 million annually in Africa. In addition to cattle, cysticerci occur in buffalo and have been reported from reindeer in Siberia, from wild game animals in Africa and from pigs in Asia and Africa (but see below).

Taenia saginata asiatica Fan, Lin, Chen and Chung, 1995, is a recently named subspecies, in which cysticerci are found in the liver and mesenteries of pigs and wild boars, as well as in cattle (and goats and monkeys), in Burma (Myanmar), China, Indonesia (western islands), Korea (Cheju Island) and Taiwan (Ito, 1992); a similar form has been reported from areas of Africa. The cysticercus has a sunken rostellum with two rows of rudimentary hooks and there are many branches to the uterus in gravid proglottides (Fan *et al.*, 1995). It has been estimated to cause an annual economic loss of $34 million in Indonesia, Korea and Taiwan (Fan, 1997). Cysticercosis can also occur in humans, as with *T. solium*. In Taiwan, cysts of *T. s. saginata*, as well as *T. s. asiatica*, can develop in pigs as well as in cattle.

PREVENTION AND CONTROL
Personal protection is by thorough cooking of all beef and pork (above 56°C.) or by freezing at −10°C. for 10 days. Meat

inspection is the most important public-health measure possible. The most heavily infected muscles for inspection may vary from region to region but usually include the heart, masseters, shoulder muscle and tongue, and also the liver of cattle or pigs in Asia. The cysts can be easily recognized in 'measly beef' (or pork) about 6 weeks after infection.

Infection rates have been reduced somewhat in recent years in eastern Europe and East Africa by sanitation measures, and mass diagnosis and treatment campaigns have been tried in Russia.

ZOONOTIC ASPECTS
In the strict sense this is an obligatory cyclo-zoonotic infection, the life cycle necessarily involving both cattle (or pig) and humans (sometimes termed a euzoonosis or an anthropozoonosis). However, there is no animal reservoir host of the adult tapeworms, which occur only in humans.

Taenia solium
Linnaeus, 1758

SYNONYM
Taenia cucurbitina Pallas, 1766.

DISEASE AND POPULAR NAME
Taeniasis or taeniosis solium; pork tapeworm infection.

LOCAL NAMES
As for *T. saginata*.

GEOGRAPHICAL DISTRIBUTION
Taenia solium infection has a cosmopolitan distribution in countries where pork is eaten raw or undercooked. It is most common in Africa, Central and South America (particularly Mexico and Chile) and China. Prevalences fell greatly in eastern European countries but with less efficient control are beginning to rise again.

LOCATION IN HOST
The scolex is embedded in the mucosa of the jejunum, with the rest of the tape extending through the ileum.

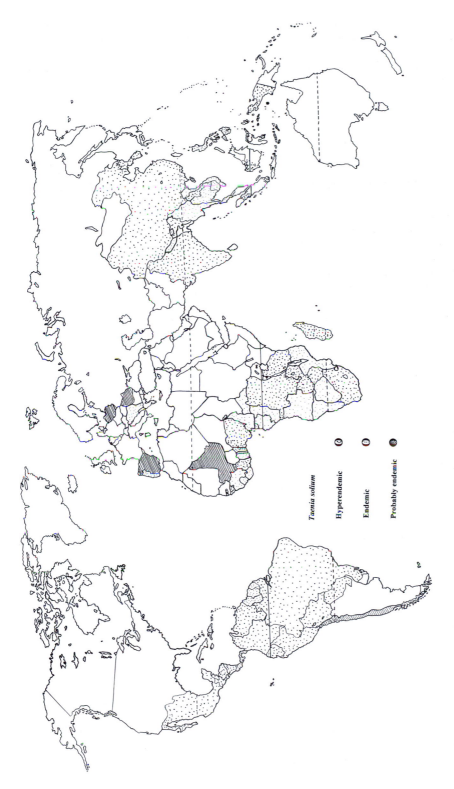

Map 5. Distribution of *Taenia solium* (and cysticercosis) on a country basis.

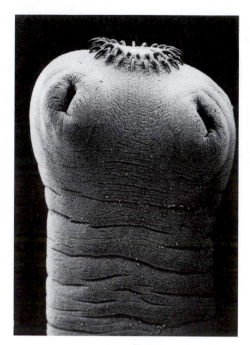

Fig. 35. Stereoscan photograph of the scolex of
T. solium.

MORPHOLOGY

Taenia solium is a long tapeworm, 2–3 m
in length and having up to 4000 proglottides (usually around 1000). The scolex
measures 1 mm in diameter with four large
suckers and a conspicuous rostellum with
two rows of alternating large and small
hooks. There are 25–30 of these hooks, the
large hooks measuring about 170 µm in
length and the short ones about 130 µm
(Fig. 35). The shape of the hooks is characteristic of the family Taeniidae. The neck
region is thin and measures 5–10 mm.

The mature proglottides are roughly
square (12 mm × 10 mm) (Fig. 33) and are
superficially identical to those of *T. saginata*. The gravid proglottides are about
12 mm long by 6 mm wide. Eight to ten are
usually passed in the faeces each day, often
in a short chain. The uterus ends blindly,
as in all cyclophyllidean tapeworms, and
when it becomes filled with eggs (up to
90,000) it has branched lateral extensions.
There are 7–13 main branches and this is
the feature used to differentiate the gravid
proglottides in faeces from those of *T. sagi-*

nata (which have 15–32 main branches).
There are usually one to three tapeworms
present but there may be as many as 25.

LIFE CYCLE

The eggs are roughly spherical and measure
47–77 µm in diameter (Fig. 123). They have
an outer vitelline layer, which is often lost,
and then a thick brown embryophore made
up of keratin blocks, giving it a striated
appearance (the true outer eggshell is lost).
Inside there is an embryo, termed an oncosphere or hexacanth, which has six hooklets.
The eggs are morphologically identical to
those of *T. saginata*.

Eggs may burst free from the proglottid,
whether in the gut or on the ground, and
can survive on soil for weeks. Often, however, the pig, which acts as the intermediate
host, ingests the gravid proglottid in human
faeces. The cement substance between the
embryophore blocks is dissolved by the gastric secretions and the oncosphere hatches
in the duodenum. It penetrates through the
intestinal wall with the aid of the hooklets
and enters the venous capillaries (or the
mesenteric lymph vessels) in about 30 min.
The embryos are carried by the circulation
until they reach the voluntary muscles,
where they lose the embryonic hooks and
develop into cysticerci (known to veterinarians as 'cysticerci cellulosae') or bladder-
worms in 60–75 days. Cysts in pigs are
commonly found in the heart muscle (in
80% of infected animals), masseters (50%),
diaphragm (50%) and tongue (40%).
Cysticerci may also be found in the liver,
kidneys, brain and eyes. The fully formed
cysticerci are ovoid and white in colour
and measure about 8 mm × 5 mm. They are
thus easily visible to the naked eye as white
dots and give rise to the condition known
as 'measly' pork. Each cyst consists of a
fluid-filled bladder with a minute protoscolex invaginated into the lumen; the
protoscolex has four suckers and two rows
of hooks (Fig. 36a,b).

Humans can become infected with cysticerci from ingestion of eggs (or possibly
occasionally by retroinfection of gravid
proglottides), similarly to pigs; this is discussed on p. 81.

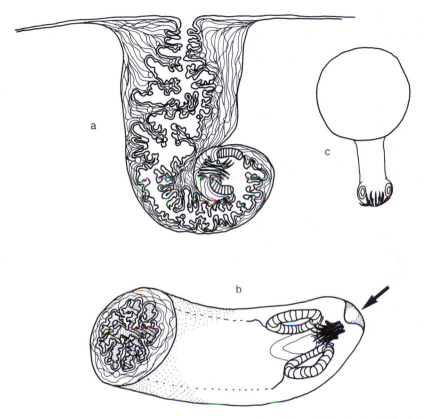

Fig. 36. The invaginated protoscolex of a cysticercus of *T. solium*. That of *T. saginata* is identical apart from the absence of hooks. (a) In section. (b) In solid view, arrow indicates beginning of evagination. (c) Whole cysticercus after invagination in stomach of new host.

Human infection with the adult tapeworms occurs through eating raw or inadequately cooked pork. The protoscolex invaginates in the duodenum (Fig. 36b, c), and attaches to the mucosa of the small intestine, and the worm matures in 5–12 weeks.

CLINICAL MANIFESTATIONS AND PATHOGENESIS
Usually the presence of an adult tapeworm causes no distinct clinical symptoms or signs. Sometimes vague abdominal pain, with diarrhoea or constipation, is found. Excessive appetite is also occasionally reported, with loss of weight and weakness. Symptoms may be psychological in origin or perhaps due to toxic waste products produced by the worm.

There is usually slight traumatic damage to the mucosa at the site of attachment of the scolex, although it has been known to perforate the wall of the intestine, very rarely causing death.

There is often an eosinophilia of 10–13%.

Far more serious than the presence of an adult tapeworm of *T. solium* is human infection with cysticerci.

DIAGNOSIS
As for *T. saginata*. An immunoblot assay utilizing ES antigens is specific to adult *T. solium* infections (Williams *et al.*, 1999), not reacting to *T. saginata* or to cases of cysticercosis. There are also specific antibody-based dot ELISAs for diagnosis of cysticercus antigens.

TREATMENT
The theoretical risk with *T. solium* infection that regurgitation of proglottides

caused by chemotherapy will lead to hatching of the eggs and subsequent cysticercosis does not appear to be important in practice. None the less, it may be advisable to give an antiemetic and follow treatment with a saline purge.

Praziquantel at 5–10 mg kg^{-1} in a single oral dose is usually completely effective against adult worms.

Niclosamide at an oral dose of 2 g for an adult given in a divided dose over 2 days is effective and causes only minor side-effects, although syncope has been reported. It appears to disturb mitochondrial phosphorylation.

EPIDEMIOLOGY

Infection with *T. solium* is nowhere near as common as with *T. saginata,* presumably because pork is not so often eaten undercooked as beef. In Bali, however, 'lawal', a dish of often uncooked spiced pork is popular and taeniasis is common (although this is probably due to *T. saginata asiatica*). In many areas the recorded infection rate in pigs (and sometimes also the cysticerci rate in humans) is very much higher than the recorded infection rate of adult tapeworms in humans would indicate and it is likely that gravid proglottides are sometimes mistaken for those of *T. saginata.*

Unhygienic disposal of human faeces is the primary means of dissemination; the eggs surviving on pastures for many weeks. In a rural area of Mexico many households (38%) have pigs and all eat pork (often measly or 'granos' pork). There are poor personal and household standards of hygiene and pigs routinely eat human faeces (Sarti *et al.*, 1992, 1994).

It is not known how long cysticerci can survive in the pig, but, since degenerated cysts are rare, it is probable that they remain viable throughout the lifetime of the animal.

Estimated human infection rates in areas of various countries are: Brazil 13%, Bulgaria 1.4% (0.7% in 1989), Cambodia 2.2%, Chile 0.1% (0.7% in 1977), China (Shandung Province) 0.3%, Guatemala 3.5%, Honduras 0.3 (large-scale survey)–17%, India (Uttar Pradesh) 2.0%, Indonesia (Bali) 7.1%, (Irian Jaya) 3–42.7%, (Sumatra) 9.5%, Mexico 1.5%, Nigeria (plateau) 3.8%, (eastern) 8.6%, (northern) 11.5%, Peru 3.0% (8.6% in chicharroneros or pork sellers), Reunion 1.4% and Zimbabwe 12%. Cysticerci rates in pigs are: Cameroon 24.6%, Colombia 26%, Egypt 0.1%, Honduras 4.0%–27%, India (Andhra Pradesh) 4.5–8.0%, (Karnataka) 7.0%, (Uttar Pradesh) 9.3–15.5%, (Assam) 27.5%, Indonesia (Bali) 13%, Mexico 4–33%, Nigeria (northern) 3.3%, (eastern) 20%, Tanzania 13.3% and Togo 17%.

PREVENTION AND CONTROL

Thorough cooking of pork and pork products is essential. Cysticerci are killed by a temperature of 45–50°C, but may survive in large pieces of meat if the centre does not reach that temperature. Deep-freezing at −10°C for 4 days kills all cysts, but they can survive for 70 days at 0°C. Pickling and salting is not usually effective. At 18–20°C, cysts can survive the death of the host for up to 4 weeks.

Inspection of meat at the abattoir is important; the underside of the tongue can be examined in life and the intercostal and cervical muscles after slaughter.

ZOONOTIC ASPECTS

Humans are the only definitive hosts for the adult tapeworms. Both humans and pigs are necessary for the complete life cycle. Cysticerci can develop in wild boars and have been found in the lar gibbon (*Hylobates lar*), in which adult tapeworms will also develop experimentally. Cysts have also been reported from sheep, dogs and cats but these may not be those of *T. solium.*

Cysticercosis

In addition to infection with adult *Taenia solium,* human infection with the cysticercus stage normally found in pigs can also occur and is the cause of an important and serious disease.

SYNONYM

Taenia solium cysticercosis, cysticercus cellulosae (in pigs).

DISEASE AND LOCAL NAME
Cysticercosis; bladder-worm infection.

GEOGRAPHICAL DISTRIBUTION
All areas where adult *T. solium* infection occurs. Estimated cysticercosis infection rates in some endemic areas are: Benin 4.0%, Brazil (São Paulo) 0.27%, (Minas Gerais) 18.3%, China (Shandung Province) 0.7%, Ecuador 14.4%, Guatemala 3.5%, Indonesia (Irian Jaya) 17–43%, Madagascar (large-scale survey) 18%, Peru 6–10% in endemic areas, Reunion 8.2%, South Africa (Transkei) 5.5–13.5% and Togo (north) 2.4%. Other endemic areas are Colombia, India, Korea, Mexico, New Guinea, West Africa and Zimbabwe.

MORPHOLOGY
The fully developed cysticercus measures 10 mm × 5 mm with an opaque invaginated scolex (protoscolex) with four suckers and hooks and a fluid-filled bladder; it is identical to the cyst normally found in pigs. Development to the infective stage usually takes 9–10 weeks. A characteristic feature, apparent in sections of most cestode tissues, is the presence of numerous calcareous corpuscles.

TRANSMISSION
This is by the accidental ingestion of eggs of *T. solium* which have been passed in human faeces, presumably on vegetables or in water. In Indonesia, very young children may have cysts, apparently from ingesting eggs on sweet potatoes, but rarely have adult tapeworms below the age of 5 years (Simanjuntak *et al.*, 1997). About 25% of patients with cysticercosis also harbour an adult tapeworm and this led to the belief that autoinfection may follow the regurgitation of proglottides into the stomach, caused by antiperistalsis; however, there is no proof of this. It has been shown experimentally that oncosphere (hexacanth) larvae in eggs must pass through the stomach before they can excyst and the usual course of self-infection is likely to be from anus to fingers to mouth or from eggs on vegetables or perhaps in water.

CLINICAL MANIFESTATIONS
Clinical disease is usually caused by the presence of cysts in the brain (Plate 9). The incubation period from ingestion of eggs to the development of symptoms of cerebral cysticercosis is normally 5–15 years, although it can be much less.

Characteristic nervous manifestations are epilepsiform attacks of the Jacksonian type, but minor symptoms are also very frequent. Cysticerci scattered throughout the brain may produce a variety of symptoms, motor, sensory or mental, with the resulting classical features of any focal lesion, and various focal symptoms and signs may occur in the same patient. The most frequent of these are transient monoplegic paraesthesia, localized anaesthesia, visual and aural symptoms, aphasia and amnesia. Convulsions and seizures are common (1.5% of cysticercosis patients in Benin, 9.5–14.2% in Brazil, 14.4% in Ecuador), but there may be unconsciousness without convulsions, and headaches can be severe. There is some evidence that in Latin America cases of neurocysticercosis have fewer subcutaneous cysts than similar cases in other parts of the world.

PATHOGENESIS
This depends very much on the localization of the cysts in the body. They are normally spread throughout the body roughly in proportion to the weight of each organ, the most important serious effects being caused by cysts in the central nervous system.

DIAGNOSIS
Clinical and parasitological. Palpable subcutaneous nodules can sometimes be felt and diagnosis confirmed by biopsy (Fig. 37), although the hooks are not always seen in tissue sections.

Radiological. X-rays will only detect old cysts that have calcified (Fig. 38). CT and MRI scans are helpful, particularly for neurological cases, and portable ultrasound has been useful in the field (Macpherson, 1992).

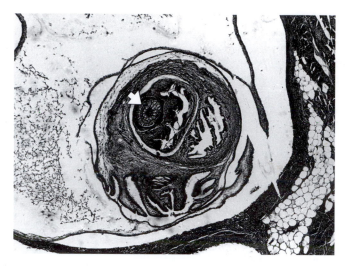

Fig. 37. Section of cysticercus in human muscle. Arrow points to the hooks.

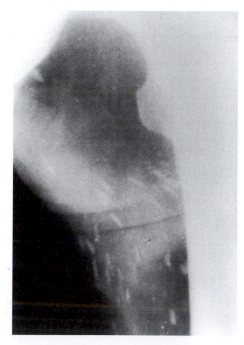

Fig. 38. Radiograph of the thigh region of a young adult with numerous calcified cysticerci (these can be visualized while still living by CT or ultrasonography (US) scans).

Serological. There have been numerous recent studies and an ELISA using recombinant antigens was found to be both sensitive and specific (Hubert *et al.*, 1999). A Western blot technique, using commercially available affinity purified glycoprotein antigen strips, is even more sensitive.

TREATMENT

Treatment with praziquantel at 50 mg kg^{-1} daily for 10–15 days has some effect while the cysts are still alive (treatment at double this dose for 21 days has been used in nonresponding cases). Albendazole at 15 mg kg^{-1} daily for 30 days and flubendazole at 40 mg kg^{-1} daily for 10 days have also been used, with variable results..

Neurocysticercosis may need to be treated with anti-inflammatory agents and anticonvulsants.

EPIDEMIOLOGY

It has been estimated that in Latin America, where about 75 million people live in endemic areas there are 0.4 million symptomatic cases, with 24,000–39,000 cases in Peru in highland and high jungle areas (Bern *et al.*, 1999); in a survey of soldiers in Mexico City, 14.7% were infected (they often ate pork from street vendors).

Taenia crassiceps (Zeder, 1800) Rudolphi, 1810, is a tapeworm of dogs and wild carnivores with cysticerci in various rodents, and human cases have been reported from Canada and the USA. The cysticercus ('cysticercus longicollis') in the intermediate host is unusual, as it multiplies by a process of asexual budding and produces many hundreds of new cysticerci. In a recent patient who also had AIDS, there was a painful spreading tumour in the subcutaneous tissues containing a tapioca-like material with numerous cysticercus-like small vesicles and with a marked granulomatous reaction (Francois *et al.*, 1998).

Small tapeworm cysts (up to 1 mm) were recovered post-mortem from all the deep organs of a man in the USA who died with Hodgkin's lymphoma (Connor *et al.*, 1976). These might be multipying metacestodes of an animal taeniid, such as *T. crassiceps*, or aberrant cysticercoids of *Hymenolepis nana,* which behave similarly in immunosuppressed mice (Lucas *et al.*, 1979).

Taenia multiceps
Leske, 1780

SYNONYMS
Multiceps multiceps (Leske, 1789) Hall, 1910; *Coenurus cerebralis* (Batsch, 1780) Rudolphi, 1808 (larvae); *Multiceps gaigeri* Hall, 1916 (larvae in goats).

DISEASE
Coenurus infection; cerebral coenuriasis or coenuriosis; multicepsosis (adults in carnivores).

MORPHOLOGY AND LIFE CYCLE
The adult taeniid tapeworm is a natural parasite of dogs and wild Canidae. The strobila measures 40–60 cm and the scolex has a rostellum with two rows of hooks (large hooks measuring 150–170 µm, small ones 90–130 µm) of typical taeniid shape. The gravid proglottid has 18–26 small branches to the uterus and is passed in the dog's faeces. The eggs are identical to those of *Echinococcus* in dogs or human *Taenia* and measure 31–36 µm in diameter; when ingested by a suitable intermediate host, the oncosphere is liberated and bores through the wall of the intestine. It is then carried by the blood (or lymph) and normally develops only in the brain or spinal cord. Once lodged, the embryo grows into a bladder-worm stage, known as a coenurus. This differs from a cysticercus in measuring about 3 mm in circumference and in having as many as 100 protoscolices invaginated from the wall into the central cavity. Each protoscolex measures 3 mm in length and has 26–36 hooklets in two rows.

The normal intermediate hosts are sheep and goats, in which the coenurus in the brain is known as a 'gid worm', producing the 'staggers', but development may also occur in cattle, horses and other ruminants, as well as humans.

CLINICAL MANIFESTATIONS AND PATHOGENESIS
In the majority of human cases from temperate countries, including Australia, France, Great Britain, Russia, South Africa and the USA (six cases), the coenurus has been in the brain. However, in many cases from tropical Africa; in Ghana, Nigeria, Senegal and Uganda, a cyst often presents as a subcutaneous or intramuscular nodule, diagnosed as a lipoma, ganglion or neurofibroma (Fig. 39). A papillary oedema with punctiform haemorrhages occurs about a month before the onset of clinical signs. Symptoms include headache and vomiting. In many human cases (over 50%) cysts are sterile, without the presence of protoscolices, which makes diagnosis difficult. There is no clinical way of differentiating infection with this parasite from cases of cysticercosis or echinococcosis (apart from imaging techniques).

A fatal cerebral case in a Nigerian resulted in intermittent seizures, dizziness, headaches and blindness. At autopsy numerous cysts measuring 0.5–2.0 cm were found in both cerebral hemispheres (Malomo *et al.*, 1990).

Treatment has been with praziquantel but concern has been expressed that it might cause inflammation.

In Uganda, cases in the eye may be due to ***Taenia brauni*** (Setti, 1897), with dogs and wild carnivores as normal definitive hosts and rodents as intermediate hosts (Fig. 40).

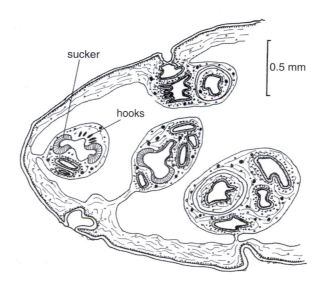

sucker

hooks

0.5 mm

Fig. 39. Section of a portion of a coenurus cyst removed from the neck of a child.

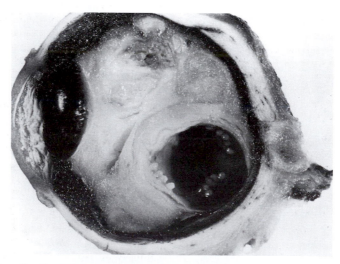

Fig. 40. Sagittal section through an eye with a coenurus in the vitreous chamber from Uganda (possibly of *Taenia brauni*).

Taenia serialis (Gervais, 1847) is a tapeworm of the dog and other carnivores with coenuri in herbivorous mammals (rabbits and hares) and primates in Africa (Senegal, South Africa and Uganda), the Americas (Brazil and the USA) and Europe (France and the UK). Six cases have been reported from the USA, usually in nervous tissue and sometimes with extensive involvement (Ing *et al.*, 1998). One case was treated with praziquantel but this caused marked inflammation. Intramuscular cysts in a man in Nigeria were ascribed to ***Taenia glomeratus*** Railliet and Henry, 1915.

Adults of ***Taenia longihamatus*** Morishita and Sawada, 1966, have been recovered from the intestine of humans in Japan and Okinawa, probably from ingesting cysts in rabbits.

Echinococcus granulosus
(Batsch, 1786) Rudolphi, 1805

SYNONYMS
Taenia echinococcus Von Siebold, 1853 and many others.

DISEASE, POPULAR AND LOCAL NAME
Cystic echinococcosis (CE); hydatid disease. Espespes (Turkana).

GEOGRAPHICAL DISTRIBUTION
Echinococcus granulosus is found in most sheep- and cattle-raising areas of the world (Table 4) and there are also wild carnivore/wild herbivore cycles. Most human cases occur in the countries bordering the Mediterranean (European, Asian and North African), sub-Saharan Africa (East Africa, Nigeria and South Africa), South America (Argentina, Bolivia, Brazil, Chile, Peru and Uruguay), eastern Europe and Eurasia (Bulgaria, Central Asian Republics, Poland, Romania and Russia) and in Asia (Bangladesh, north-western and central China, northern India and Nepal). It was introduced into the western USA (Arizona, California, New Mexico and Utah) about 60 years ago and is important in Australia.

LOCATION IN HOST
The larval cysts (hydatid cysts) are found in various sites in humans, principally the liver and lungs.

MORPHOLOGY
The adult tapeworm becomes attached to the small intestine of dogs and other carnivores and comprises a scolex, neck and 3–5 proglottides. It is always less than 1 cm in length, usually 3–8.5 mm. The spherical scolex has a rostellum with 28–40 hooks in two rows (with large hooks measuring 30–40 μm in length and small hooks 22–34 μm) and four suckers.

The first one or two proglottides are immature, the penultimate sexually mature, with both male and female organs, and the last gravid, with a uterus filled with eggs. The gravid proglottid measures 2.0 mm × 0.5–1.0 mm, more than half the length of the whole tapeworm, and contains about 5000 eggs. In the mature proglottid there are usually 45–60 follicular testes scattered throughout. The cirrus sac is well developed and the common genital pore opens, irregularly alternating, on the lateral margin. The principal morphological features are shown in Fig. 41 and the differences between the species that occur in humans in Table 5.

The egg measures 30–37 μm in diameter and is indistinguishable from that of *Taenia* species found in the dog. It can survive for 6–12 months on soil and is the infective stage for humans.

LIFE CYCLE
The gravid proglottides disintegrate in the intestine and the eggs are passed out in the faeces of the dog. Eggs can live for 200 days in the environment at 7°C, 50 days at 21°C but only a few hours at 40°C. They are ingested on pasture by the intermediate host, which is usually sheep in the strain transmissible to humans, but may be other herbivores coming into contact with dogs such as cattle, buffalo, goat, pig or camel. Ingested eggs hatch in the duodenum, the embryophore being digested by the action of pancreatin and trypsin, and the contained oncosphere probably being activated by the action of bile salts. The released oncosphere uses the hooklets to penetrate the mucosa and reach a blood-vessel. It is carried by the bloodstream to all parts of the body but settles most frequently in the liver (in up to 76% of cases), due to capillary filtering. Arrived at its final destination, the hooklets disappear and a small cyst forms. The cyst (metacestode stage) measures about 1 mm in diameter after 1 month and 10–55 mm after 5 months, by which time brood capsules and protoscoleces are forming. The cyst wall consists of an external, anucleate, laminated cuticular membrane (composed of a chitin-like substance), about 1 mm thick, and an inner

Table 4. Estimates of percentage prevalence of hydatid cysts in humans and domestic animals and of adult *Echinococcus granulosus* in dogs in various countries.

| Country | Hydatid cysts (%) | | Adults in dogs |
	Humans	Sheep and cattle	
Argentina			
La Pampa	0.03		
Chaco	0.019		2.3
Australia	170 cases in		10.2
	3 years		48–93 (wild)
Azerbaijan	0.0014	20	15
Bulgaria	0.003–0.006	32	7
Chile	0.009	5–22	8
China			
Xinjiang	0.044	10–89	10–40
	6.8–18.2 locally		
Gansu	12 locally	2 (4 in yaks)	7–27
Ningxa			56
Quinghai	7.6 locally	22–80	11–47
Germany			
Bavaria	0.0011		
India		60	
Iraq		10	20–56
Iran	3	2–7	3–63
Israel	0.01		8
Italy			
North	0.002		
Sardinia	0.017	50	
Jordan	0.0029		9.4
Kazakhstan	0.0044		
	0.015 locally		
Kenya	10–16	5–30	10–72
Kuwait	0.0036		
Libya	0.0017–2	16 (48 in camels)	30
Morocco		5–45	33
Nepal			
Kathmandu			1.8–5.7
Peru	0.009		8–46
Southern Sudan	0.5–3.5		
Switzerland	0.0004		
Tanzania			
Maasailand	0.011		30
Tunisia	0.057–3.5		
Turkey	3 (Izmir)	50	8–29
Uruguay			
USA			
Florida	0.0056	60	13.2
Mid-Wales	0.0023	13	9.2

germinal layer, 10–25 µm thick, with many nuclei (Fig. 42). The germinal layer forms small masses, which give rise to the brood capsules. These enlarge and 5–20 small buds, about 0.1 mm in diameter, appear on the inner surface of their walls. They develop into invaginated protoscolices with four suckers and a double row of hooks. Many small brood capsules and freed protoscolices are released into the fluid of the original cyst and, together with calcareous bodies, form the 'hydatid sand' (Fig. 43). In

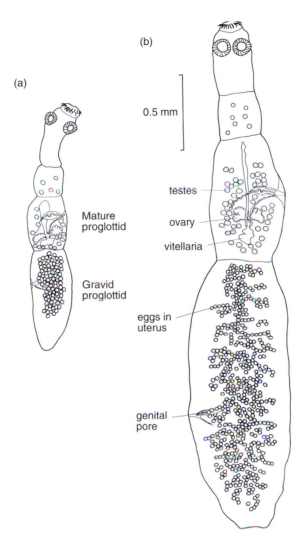

Fig. 41.　Diagrams of adult (a) *E. multilocularis* and (b) *E. granulosus.*

addition to the sand grain-like proto-scolices, there may be many large, thin-walled, daughter cysts inside the outer hydatid cyst. The host tissues, especially in the liver, form an adventitious fibrous wall around the cyst. Fertile cysts may vary in size from 10 to 300 mm. The cyst cavity is filled with a bacteriologically sterile fluid, which is clear or slightly yellowish, with a specific gravity less than 1.012. The fluid contains salts (with a higher concentration of sulphur than in other parasitic cysts) and enzymes, plus a little protein and toxic sub-stances.

The cysts are ingested in offal by dogs and the adult worms become mature in the intes-tine of the carnivore in 6–7 weeks. There may be many thousands of worms in wild carnivores in tropical Africa and Australia but usually only a few hundred in domestic dogs (Macpherson and Craig, 2000).

CLINICAL MANIFESTATIONS
These depend very much on how many hydatid cysts are present and where they are found. Cysts are usually single and in about 50% of infected adults are in the right lobe of the liver towards its lower

Table 5. Differences between *Echinococcus* species.

	E. granulosus	*E. multilocularis*	*E. oligarthrus*
Length of adult	3.0–6.0 mm	1.2–3.7 mm	2.2–2.9 (2.5) mm
Size of gravid segment	More than half body length	Less than half body length	More than half body length
Position of genital pore in gravid segment	Behind midline	On or anterior to midline	Anterior to midline
Average number of testes	56 (45–65)	22 (16–26)	29 (14–46)
Number of testes anterior to genital pore	15.8 (9–23)	2.3 (0–5)	8.9 (3–14)
Shape of ovary	Bilobed or kidney-shaped	Two lobes united by a fine tube	Two lobes united by a fine tube
Shape of uterus	Branching of central column (12–15 lateral branches)	No side-branching of central column	No side-branching of central column
Number of rostellar hooks	32 (28–40)	28 (20–36)	35 (26–40) (larger hooks than the others)
Number of segments	3–4	3–5	3
Position in intestine	Middle and lower third ileum	Upper and middle jejunum	Upper and middle jejunum
Usual definitive hosts	Dog, coyote, dingo, wolf, hyena, jackal	Red fox, Arctic fox, cat (dog)	Puma, bobcat, jaguarundi
Usual intermediate hosts	Ruminants	Microtine rodents and insectivores	Agouti
Time for development to maturity in final host (i.e. eggs in faeces)	48–61 days	30–35 days	?
Structure of cyst	Usually a thick-walled hydatid cyst	Thin-walled multilocular, with many small interconnected cysts	Polycystic hydatid
Rate of development	Slow. Adapted to long-lived intermediate hosts. Protoscolices after 1–2 years	Rapidly developing. Adapted to short-lived intermediate hosts. Infective protoscolices after 2–3 months	Probably rapidly developing

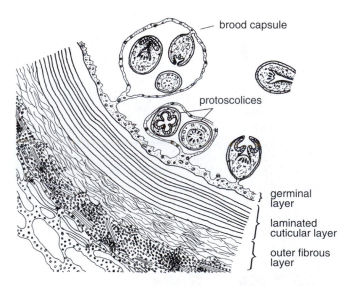

Fig. 42. Section of a portion of an early hydatid cyst of *E. granulosus* (the outer fibrous layer consists of host tissues).

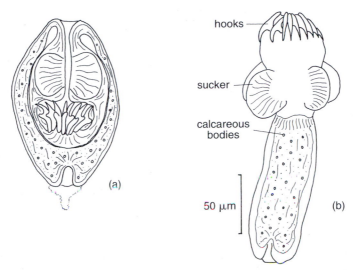

hooks

sucker

calcareous
bodies

50 μm

(a)

(b)

Fig. 43. Protoscolex of *E. granulosus* free inside a cyst ('hydatid sand'). (a) Invaginated as in cyst. (b) Evaginated in gut of a new definitive host (dog).

surface, while the lungs are involved in up to 40% of cases. In children cysts are sometimes diagnosed more often in the lungs than in the liver.

Symptoms and signs are those of slowly increasing pressure in the area of the cyst, resembling a slowly growing tumour. The incubation period is usually at least 5 years and, except for cysts in the brain or orbit, symptoms rarely appear before adolescence and sometimes not for 20 years after exposure (Fig. 44). In a proportion of cases (possibly up to 60%; Eckert *et al.*, 2000) the presence of the hydatid never becomes apparent during life and the cysts eventually calcify and are only diagnosed at autopsy.

If a cyst ruptures, allergic reactions, such as pruritus and an urticarial rash, occur. If the patient has been previously sensitized by slow leakage of antigenic

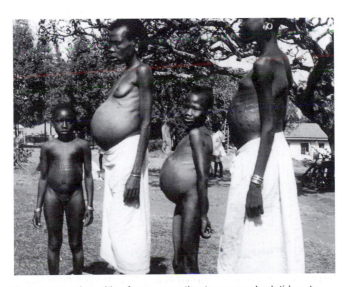

Fig. 44. Group of Turkana people waiting for an operation to remove hydatid cysts.

material from the cyst, there may be acute anaphylactic shock, with gastrointestinal disturbances, dyspnoea and cyanosis. Death may result from pulmonary oedema caused by the shock of a cyst rupturing in the lung, the severity of the effect possibly being potentiated by anaesthesia. In a few cases the anaphylactic shock reaction provides the first intimation of disease.

Eosinophilia is present in less than a quarter of cases of hydatid.

PATHOGENESIS

The pathology caused by the presence of a single unilocular cyst depends very much on its site in the body.

In over 90% of liver cysts, the oncosphere is trapped in the central veins of the hepatic lobules; only occasionally does it lodge in the portal vein. The resultant cyst may be deep or superficial and it causes compression of the liver cells, which can lead to biliary stasis and cholangitis. The cholangitis arises because of secondary infection, sometimes following the rupture of a cyst into the biliary tract. Because of compression, the cyst may take many shapes and often gives the mistaken impression of being multivesicular with many finger-like processes.

Lung cysts are more spherical than those in the liver because of the spongy nature of the pulmonary tissues (Fig. 45). The cysts are always intracapsular and their rupture may result in protoscolices being coughed up in the sputum. Sometimes only hooks can be seen, which can be recognized microscopically. The presence of bile in the sputum is suggestive of a hepatic cyst that has ruptured through the diaphragm. Haemoptysis (blood in the sputum) can result from rupture of the pulmonary capillaries.

About 3% of hydatid cysts occur in the brain or spinal cord. The cysts are usually small and cause symptoms earlier than in other sites. Most brain cysts are in the white matter and are surrounded by a thin adventitious layer.

Osseous cysts, which form 1–2% of the total, grow very slowly and have no wall as they do not elicit any host reaction. As a

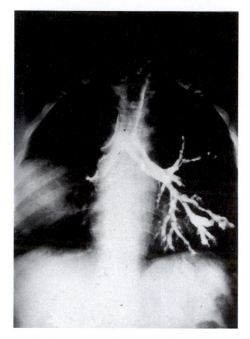

Fig. 45. Bronchogram showing blockage of bronchus caused by a cyst of *E. granulosus.*

result, many small cysts form, which destroy the cancellous bone, long bones sometimes collapsing without warning.

Renal cysts sometimes occur and, if they burst into the kidney pelvis, may become secondarily infected, but these and pancreatic cysts are usually silent. Splenic cysts are often palpable and cause pain and discomfort in the left upper quadrant.

DIAGNOSIS

Clinical and parasitological. Symptoms of a slow-growing tumour if accompanied by eosinophilia in a patient from an endemic area are suggestive of a hydatid. Occasionally, the hydatid 'thrill' can be elicited by tapping an abdominal cyst. Protoscolices or hooks may be found in the sputum following rupture of a pulmonary cyst. Needle aspiration is not to be advocated because of the danger of producing secondary infection or anaphylactic shock, but sometimes protoscolices are found unexpectedly on a subsequent stained smear.

Radiological. The cavity of a cyst usually shows up as a characteristic shadow on X-ray, although cysts in the lungs cannot always be differentiated from tumours unless they become detached and float free. The water-lily sign (sign of Camelotte) is caused by air filling the space between ecto-cyst and pericyst, and the characteristically shaped air cyst containing debris shows up on X-ray. In the last few years many new and more accurate non-invasive techniques have been used. CT is widely used (Fig. 46) and both CT and MRI can be used for diagnosing deep-seated cysts and also for estimating the size of cysts (this can be useful for evaluating chemotherapy). Thin, ring-shaped or crescentic calcifications surround the cysts in 5–10-year-old infections. Completely calcified cysts are not likely to be pathogenic if causing no symptoms. Ultrasonography (US) is another cheaper technique that can be very helpful for diagnosis of liver cysts and a portable apparatus can be employed in the field, making it particularly useful for epidemiological surveys in remote areas.

Immunodiagnosis. The indirect haemagglutination (HA) test with cyst fluid as antigen has been used for the last 25 years and gives a sensitivity of about 80%. More recently, ELISA and dot ELISA techniques, using hydatid cyst fluid (fraction B, containing an antigen of 8 kDa) as antigen, give over 90% specificity and sensitivity and a commercial ELISA kit is available (LMD Laboratories, Carlsbad, California). Immunoglobulin G4 (IgG4) subclass antibodies appear to be most important in serodiagnosis. *E. granulosus* can be differentiated from *E. multilocularis* infections by Western blotting using specific antigens and the test does not cross-react with any other parasitic infection or other condition (Ito *et al.*, 1999).

TREATMENT

Surgery. This is still the most common form of treatment, particularly when the cysts are large and in a site such as the brain or heart. Great care must be taken that the cyst wall does not burst, as released living protoscolices can be carried to new sites by the bloodstream and form new cysts (Plate 10). The cyst cavity can be sterilized with an injection of 0.5% silver nitrate or 2% formalin. For further safety an exposed portion of the cyst can be deep-frozen before removing the sterilized contents. The laminated membrane of the parasite usually separates readily from the fibrous host tissue reaction. No attempt should be made to remove the adventitious fibrous layer in the liver, because of the serious danger of bleeding. If the cyst is too large for closure of the cavity to be possible, marsupialization may be necessary.

Pulmonary cysts are preferably removed by enucleation of the intact cyst by making

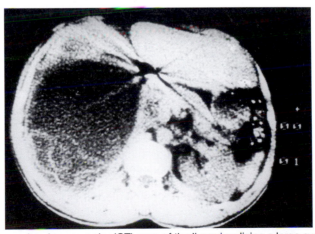

Fig. 46. A computer-assisted tomography (CT) scan of the liver visualizing a large cyst of *E. granulosus*.

an incision through the adventitia, aided by increasing the intrapulmonary pressure with an inflated cuff tube in the trachea. Cysts in the long bones are very difficult to deal with and may call for amputation.

Removal of a cyst is followed by a recurrence in up to 25% of cases, possibly caused by release of protoscolices during operation, but more probably by increase in size of another small silent cyst when the first is removed. Mortality is about 2% in primary operations but is much higher if another operation is required.

Percutaneous aspiration under US guidance, followed by irrigation with hypertonic (20%) saline, has been used for liver cysts causing obstructive jaundice and endoscopy for evacuating biliary cysts and for irrigating the main liver cyst. Similar guided percutaneous aspiration of liver cysts in general, followed by injection of 95% sterile ethanol, puncture, aspiration, injection and reaspiration (PAIR) and then a course of chemotherapy is proving to be an alternative to surgery.

Chemotherapy. This is with albendazole or mebendazole at high dosages over a long period; the former is slightly more effective as it is absorbed better. Albendazole is given at 10 mg kg^{-1} daily and mebendazole at 50 mg kg^{-1} daily, both for at least 3 months. Prognosis is uncertain but about one-third of patients appear to be cured and about two-thirds improved. Side-effects are common while the drugs are in use, including possible liver toxicity. The drugs will probably be of use before and after surgery (to prevent the growth of new cysts). Praziquantel is also being evaluated but its effectiveness has not been proved (Craig, 1994); however, there is evidence that it has a synergistic effect when used at 25 mg kg^{-1} week^{-1} for 7–14 days and then 40–50 mg kg^{-1} once a week for 8 weeks together with albendazole.

EPIDEMIOLOGY

Although echinococcosis is not a common disease in most endemic areas, its serious nature and the difficulty of cure make it an important public health problem in many countries.

Four species of *Echinococcus* are generally recognized (*E. granulosus*, *E. multilocularis*, *E. oligarthrus* and *E. vogeli*) but the characteristics of *E. granulosus* differ greatly in various parts of the world and in different intermediate hosts (Thompson and Lymberry, 1995; Thompson *et al.*, 1995; Eckert and Thompson, 1996; Lymberry and Thompson, 1996). These are usually designated as strains, but with sequence data from mitochondrial and nuclear genes the molecular distances between some strains can be greater than between the recognized species (Bowles *et al.*, 1995).

The principal strains are given below, with suggested specific names in square brackets (Rausch, 1995; Thompson *et al.*, 1995):

1. Dog/sheep (also goat and other herbivores) strain, which is cosmopolitan and uniform (European biotype) [*E. granulosus*].
2. Wolf/wild cervids (moose and reindeer) strain in northern Alaska, Canada, Eurasia and Scandinavia (northern sylvatic biotype) [*E. granulosus*].
3. Dog/cattle or buffalo strain is found in Asia, Europe and South Africa and is genetically very distinct from the others [*E. ortleppi*].
4. Dog/horse strain is widely distributed but does not appear to be infective to humans [*E. equinus*].
5. Dog/pig (and camel?) strain in North and East Africa and the Middle East, eastern Europe, Russia and Mexico is also probably not infective to humans [*E. suis?*].
6. Dingo/marsupial strain in Australia and wild carnivore/wild suid strain in Africa are probably the same as dog/sheep strain [*E. granulosus*].

PREVENTION AND CONTROL

Personal prevention is by taking hygienic measures to avoid eggs voided from dogs being ingested, particularly by children. Control measures should include the sanitary disposal of offal following slaughter of sheep, goats and cattle, both in small abattoirs and at home (often for religous festivals), and campaigns to treat dogs (Meslin *et al.*, 2000). Dogs can be successfully treated with praziquantel (at 5 mg kg^{-1}) or the older arecoline hydrobromide, although reinfection is common. Infections in dogs can be specifically diagnosed using an ELISA for detection of coproantigens (Craig *et al.*, 1996). In sheep-rearing areas, the treatment of farm dogs is particularly important. In North African countries, there are often high infection rates in feral dogs which feed on discarded offal, and these might have to be killed.

The disease has been eliminated from Iceland in the last 100 years by a combination of treatment of dogs and public health measures, particularly by preventing offal from reaching dogs. There used to be very high infection rates and pamphlets pointing out the importance of control, first distributed in 1863, provided welcome reading matter in the long winter nights. Changes in animal husbandry, involving slaughtering of lambs rather than older sheep, so that cysts have no time to develop, also aided eradication (the last case was diagnosed in 1960). The disease was eradicated in New Zealand 50 years ago by similar measures, including compulsory dosing strips, followed by infection checks for dogs, and a successful campaign was carried out in Tasmania. Infection has returned (or was not completely eliminated) in Cyprus, which is now in the consolidation phase, and there are control campaigns under way in regions of Argentina and Chile, the Falkland Islands, northern Kenya, Extramadura (Spain) and western Australia. However, prevalences are rising in most countries of eastern Europe, as controls have been relaxed.

IMMUNOLOGY OF TAPEWORM INFECTIONS AND POSSIBILITIES FOR VACCINES

There is little or or no evidence for immunity in humans against adult tapeworms and reinfection occurs readily. Infected humans do make immune responses, however, and antibodies can be demonstrated in serum. Immunity can be demonstrated against intestinal tapeworms in rodents, but the underlying mechanisms are still not clear. Much more is known about immunity and immune responses to larval cestodes. There have been many experimental studies on taeniid metacestodes in domestic animals, such as sheep, as well as in rodents, and detailed studies have been made of hydatid disease and cysticercosis in humans. Humans infected with these parasites make strong antibody responses and these can be used in diagnosis. The antigens of hydatid cysts and the cysticerci of *T. solium* have been analysed in detail; two (antigen 5 and antigen B) can be used as diagnostic antigens for both conditions. The immunological relationships between hydatid cysts and the host are complex. There is evidence for antiparasite responses, and for specific and non-specific immune suppression. Established cysts can survive in hosts that are resistant to incoming larvae (concomitant immunity) and evidence from animal studies suggests that resistance operates against larvae at an early stage, particularly invading oncospheres and developing cystic stages. Fully developed cysts are surrounded by thick protective layers and possess a variety of defensive mechanisms that reduce the effectiveness of host responses (e.g. inactivation of complement).

Recombinant vaccines have been developed that provide protection against the cysts of *Taenia ovis* in sheep, *T. solium* in pigs and *E. granulosus* in sheep. The antigen Eg95, a specific protein on the oncosphere coat of *E. granulosus* has been expressed as a fusion protein with soluble glutathione-*S*-transferase (GST) from a schistosome. Purified and injected into sheep, this fusion protein gave 98% protection against subsequent egg infection for at least 12 months in field trials in Argentina and Australia. The vaccine, which is stable for over 1 year, protects against the establishment of cysts in sheeps; human trials are also envisaged. A similar vaccine against the larvae of *T. ovis*, which is of veterinary importance with a cycle involving dogs and sheep, is already commercially available, with 98% protection against natural infections in pastures, and is also likely to have future relevance for human tapeworm infections (Lightowers *et al.*, 2000).

Echinococcus multilocularis
(Leuckart, 1863) Vogel, 1955

SYNONYMS
Echinococcus alveolaris Klemm, 1883; *E. sibiricensis* Rausch and Schiller, 1954; *Alveococcus multilocularis* Abuladse, 1959.

DISEASE
Alveolar echinococcosis (AE).

GEOGRAPHICAL DISTRIBUTION
Infection in animals is principally holarctic and occasional human cases occur in Austria (Tyrol), central Europe, southern Germany, Switzerland, Belarus, Russia (northern tundra areas, Caucasus and Siberia), Ukraine, Central Asiatic Republics, China, Alaska (and nine other states in the USA), Canada, Bering Sea islands, Japan (Hokkaido and Rebun) and north-western Pacific.

MORPHOLOGY
The adult tapeworms are one-third to one-half the size of E. granulosus; other differences are shown in Fig. 41 and listed in Table 5.

LIFE CYCLE
This is similar to that of *E. granulosus* except that adult tapeworms are found in about seven species of wild carnivore, principally the Arctic (*Alopex lagopus*) and red (*Vulpes vulpes*) fox, and occasionally the dog and cat, while the usual intermediate hosts are the field mouse in Europe and the field or red-backed vole and lemming in Alaska and Siberia (and possibly 27 other species of rodent). On Rebun Island, Japan, the cat and red fox act as hosts for *E. multilocularis* but cannot be infected with *E. granulosus*.

When natural hosts, such as the vole (*Microtus*) ingest eggs on vegetation passed out by the definitive host, growth of the cyst in the liver is rapid, with extensions from the germinal membrane invading the adventitia and forming numerous, minute, interconnected, secondary vesicles in about 9 days. By 150 days the alveolar vesicles are almost filled with protoscolices and the weight of the liver may exceed that of the rest of the body (Fig. 47). This rapid growth is an essential adaptation to a short-lived intermediate host. In the winter, when the hosts are hibernating, the cysts stop developing. It is probable that when they continue growing in the spring they impair the vitality of the animal, so that it is more easily caught by a carnivore. Infected rodents rarely live for more than 5–6 months. Ingested protoscolices take 26–28 days to develop into mature adults in the intestine of the carnivores.

CLINICAL MANIFESTATIONS
Cysts resemble a slowly growing malignant growth in the liver, making this the most

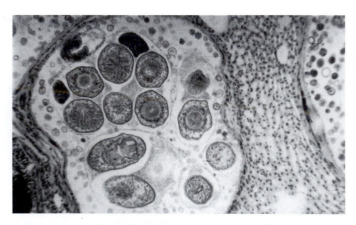

Fig. 47. Section of alveolar cyst of *E. multilocularis* from a liver of vole. The wall is thin and protoscolices are embedded in a semi-solid matrix (cysts in humans are almost always sterile without protoscolices).

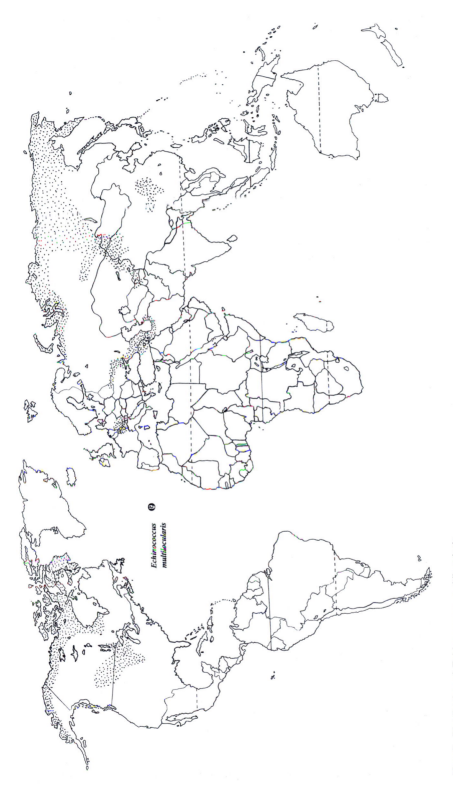

Echinococcus multilocularis

Map 6. Distribution of *Echinococcus multilocularis*.

dangerous helminth infection of humans. There are no symptoms due to pressure effects, because of the absence of a thick-walled hydatid cyst surrounded by a fibrous host reaction, although there is an outer laminated cyst layer, which appears to protect the parasite from host immune responses.

The parasite destroys the liver paren-chyma, bile-ducts and blood-vessels, result-ing in symptoms of biliary obstruction and portal hypertension; necrosis of the cyst, with abscess formation may also occur. Hepatomegaly is often the first sign of infec-tion. There may be wasting in the later stages and the condition is often mistaken for a car-cinoma. The cysts often metastase via the bloodstream to form new cysts, particularly in the lungs and brain. Clinical symptoms may not appear for 10–15 years after infec-tion but in untreated cases there is 94% fatality within 10 years. There is an eosinophilia of over 5% in 15–20% of patients.

PATHOGENESIS

In humans the multilocular or alveolar cysts form pseudo-malignant growths with a spongy mass of proliferating vesicles embedded in a dense fibrous stroma, almost always in the liver. They differ from the hydatid cyst by the thinness of the outer layer, by exogenous budding and usually by the absence of protoscolices. The germina-tive membranes are hyperplastic and folded on themselves and the vacuole is filled with a gelatinous matrix rather than with fluid. The germinal layer is often absent in human infections, so that there are no protoscolices present in 85% of cases, and many cysts atrophy and disappear. Calcified cysts may be found in Inuit at autopsy, undiagnosed during life. The relatively slow growth and few germinal cells indicate that humans are not very suitable hosts.

In humans cysts cause necrosis of the surrounding liver tissue with an oblitera-tive endarteritis. The outer zone consists of an inflammatory response, with the pres-ence of giant cells and jaundice, and ascites might result from portal hypertension. Cysts sometimes metastase and secondary

cysts may be present in the lymph glands, lungs and brain – almost always fatal.

In patients susceptible to disease, there is a specific lymphoproliferative host response to cyst antigens containing pre-dominantly CD8+ cells and a T-helper (Th2) cell response develops slowly, with a still unknown functional potential of inter-leukin 5 (IL-5). In a proportion of cases the symptomless cysts become calcified and contain no living cells and there is a marked host response containing primarily CD4+ T cells in the periparasitic granuloma (Gottstein and Felleisen, 1995).

DIAGNOSIS

As for *E. granulosus*. US can be helpful. Serological tests using antigen obtained from protoscolices (Em2 or Em18) are extremely specific. Early diagnosis is very important in determining the success of surgery.

TREATMENT

Surgical resection of the liver is very difficult and prognosis is rather poor; however, about 90% of non-resectable patients die within 10 years. Liver transplantation has been attempted in patients with advanced infec-tions (mortality rate of 30%).

Very long-term chemotherapy with albendazole ($10–15$ mg kg^{-1} day^{-1}) or mebendazole (50 mg kg^{-1} day^{-1}) inhibits the growth of cysts and prevents the occur-rence of metastases. Patients have a better quality of life and greater longevity, although disease may recur, as both these drugs appear to be parasitostatic, not para-sitocidal. Albendazole is better absorbed but can occasionally be hepatotoxic, while there should be breaks – say, every 28 days – with both drugs to prevent leucopenia (Tornieporth and Disko, 1994).

EPIDEMIOLOGY

Prevalence rates in various countries (per 100,000 population) are: Alaska 7–98, China (Gansu) 2200, Central Europe 0.02–1.4, Germany (Bavaria) 0.6, northern Siberia 170, northern Russia in general 10, Switzerland 0.18. There can be high infec-tion rates with adult tapeworms in the red fox: Austria 3.6%, Czech Republic 10.6%, Germany 18.4%, Japan (Hokkaido) 52–67%, Poland 2.6%, Slovakia 10.7% and Switzerland 35%.

The life cycle of *E. multilocularis*, involving wild carnivores and rodents, usually involves ecosystems separate from humans so that human infection is much less likely than with *E. granulosus*. However, the distribution appears to be spreading in Europe, Japan and North America (Eckert *et al.*, 2000). In Arctic regions 50% of tundra voles (*Microtus oeconomus*) may be infected at some time of the year and 100% of Arctic foxes may have up to 200,000 adult tapeworms. Many human infections are reported from fur trappers, who ingest eggs when skinning wild canids. Eggs may also be ingested on salad vegetables during Arctic summer, as they can withstand very low temperatures (240 days at −18°C: a temperature as low as −70°C is necessary to be sure they are killed). In Alaska and areas of Russia over 50% of dogs are infected.

In woodland and agricultural areas of central Europe, human infection is thought to be primarily from eating fruits, berries and vegetables (wild strawberries, cranberries, fallen apples and lettuce) picked off the ground and contaminated with faeces from foxes or dogs.

PREVENTION AND CONTROL

Thorough washing of fruit and vegetables likely to become contaminated. Chemotherapy of dogs is possible, as for *E. granulosus*.

Echinococcus oligarthrus
(Diesing, 1863) Lühe, 1910

This species is in many features intermediate between the other two (see Table 5). Adults occur in the jaguarundi (*Felis yagouaroundi*) in Panama, the puma (*Puma concolor*) in Panama and Brazil and the bobcat (*Lynx rufus*) in Mexico. The intermediate hosts are agoutis (*Dasyprocta aguti*). It is an infection of tropical sylvatic areas and identified human cases have been reported from Brazil (Minais Gerais),

India, Panama, Surinam and Venezuela; characteristic cysts have also been reported from Argentina, Chile, Costa Rica, Mexico, Nicaragua and Uruguay (these might have been due to *E. vogeli* but are outside the host range of the bush dog, its natural definitive host).

Cysts in humans are usually in the liver (80% of cases), with most of the remainder in the lungs, although there have been two orbital infections. Clinically, cysts in the liver have caused abdominal pain, hepatosplenomegaly, marked weight loss and fever, with the presence of hard, round, masses. Ascites and obstructive jaundice can also occur. Portal hypertension is found in about 25% of cases and often results in death following biliary drainage or partial hepatectomy. The cysts are of the hydatid type but form polylobed masses (polycystic echinococcosis (PE) spilling into the peritoneal cavity (Plate 11); the rostellar hooks are larger than those of other species.

Treatment is with albendazole at 10 mg kg^{-1} daily for 2–8 months and has given encouraging results in most cases. Side-effects stop when treatment is finished.

Echinococcus vogeli
Rausch and Bernstein, 1972

Adults of this species are found in the bush dog (*Spetheos venaticus*), with cysts in the paca (*Cuniculus paca*), in South and Central America. Human cases have been reported from Argentina, Brazil (Amazon), Ecuador and Surinam. Infection is very rare in humans, partly because the bush dog avoids human habitations, and may result from dogs that have been fed on the viscera of pacas. The polycystic hydatid cysts (causing PE) are similar to those of *E. oligarthrus* but the outer membrane is thicker and the rostellar hooks on the protoscolices are smaller and morphologically distinct. Clinical effects are similar also, with both exogenous budding of cysts into the peritoneal cavity which grow in other organs and also endogenous budding with daughter cysts inside the main cyst. Treatment with albendazole at 10 mg kg^{-1} daily for up to 10 months has some effect.

Family Hymenolepididae

Hymenolepis nana
(Von Siebold, 1852) Blanchard, 1891

SYNONYMS
*Taenia   nana   Von   Siebold,   1852;
Hymenolepis   fraterna   Stiles,   1906;
Vampirolepis nana.*

DISEASE AND POPULAR NAME
Hymenolepiasis or hymenolepiosis nana;
dwarf tapeworm infection.

GEOGRAPHICAL DISTRIBUTION
Cosmopolitan, particularly in children.

LOCATION IN HOST
The adults inhabit the lumen of the upper
three-quarters of the ileum, with the scolex
embedded in the mucosa. There may be
many thousands of tapeworms present in a
heavy infection.

MORPHOLOGY
Hymenolepis nana is a very short tapeworm,   measuring   15–40 mm   ×
0.5–1.0 mm, and has approximately 200
proglottides.

The scolex is spherical, about 0.3 in
diameter (one-third the size of that of

Taenia solium) and has a short retractile
rostellum with a single row of 20–30 small
hooks and four round suckers or acetabula.
The hooks are spanner-shaped, which is
typical of the family Hymenolepidiidae.
The neck region is long and slender (Fig.
48). Mature proglottides are broader than
long (0.22 mm × 0.85 mm), with a single
common genital pore on one side of the
strobila or chain.

There are three round testes, which lie
in the posterior part of each proglottid. The
bilobed, coarsely granular, ovary lies posteriorly between the testes with the compact
vitelline gland behind it (Fig. 49). The
gravid uterus forms a sac filled with
80–200 eggs.

LIFE CYCLE
This is the only known human tapeworm
that does not require an intermediate host.

The gravid proglottides are usually broken up in the colon so that free eggs are
found in the faeces. The eggs measure
30–47 μm (Fig. 123). They are spherical or
ovoid and are enclosed in two transparent
membranes, the inner of which, the
embryophore, is lemon-shaped and has
polar thickenings, from which arise 4–8
slender filaments (these are not always evi-

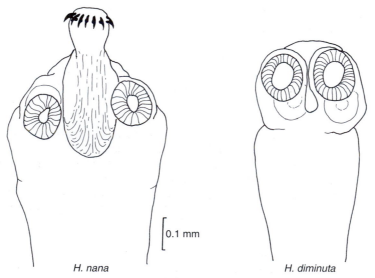

0.1 mm

H. nana   *H. diminuta*

Fig. 48. Diagrams of the scolices of *Hymenolepis nana* and *H. diminuta* (see also Fig. 33).

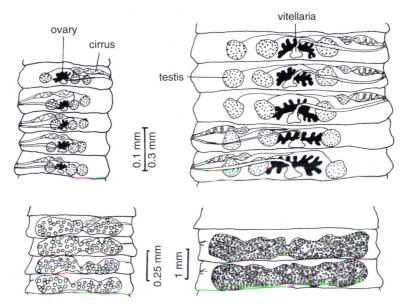

Fig. 49. Mature proglottides of *H. nana* (left) and *H. diminuta* (right). Note the different scales – the proglottides of *H. diminuta* are comparatively much larger than shown.

dent when the eggs are preserved). The enclosed oncosphere measures about 18 μm in diameter and has the usual six hooklets. The egg is immediately infective.

When ingested by another person, the oncosphere is liberated in the small intestine and penetrates a villus by means of the hooklets. It then loses the larval hooklets and becomes a tailless cysticercoid (sometimes known as a cercocystis) in about 90 h. This stage re-enters the intestinal lumen after 4 days and develops into a tapeworm with mature proglottides in 10–12 days (Fig. 50). Eggs are passed in the faeces about 30 days after infection.

Autoinfection is possible, eggs and freed oncospheres having been obtained by intestinal aspiration from an infected child. This accounts for reports of infections lasting many years although, in children removed from an endemic area, the adult tapeworms live for only a few months.

CLINICAL MANIFESTATIONS AND PATHOGENESIS
In most cases no symptoms can be attributed to a light infection but the presence of more than 2000 worms results in enteritis,

with abdominal pain, diarrhoea, irritability, loss of appetite, vomiting and dizziness, presumably due to systemic toxaemia caused by the waste products or to allergic responses. Epileptoid fits have been reported from children. Necrosis of the mucosa has been found in rats but has not been demonstrated to occur in humans.

An eosinophilia of up to 15% occurs in about 7% of infected individuals.

DIAGNOSIS
This is by the identification of eggs in the faeces (p. 254 and Fig. 123).

TREATMENT
Praziquantel at a single dose of 15 mg kg^{-1} has about 80% effectiveness; the presence of cysticercoids in the tissues may necessitate re-treatment.

Niclosamide can be given at 60–80 mg kg^{-1} for 5 days and perhaps repeated 10 days later.

EPIDEMIOLOGY
H. nana is more common in children than in adults, particularly children from institutions

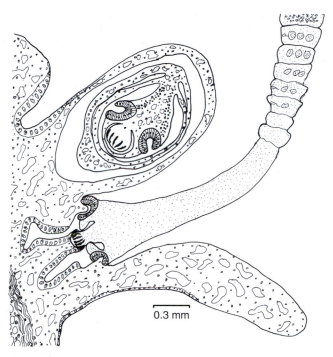

0.3 mm

Fig. 50. Diagrammatic section of adult and cysticercoid of *H. nana* in a villus of the ileum. In heavy iinfections the mucosal lining may become abraded.

in tropical countries. Estimates in children in regions of various countries are: Argentina 10–15%; Bahrain 3%; Brazil (Amazon) 11%, (Minais Gerais) 7%, (Rio) 1.4%, (Sao Paulo) 9–15%; Chile 0.4–4%; Côte d'Ivoire 1–7%; Egypt 6–20%; Ethiopia 0.6–1%; Honduras 8%; India 1–12%; Japan 2.3%; Mexico 3–5%; Nepal 7%; Pakistan 7–18%; Peru 23%; Romania 5%; Sudan 7–10%; Tunisia 2%; Turkey 6–14%; Uganda 0.5%; Venezuela 6–12%; Zimbabwe 21%. Large-scale estimates in the general population are: Albania 1.5%; Australia (aboriginals) 55%; Bolivia 9%; Cuba (overall) 0.008%; Dominican Republic 2%; Ecuador 3–4%; Egypt (Cairo) 0.2%; Iraq 7%; Kenya 5%; Korea 0.03–0.4%; Madagascar 9%; Mexico 5%; Namibia 1%; Nigeria (Plateau) 0.3–3%; Russia (Siberia) 0.1%; Saudi Arabia 0.4–3%; Senegal 1.5%; Turkey 0.6–2%; Venezuela 2%.

The eggs are not resistant to heat or desiccation and are viable for a maximum of 11 days. Infection is often from hand to mouth, although it may also be by food or water.

PREVENTION AND CONTROL

Hygienic measures are not always immediately effective and eradication has been very difficult in the past. As the eggs have so little resistance to desiccation, measures can be directed against direct hand-to-mouth transmission and to cleaning of clothes and bed-linen. The much improved chemotherapy available in the last few years makes control considerably easier.

ZOONOTIC ASPECTS

The role of animals in the spread of human infection is not clear. A morphologically identical parasite, *H. nana* var. *fraterna*, is common in rats and mice and often has as intermediate hosts either fleas (*Xenopsylla cheopis*, *Ctenocephalides canis*) or beetles (*Tenebrio molitor*, *Tribolium confusatum*). However, the rodent variety differs physiologically and does not usually cause infection in humans. The situation is further complicated because the human tapeworm can also develop in insects and these are subsequently infective when ingested, and possibly rodents sometimes act as reservoir hosts of the human strain without the presence of an intermediate host.

Hymenolepis diminuta
(Rudolphi, 1819) Blanchard, 1891

SYNONYMS

Taenia diminuta Rudolphi, 1819; *Taenia flavopunctata* Weinland, 1858; *Taenia minima* Grassi, 1886.

DISEASE AND POPULAR NAME
Hymenolepiasis or hymenolepiosis diminuta; the rat tapeworm.

GEOGRAPHICAL DISTRIBUTION
This is a common and cosmopolitan parasite of rats, mice and wild rodents in many parts of the world. It is an occasional parasite of humans, most cases being reported from children. In a few countries infection in children is not uncommon (1.9% in the New Guinea highlands; 1.3% in India (Uttar Pradesh); 0.4% in Morocco (Agadir); 0.05–0.1% in Turkey).

LOCATION IN HOST
Adults are found in the upper three-quarters of the ileum, with the scolex usually embedded in the mucosa. However, in rats it has been shown that the tapeworm moves backwards and forwards in the intestine and this may be generally true of this and other tapeworms in humans.

MORPHOLOGY
In spite of its name this species is considerably larger than *H. nana*. The entire tapeworm measures 300–600 mm × 4 mm and has 800–1000 proglottides. The scolex (0.2–0.4 mm in diameter) is spherical and has four small suckers and a retractable rostellum; but no hooks (Fig. 48).

The mature proglottides are broader than long and measure 0.75 mm × 0.25 mm

(Fig. 49). The reproductive organs are similar in structure to those of *H. nana*, although the three testes are more widely separated.

The egg is slightly ovoid and has a thick yellow outer shell and a thin colourless inner membrane (embryophore), with a granular intermediate layer. There are no polar filaments. The egg measures 60–80 μm in maximum diameter (Fig. 123).

LIFE CYCLE
For further development, the eggs passed in the faeces need to be ingested by an insect intermediate host. They can survive in the environment for about 1 week.

The most important intermediate hosts are flour beetles (*Tribolium confusatum* and *Tenebrio molitor*) and rat fleas (*Xenopsylla cheopis* and *Nosophyllus fasciatus*). When ingested, often on contaminated grain, the oncosphere larva inside the egg develops into a tailed, solid, cysticercoid larva in the body cavity of the insect. If the infected insect is ingested by a rat (or a child), the liberated cysticercoids attach to the intestinal mucosa and the worm matures in 18–20 days. There is not the invasive tissue phase characteristic of *H. nana*.

Infection in children appears to cause no clinical symptoms apart from diarrhoea. Some cases have been referred for neuropsychiatric problems but these may be coincidental. Diagnosis is by finding the characteristic eggs in the faeces, and treatment is as for *H. nana*; repeated doses have proved necessary in some cases. A single dose of 500 mg of niclosamide is an older treatment.

Although *H. diminuta* has little direct medical importance, it is of great scientific interest as a laboratory model, and is being used in many research studies on the physiology, biochemistry and immunology of cestodes and for chemotherapeutic screening tests.

Drepanidotaenia lanceolata (Bloch, 1782) Railliet, 1892, is a hymenolepid parasite of water-birds with cysticercoids in copepods and with a single case in a boy in Germany.

Family Dipylididae

Dipylidium caninum
(Linnaeus, 1758) Railliet, 1892

SYNONYMS, DISEASE AND POPULAR NAME
Taenia canina L., 1758 and many others;
dipylidiasis or dipylidiosis; double-pored
dog tapeworm.

GEOGRAPHICAL DISTRIBUTION
This is a very common and cosmopolitan
parasite of dogs and cats and is found
sporadically in humans; a few hundred
cases having been reported, almost all in
children. Recent reported cases in children
and infants have been from Austria,
Bulgaria, Chile, China, India, Italy, Japan,
Russia, Sri Lanka and the USA.

MORPHOLOGY
Dipylidium caninum is a short tapeworm
measuring 200–400 mm × 2.5–3 mm and
has 60–175 proglottides. The scolex measures about 0.37 mm, has four prominent
suckers, a retractable rostellum and 30–150
thorn-shaped hooks in 3–4 rows. Mature
proglottides are longer than broad. The
genital organs are in two sets, one set each
side of the midline. The two common genital pores open at the centre of both lateral
margins.

The gravid proglottides are filled with
eggs in egg capsules (Fig. 124), each containing up to 20 eggs, proglottides are
passed in the faeces. In shape, the proglottides are an elongate oval, measuring
12 mm × 2.7 mm, and are very active when
passed; frequently they are mistaken for
trematodes when seen in the faeces of dogs
or children.

LIFE CYCLE
The egg capsules are liberated on the
ground or stick to the anal hairs of dogs.
They cannot survive drying for more than
1–2 days and live only 1–2 minutes in
water. The eggs are ingested by the larval
stages of ectoparasitic insects, such as
Ctenocephalides canis or *C. felis* (the dog
and cat fleas) and develop in the body
cavity into tailed cysticercoids in about 18
days.

Human infection is presumably from
ingestion of fleas and is almost always in
children. There is no definite pathogenesis
associated with this species and treatment
is with praziquantel (25 mg kg^{-1} in a single
oral dose). Diagnosis is by finding the
mobile, gravid, barrel-shaped, proglottides
(with remains of double organs or pores) or
egg capsules in the faeces (Fig. 124).

Very occasional human tapeworms

Bertiella studeri (Blanchard, 1891) Stiles and Hassall 1902 and *B. mucronata* (Meyner, 1895) Stiles and Hassall, 1902 (family Anoplocephalidae)

These are parasites of monkeys with cysticercoids in oribatid mites. About 60 cases
of *B. studeri* in humans, mostly in children,
have been reported from Equatorial Guinea,
India, Indonesia, Japan, Kenya, Malaysia,
Mauritius, Nigeria, Philippines, Sri Lanka,
Thailand and Yemen and of *B. mucronata*
in Argentina, Brazil, Cuba and Paraguay
(Denegri and Perez-Serrano, 1997). A chain
of thick, very broad proglottides passed in
the faeces usually provides the first evidence of infection. A woman in Equatorial
Guinea had suffered abdominal discomfort
for 6 years before proglottides were passed
and she was cured by 40 mg kg^{-1} of praziquantel (Galan-Puchades *et al.*, 1997).

Inermicapsifer madagascariensis (Davaine, 1870) Baer, 1956 (syn. *I. cubensis*) (family Anoplocephalidae)

This is a small tapeworm (5 cm) of rodents
and hyraxes with cysticercoids presumably
in mites. Human cases have occurred in
Cuba, Comoros Islands, Congo, Kenya,
Madagascar, South Africa, Venezuela,
Zambia and Zimbabwe. It is not uncommon in children around Havana, Cuba, and
is probably more common in East Africa
than reported.

Mathevotaenia symmetrica (Baylis,
1927) Akhumian, 1946, is widely distributed in rodents in Thailand, with cysticer-

coids in flour beetles and moths (and one case in a human).

Mesocestoides lineatus (Goeze, 1782) Railliet, 1893 and *M. variabilis* Mueller, 1927 (family Mesocestoididae)

M. lineatus is a parasite of carnivores probably with an arthropod as the first intermediate host and amphibians, reptiles, small mammals and birds as second (with a modified cysticercoid known as a tetrathyridium, of the plerocercoid type). Human cases have been reported from China (two cases), Japan (12), Korea (one) and Sri Lanka (one). The man infected in Korea ate raw chicken viscera and passed 32 worms after treatment with niclosamide. *M. variabilis* has a similar life cycle and human cases have been reported from Greenland and the USA (6 cases).

Raillietina spp. (family Davaineidae)

Species found in humans include *R. asiatica* (Von Linstow, 1901) Stiles and Hassall (a single case in Russia, a doubtful case in Iran); *R. celebensis* (Janicki, 1902) Fuhrmann, 1924, a parasite of rats and mice with cysticercoids in ants (a few cases in children from Australia, China, Japan, Moorea, Philippines, Tahiti and Taiwan); *R. garrisoni* Tubangui, 1931 (one case in a child in the Philippines); *R. madagascariensis* (Davaine, 1869) Joyeux and Baer, 1919, a common parasite of rats in Asia with cysticercoids probably in cockroaches (human cases from Comoros, Indonesia, Mauritius, Philippines and Thailand); *R. siviraji* Chandler and Pradatsundarasar, 1957, a common parasite of rats in Thailand (and with a few cases in children). *Buginetta* (= *R.*) *alouattae* Spaskii, 1994 is found in South American monkeys and occasionally humans.

References

Beaver, P.C. and Rolon, F.A. (1981) Proliferating larval cestode in a man in Paraguay: a case report and review. *American Journal of Tropical Medicine and Hygiene* 30, 625–637.

Bern, C., Garcia, H.H., Evans, C., Gonzalez, A.E., Verastegul, M., Tsang, V.C.M. and Gilman, R.H. (1999) Magnitude of the disease burden from neurocysticercosis in a developing country. *Clinical Infectious Diseases* 29, 1203–1209.

Bessenov, A.S., Movsession, S.O. and Abuladze, K.I. (1994) On the classification and validity of superspecies taxons of the cestodes of the suborder Taeniata Skrjabin et Schulz, 1937. *Helminthologia* 31, 67–71.

Bowles, J., Blair, D. and McManus, D.P. (1995) A molecular phylogeny of the genus *Echinococcus*. *Parasitology* 110, 317–328.

Chang, K.H., Chi, J.G., Cho, S.Y., Han, M.H., Han, D.H. and Han, M.C. (1992) Cerebral sparganosis: analysis of 34 cases with emphasis on CT features. *Neuroradiology* 34, 1–8.

Connor, D.H., Sparks, A.K., Strano, A.J., Neafie, R.C. and Juvelier, B. (1976) Disseminated parasitosis in an immunosuppressed patient – possibly a mutated sparganum. *Archives of Pathological Laboratory Medicine* 100, 65–68.

Craig, P.S. (1994) Current research in echinococcosis. *Parasitology Today* 10, 209–211.

Craig, P.S., Rogan, M.T. and Allan, J.C. (1996) Detection, screening and community epidemiology of taeniid cestode zoonoses: cystic echinococcosis, alveolar echinococcosis and neurocysticercosis. *Advances in Parasitology* 38, 170–250.

Denegri, G.M. and Perez-Serrano, J. (1997) Bertiellosis in man: a review of cases. *Revista do Instituto de Medecina Tropical de Sao Paulo* 39, 123–127.

Eckert, J. and Thompson, R.C.A. (1996) Intraspecific variation of *Echinococcus granulosus* and related species with emphasis on their infectivity to humans. *Acta Tropica* 64, 19–34.

Eckert, J., Conraths, F.J. and Taekmann, K. (2000) Echinococcosis: an emerging or re-emerging zoonosis? *International Journal for Parasitology* 30, 1283–1294.

Fan, P.C. (1997) Annual economic loss caused by *Taenia saginata asiatica* taeniasis in East Asia. *Parasitology Today* 13, 194–196.

Fan, P.C., Lin, C.Y., Chen, C.C. and Chung, W.C. (1995) Morphological description of *Taenia saginata asiatica* (Cyclophyllidea: Taeniidae) from man in Asia. *Journal of Helminthology* 69, 299–303.

Francois, A., Favennec, L., Cambon-Michot, C., Gueit, I., Biga, N., Tron, F., Brasseur, P. and Hemet, J. (1998) *Taenia crassiceps* invasive cysticercosis: a new human pathogen in acquired immuno-deficiency syndrome? *American Journal of Surgical Pathology* 22, 488–492.

Galan-Puchades, M.T., Frentes, M.V., Simarro, P.P. and Mas Coma, S. (1997) Human *Bertiella studeri* in Equatorial Guinea. *Transactions of the Royal Society of Tropical Medicine and Hygiene* 91, 680.

Gottstein, B. and Felleisen, R. (1995) Protective immune mechanisms against the metacestode of *Echinococcus multilocularis*. *Parasitology Today* 11, 320–326.

Hubert, K., Andriantsimahavandy, A., Michault, A., Frosch, M. and Muhlschlegel, F.A. (1999) Serological diagnosis of human cysticercosis by use of recombinant antigens from *Taenia solium* cysticerci. *Clinical and Diagnostic Laboratory Immunology* 6, 479–482.

Ing, M.B., Schantz, P.M. and Turner, J.A. (1998) Human coenurosis in North America: case reports and review. *Clinical and Infectious Diseases* 27, 519–523.

Ito, A. (1992) Cysticercosis in Asian-Pacific regions. *Parasitology Today* 8, 182–183.

Ito, A., Ma-LiAng, Schantz, P.M., Gottstein, B., Liu-Yuetlan, Chai JunJie, Abdel-Hafez, S.K., Altintas, N., Joshi, D.D., Lightowers, M.W., Pawlowski, Z.S., Ma-La, Liu, Y.H. and Chi, J.J. (1999) Differential serodiagnosis for cystic and alveolar echinococcosis using fractions of *Echinococcus granulosus* cyst fluid (antigen B) and *Echinococcus multilocularis* protoscolex (Em18). *American Journal of Hygiene and Tropical Medicine* 60, 188–192.

Khalil, L.F., Jones, A. and Bray, R.A. (1994) *Keys to the Cestode Parasites of Vertebrates.* 768 pp. CAB International, Wallingford, UK.

Lightowers, M.W., Flisser, A., Gauci, C.G., Heath, D.D., Jensen, O. and Rolfe, R. (2000) Vaccination against cysticercosis and hydatid disease. *Parasitology Today* 16, 191–196.

Lo, Y.-K., Chao, D. and Yan, S.-H. (1987) Spinal cord proliferative sparganosis in Taiwan: a case report. *Neurosurgery* 21, 235–238.

Lucas, S.B., Hassounah, O.A., Doenhoff, M. and Muller, R. (1979) Aberrant form of *Hymenolepis nana*; possible opportunistic infections in immunosuppressed patients. *Lancet* 22 Dec. (ii), 1372–1373.

Lymberry, A.J. and Thompson, R.C.A. (1996) Species of *Echinococcus*: pattern and process. *Parasitology Today* 12, 486–491.

Machnicka, B., Dziemian, E. and Zwierz, C. (1996) Detection of *Taenia saginata* antigens in faeces by ELISA. *Applied Parasitology* 37, 99–105 and 106–110.

Macpherson, C.N.L. (1992) Ultrasound in the diagnosis of parasitic disease. *Tropical Doctor* 22, 14–20.

Macpherson, C.N.L. and Craig, P.S. (2000) Dogs and cestode zoonoses. In: Macpherson, C.N.L., Meslin, F.X. and Wandeler, A.I. (eds) *Dogs, Zoonoses and Public Health*. CAB International, Wallingford, UK, pp. 177–212.

Malomo, A., Ogunniyi, J., Ogunniyi, A., Akang, A., Akang, E.E.U. and Shokunbi, M.J. (1990) Coenurosis of the central nervous system in a Nigerian. *Tropical and Geographical Medicine* 42, 280–282.

Meslin, F.X., Miles, M.A., Vexenat, J.A. and Gemmell, M.A. (2000) Zoonoses control in dogs. In: Macpherson, C.N.L., Meslin, F.X. and Wandeler, A.I. (eds) *Dogs, Zoonoses and Public Health*. CAB International, Wallingford, UK, pp. 333–372.

Muller, R. (1983) *Taenia*, taeniasis and cysticercosis. In: Feachem, R.G., Bradley, D.J., Garelick, H. and Marr, D.D. (eds) *Sanitation and Disease: Health Aspects of Excreta and Wastewater Management*. John Wiley & Sons, Chichester, UK, pp. 463–472.

Rausch, R.L. (1995) Life cycle patterns and geographic distribution of *Echinococcus* species. In: Thompson, R.C.A. and Lymberry, A.J. (eds) Echinococcus *and Hydatid Disease*. CAB International, Wallingford, UK, pp. 89–119.

Ruttenber, D.J., Weniger, F., Sorvillo, R., Murray, R.A. and Ford, S.L. (1984) Diphyllobothriasis associated with salmon consumption in Pacific coast states. *American Journal of Tropical Medicine and Hygiene* 33, 455–459.

Sarti, E., Schantz, P.M., Plancarte, A., Wilson M., Gutierrez O., I., Lopez, A., Roberts, J. and Flisser, A. (1992) Prevalence and risk factors for *Taenia solium* taeniasis and cysticercosis in a village in Morelos, Mexico. *American Journal of Tropical Medicine and Hygiene* 46, 677–685.

Sarti, E., Schantz, P.M., Plancarte, A., Wilson, M., Gutierrez, O., I., Aguilera, J., Roberts, J. and Flisser, A. (1994) Epidemiological investigation of *Taenia solium* taeniasis and cysticercosis in a rural village of Michoacan State, Mexico. *Transactions of the Royal Society of Tropical Medicine and Hygiene* 88, 49–52.

Sen, D.K., Muller, R., Gupta, V.P. and Chilana, J.S. (1989) Cestode larva (sparganum) in the anterior chamber of the eye. *Tropical and Geographical Medicine* 41, 270–273.

Simanjuntak, G.M., Margono, S.S., Okamoto, M. and Ito, A. (1997) Taeniasis/cysticercosis in Indonesia as an emerging disease. *Parasitology Today* 13, 321–322.

Smyth, J.D. and McManus, D.P. (1989) *The Physiology and Biochemistry of Cestodes.* Cambridge University Press, Cambridge, UK.

Thompson, R.C.A. and Lymberry, A.J. (eds) (1995) Echinococcus *and Hydatid Disease.* CAB International, Wallingford, UK.

Thompson, R.C.A., Lymberry, A.J. and Constantine, C.C. (1995) Variation in *Echinococcus*: towards a taxonomic revision of the genus. *Advances in Parasitology* 35, 145–176.

Tornieporth, N.G. and Disko, R. (1994) Alveolar hydatid disease (*Echinococcus multilocularis*) – review and update. In: Sun, T. (ed.) *Progress in Clinical Parasitology* Vol. 4. Norton, New York, USA, pp. 55–76.

von Bonsdorff, B. (1977) *Diphyllobothriasis in Man.* Academic Press, London, UK.

Williams, P.P., Allan, J.C., Verastegui, M., Acosta, M., Eason, A.G., Garcia, H.H., Gonzalez, A.E., Gilman, R.H. and Tsang, V.C.W. (1999) Development of a serological assay to detect *Taenia solium* taeniasis. *American Journal of Tropical Medicine and Hygiene* 60, 199–204.

3

The Acanthocephala

Members of the phylum Acanthocephala are all parasitic and show similarities in structure to both the nematodes and the platyhelminthes (Crompton and Nickol, 1985). Most species are under 1 cm in length but some may be up to 70 cm. The principal diagnostic character is the presence of an eversible proboscis armed with rows of hooks (thorny-headed worms). Acanthocephalans are pseudocoelomate animals (that is, they have a body cavity but it is not homologous to a true coelom) with separate sexes and, like cestodes, have no digestive tract. The life cycle usually involves an insect or crustacean as intermediate host. Many acanthocephalans have a low specificity for the definitive host but are not found in humans because the intermediate hosts are not likely to be ingested (e.g. cockroaches).

Two genera, both belonging to the class Archiacanthocephala, are occasional parasites of humans (Taraschewski, 2000).

Moniliformis moniliformis
(Bremser, 1811), Travassos, 1915

SYNONYMS
Echinorhynchus moniliformis Bremser, 1811; *Moniliformis dubius* Meyer, 1932.

DISTRIBUTION
Moniliformis is a very occasional human parasite. Cases have been reported from Australia, Bangladesh, Belize, Iran, Israel, Italy, Japan, Madagascar, Papua New Guinea, Russia, the USA and Zimbabwe. Infection is common and cosmopolitan in rodents and also occurs in dogs and cats.

LOCATION IN THE HOST
Adults inhabit the small intestine, the proboscis being deeply embedded in the mucosa.

MORPHOLOGY
The adult worms appear to be made up of a series of bead-like annulations, but these are only superficial. The anterior proboscis is cylindrical and has 12–15 rows of curved hooks, with 7–8 hooks per row. Females measure 10–25 cm in length, males 4–14 cm.

LIFE CYCLE
The ovoid eggs measure 70–120 μm × 30–60 μm and are passed in the faeces. The egg has three envelopes characteristic of members of the phylum and contains a spiny acanthor larva when passed. The larva inside can survive for months in soil but develops further if the egg is ingested by various beetles or cockroaches. The larvae require several weeks before they reach the infective stage. The encysted juvenile stages (cystacanths) are ingested by a mammalian host (usually the rat) and develop into adults in 5–6 weeks.

Human infection is probably usually from grain beetles and it is of interest that 15% of coprolites from grain-eating prehistoric humans in a cave in Utah (USA) contained acanthocephalan eggs, which were probably of *Moniliformis*.

CLINICAL MANIFESTATIONS AND PATHOGENESIS

The clinical manifestations have been known since Calandruccio in 1888 infected himself experimentally. Nineteen days after ingesting cystacanth larvae, he had gastrointestinal disturbances with diarrhoea, exhaustion and a ringing in the ears. Eggs appeared in his faeces about 2 weeks later. In a recent case in Florida, USA, an infant had repeated episodes of diarrhoea, accompanied by coughing and fever; after each episode an adult worm was passed in the faeces (Counselman *et al.*, 1989).

TREATMENT

Mebendazole and pyrantel pamoate have been used in recent cases with variable results.

Macranthorhynchus hirudinaceus (Pallas, 1781) Travassos, 1917

SYNONYMS AND POPULAR NAME

Taenia hirudinaceus Pallas, 1781; *Gigantorhynchus gigas* (Pallas, 1781); the giant thorny-headed worm.

DISTRIBUTION

Occasional human cases have been reported from Australia, Brazil, China, Czech Republic, Iraq, Russia and Thailand.

MORPHOLOGY AND LIFE CYCLE

These are large parasites, the female measuring 20–65 cm × 4–10 cm and the male 5–10 cm × 3.5 cm. The most important intermediate hosts are soil-inhabiting beetle larvae belonging to the family Scarabeidae. Development is similar to that of *Moniliformis*. Recent cases in China have had acute abdominal colic with multiple perforations in the jejunum (Leng *et al.*, 1983).

Macranthorhynchus ingens, normally found in the raccoon, has been reported from a child in Texas, USA (Dingley and Beaver, 1985).

Other genera (belonging to the class Palaeacanthocephala) found once or twice in humans are: ***Acanthocephalus rauschi*** Golvan, 1969 from an Inuit in Alaska, with a fish probably acting as a paratenic host; ***Pseudoacanthocephalus bufonis*** (Shipley, 1903) Southwell and Macfie, 1925, a toad parasite, with one case reported from Indonesia; ***Corynosoma strumosum*** (Rudolphi, 1802) Luhe, 1904, one human case being reported from Alaska (adults are normally found in seals with fish acting as paratenic hosts).

Bolbosoma sp., a parasite of cetaceans, has been recorded once from the jejunum of a Japanese, probably contracted from eating raw marine fish.

References

Counselman, K., Fied, C., Lea, G., Nickol, B. and Neafie, R. (1989) *Moniliformis moniliformis* from a child in Florida. *American Journal of Tropical Medicine and Hygiene* 41, 88–90.

Crompton, D.W.T. and Nickol, B.B. (eds) (1985) *Biology of the Acanthocephala*. Cambridge University Press, Cambridge, UK.

Dingley, D. and Beaver, P.C. (1985) *Macranthorhynchus ingens* from a child in Texas. *American Journal of Tropical Medicine and Hygiene* 34, 918–920.

Leng, Y.J., Huang, W.D. and Liang, P.N. (1983) Human infection with *Macranthorhynchus hirudinaceus* Travassos, 1916 [*sic*], in Guangdong Province with notes on its prevalence in China. *Annals of Tropical Medicine and Parasitology* 77, 107–109.

Taraschewski, H. (2000) Host parasite interactions in Acanthocephala – a morphological approach. *Advances in Parasitology* 42, 1–180.

4

The Nematomorpha

This phylum includes the gordiids or hair-worms, in which the adults are free-living in water and the larvae are parasitic in insects. Often adults have been found in water in a toilet bowl from an insect that fell into the water and were thought to have been passed in the faeces or urine. However, in isolated cases from many parts of the world, worms do seem to have been passed in the faeces or per urethra or have been vomited out (Uchikawa *et al.*, 1987) or removed from the eye or ear; in some cases, infection was probably acquired while swimming.

Numerous species have been implicated: *Gordius aquaticus, G. chilensis, G. gesneri, G. inesae, G. ogatai, G. perronciti, G. reddyi* (a case in India with worms in the orbit), *G. robustus* (abscess in orbit), *G. setiger, G. skorikowi, Chordodes capensis, Neochordades columbianus* (from the ear in Colombia), *Parachordodes alpestris, P. pustulosus, P. raphaelis, P. tolusanus, P. violaceus, P. wolterstoffi, Paragordius cinctus, P. esavianus* (in urethra), *P. tanganyikae, P. tricuspidatus* and *P. varius* (see Coombs and Crompton, 1991).

References

Coombs, I. and Crompton, D.W.T. (1991) *A Guide to Human Helminths.* Taylor and Francis, London, UK. pp. 177–190.

Uchikawa, R., Akune, K., Tinone, I., Akune, K., Inove, J., Kagei, N. and Sato, A. (1987) A human case of hair worm (*Gordius* sp.) infection in Kagoshima, Japan. *Japanese Journal of Parasitology* 36, 358–360.

5

The Nematodes

The nematodes are unsegmented pseudo-coelomate worms, usually cylindrical but tapering at the anterior and posterior ends. As a group they are remarkably uniform in structure, although differing in size and habitat. Their uniformity is partly imposed by high internal hydrostatic pressure and has resulted in fewer external protruberances than are found in most invertebrates. They are probably one of the most abundant and widespread of all animal groups, occurring in the sea, fresh water and soil and as parasites of vertebrates, invertebrates and plants.

Species parasitic in humans (63 species in total here) vary in size from threadlike objects just visible to the naked eye (*Strongyloides*, *Trichinella*), to elongate stringlike worms attaining a length of 50 cm (*Dracunculus*).

The outer layer of the body forms a multilayered proteinaceous cuticle. It contains collagen fibres arranged in a trellis-like pattern, thus allowing some contraction and extension of the body. The surface of the living worm is biologically inert (in contrast to that of trematodes and cestodes) and the main antigenic stimulus to the host occurs at various orifices with the production of excretory and secretory (ES) antigens.

During the life history the cuticle is shed periodically, the process being termed a moult or ecdysis. There are four moults during development from ovum to adult, and in the majority of phasmidian species the third-stage larva is responsible for infection of a new host. The geographical distribution, location in the body and life cycles of nematodes of most medical importance are summarized in Tables 6 and 7.

All nematodes are dioecious and the features typical of the male and female phasmid nematode are shown in diagrams of the pinworm, *Enterobius* (Fig. 51).

Classification
(mainly based on Anderson *et al.*, 1974–1983)

KEY: M = mammal, B = bird, R = reptile, A = amphibian, F = fish.

PHYLUM NEMATODA
Elongate, bilaterally symmetrical, cylindrical parasites. Unsegmented, with a gut and anus. Pseudocoelomate. Sexes separate. With four larval stages.

CLASS SECERNENTEA ('Phasmidia')
These have the presence of small sensory structures on the tail end (phasmids) and a characteristic excretory system. With numerous caudal papillae.

Order Rhabditida (MBRA)
Family Strongyloididae
Free-living and parasitic generations can alternate. The parasitic females are parthenogenetic. Small buccal capsule without teeth. Oesophagus of free-living adults and of first-stage larva with posterior bulb (rhabditoid).
Strongyloides

Order Strongylida (MBRA, occasionally F)
Male with cuticular copulatory bursa supported by rays and with two similar

Table 6. Outline of nematode life cycles.

1. Direct cycle: no intermediate host required

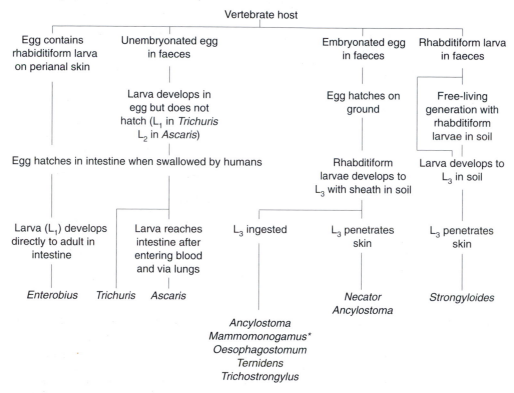

Vertebrate host

Egg contains rhabditiform larva on perianal skin	Unembryonated egg in faeces	Embryonated egg in faeces	Rhabditiform larva in faeces
	Larva develops in egg but does not hatch (L$_1$ in *Trichuris* L$_2$ in *Ascaris*)	Egg hatches on ground	Free-living generation with rhabditiform larvae in soil
Egg hatches in intestine when swallowed by humans		Rhabditiform larvae develops to L$_3$ with sheath in soil	Larva develops to L$_3$ in soil
Larva (L$_1$) develops directly to adult in intestine	Larva reaches intestine after entering blood and via lungs	L$_3$ ingested	L$_3$ penetrates skin	L$_3$ penetrates skin
Enterobius *Trichuris* *Ascaris*		*Ancylostoma Mammomonogamus* Oesophagostomum Ternidens Trichostrongylus*	*Necator Ancylostoma*	*Strongyloides*

2. Indirect cycle: intermediate host required

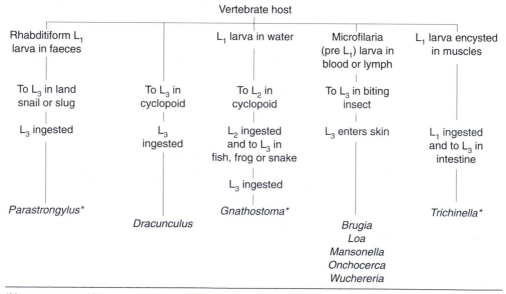

Vertebrate host

Rhabditiform L$_1$ larva in faeces		L$_1$ larva in water	Microfilaria (pre L$_1$) larva in blood or lymph	L$_1$ larva encysted in muscles
To L$_3$ in land snail or slug	To L$_3$ in cyclopoid	To L$_2$ in cyclopoid	To L$_3$ in biting insect	To L$_3$ in muscles
L$_3$ ingested	L$_3$ ingested	L$_2$ ingested and to L$_3$ in fish, frog or snake	L$_3$ enters skin	L$_1$ ingested and to L$_3$ in intestine
		L$_3$ ingested		
*Parastrongylus**	*Dracunculus*	*Gnathostoma**	*Brugia Loa Mansonella Onchocerca Wuchereria*	*Trichinella**

*Humans are accidental or aberrant hosts.

Table 7. Nematodes of medical importance.

	Species	Mode of infection and infective Stage	Site of adult	Geographical distribution
Directly contaminative	*Enterobius vermicularis*	Mouth (L_1 in eggs)	Large intestine	Cosmopolitan
Sometimes	*Strongyloides stercoralis*	Skin (L_3)	Small intestine	Africa, Asia, America, Pacific
Soil-transmitted (geohelminths)	*Strongyloides stercoralis*	Skin (L_3)	Small intestine	Africa, Asia, America, Pacific
	Necator americanus	Skin (L_3)	Small intestine	Africa, Asia, America, Pacific
	Ancylostoma duodenale	Mouth or skin (L_3)	Small intestine	Asia, Africa, Middle East, Pacific
	Trichostrongylus spp.	Mouth (L_3)	Small intestine	Asia, Middle East, Africa
	Ascaris lumbricoides	Mouth (L_2 in egg)	Stomach and small intestine	Cosmopolitan
	Trichuris trichiura	Mouth (L_1 in egg)	Caecum	Cosmopolitan
Aberrant infections	*Ancylostoma* spp. (dermal larva migrans)	Skin (L_3)	Larvae in skin	Africa, America, Asia, Pacific
	Toxocara, etc. (visceral larva migrans)	Mouth (L_2 in egg)	Larvae in liver, eye, brain	Cosmopolitan
Insect-transmitted	*Onchocerca volvulus*	*Simulium* skin (L_3)	Subcutaneous	Africa, Yemen, Central and South America
	Wuchereria bancrofti	*Culex, Anopheles* and *Aedes* skin (L_3)	Lymphatics	Asia, Africa, South America, Pacific
	Brugia malayi	*Mansonia* skin (L_3)	Lymphatics	South-East Asia
	Loa loa	*Chrysops* skin (L_3)	Subcutaneous	Africa (rain forest)
	Mansonella perstans	*Culicoides* skin (L_3)	Peritoneal cavity	Africa, South America
	Mansonella streptocerca	*Culicoides* skin (L_3)	Peritoneal cavity	Africa (rain forest)
	Mansonella ozzardi	*Culicoides, Simulium* skin (L_3)	Peritoneal cavity	South America, West Indies
Crustacean-transmitted	*Dracunculus medinensis*	Cyclopoids mouth (L_3)	Subcutaneous	Africa, Middle East, [India, Pakistan]
Aberrant infection	*Gnathostoma spinigerum*	Cyclopoids mouth (L_2)	Subcutaneous	South-East Asia
Snail-transmitted Aberrant infection	*Parastrongylus cantonensis*	Misc. snails and crustaceans mouth (L_3)	Larvae in meninges	Pacific
	Parastrongylus costaricensis	Misc. snails and crustaceans mouth (L_3)	Larvae in mesenteric arteries	Americas, Japan, Africa (?)
Meat-transmitted Accidental infection	*Trichinella spiralis*	Mouth (L_1)	Small intestine	Cosmopolitan
Fish-transmitted Aberrant infection	*Anisakis*	Mouth (L_3)	Intestine	Europe, Japan
Accidental infection	*Aonchotheca philippinensis*	Mouth (L_1)	Small intestine	Philippines, Thailand

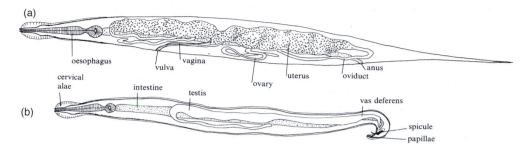

Fig. 51. Diagram of (a) a female (8–13 mm long) and (b) male (2.5 mm long) *Enterobius vermicularis* to illustrate typical nematode features (oesophagus = pharynx).

spicules. Oesophagus club-shaped posteriorly, but without definite bulb (rhabditoid in first-stage larva). Mouth without lips. Direct life cycle usually includes two free-living and feeding larval stages (except in superfamily Metastrongyloidea).

SUPERFAMILY ANCYLOSTOMATOIDEA (M)
Family Ancylostomatidae
Buccal capsule well developed, usually with ventral teeth or cutting plates. Caudal bursa of male usually supported by rays.
Ancylostoma, Necator

SUPERFAMILY STRONGYLOIDEA
Buccal capsule globular, strongly developed and cuticularized.

Family Chabertiidae (M)
Mouth surrounded by leaf crown.
Oesophagostomum, Ternidens

Family Syngamidae (MB)
Leaf crown rudimentary. Male and female attached.
Mammomonogamus

SUPERFAMILY TRICHOSTRONGYLOIDEA (MBRA)
Family Trichostrongylidae (MB)
Filiform worms with the buccal capsule absent or feebly developed. Caudal bursa with reduced or absent dorsal lobe.
Trichostrongylus

SUPERFAMILY METASTRONGYLOIDEA (M)
Family Angiostrongylidae (M)
Filiform with reduced buccal capsule. Caudal bursa of male usually asymmetrical and may be reduced. Parasites of repiratory or circulatory system. Require an intermediate host.
Parastrongylus

Order Ascaridida (MBRAF)
Large stout intestinal worms. Mouth usually with three lips. Oesophagus without valvular apparatus and not divided into two portions. Male and female similar in size. Male with equal spicules. Life cycle either direct or indirect with intermediate host.

SUPERFAMILY ASCARIDOIDEA
Family Ascarididae
Direct life cycle.
Ascaris, Toxocara, Toxascaris

Family Anisakidae
Indirect life cycle.
Anisakis, Pseudoterranova

Order Oxyurida (MBRAF)
Small stout nematodes. Oesophagus with posterior bulb with valvular apparatus. Female with long pointed tail. Direct life cycle, with two moults in egg. Female with large embryonated eggs, often flattened on one side. Parasites of colon or rectum.

SUPERFAMILY OXYUROIDEA
Family Oxyuridae
Enterobius

Order Spirurida (MBRAF)
Oesophagus in two parts, anterior muscular and posterior longer part glandular. Indirect life cycle with larvae in arthropods.

SUPERFAMILIES GNATHOSTOMATOIDEA, GONGYLONEMATOIDEA, THELAZOIDEA, HABRONEMATOIDEA, PHYSALOPTEROIDEA ('Spirurids')
Filiform. Mouth usually has two lips. Female longer than male, with vulva in the anterior region. Spicules of male very unequal. Mainly non-intestinal.
Gnathostoma, Gongylonema, Thelazia, Habronema, Physaloptera

SUPERFAMILY FILARIOIDEA (MBRA) ('Filariae')
Family Onchocercidae
Filiform. Mouth usually without lips. Female longer than male with vulva in anterior region and double uterus. Spicules very unequal in male. Non-intestinal parasites. Usually ovoviviparous, with larvae in bloodsucking insects (or arachnids).
Wuchereria, Brugia, Loa, Onchocerca, Mansonella, Dirofilaria

SUPERFAMILY DRACUNCULOIDEA (MBRF)
Family Dracunculidae
Similar in structure to filariae but females very much longer than males, with vulva and anus atrophied in gravid female and single uterus. Ovoviviparous with larvae in copepods.
Dracunculus

CLASS ADENOPHOREA ('Aphasmidia')
Phasmids absent. Caudal papillae absent or few in male. Oesophagus usually forming a stichosome. First-stage larvae, often with stylet and infective to final host.

Many members are parasites of plants and insects.

Order Enoplida (MBRAF)
SUPERFAMILY TRICHINELLOIDEA
Family Trichuridae
Sexes separate. Anterior region of body much thinner than posterior. Vulva near end of oesophagus. Male with single spicule.
Trichuris, Aonchotheca, Calodium, Eucoleus

Family Trichinellidae
Sexes separate. Anterior region of body slightly thinner than posterior. Male with single or no spicule. Female with one ovary and uterus, vulva near middle of oesophagus. Ovoviviparous.
Trichinella

SUPERFAMILY DIOCTOPHYMATOIDEA
Family Dioctophymidae
Male tail modified to form ventral sucker. Well-developed oesophagus.
Dioctophyma, Eustrongylides

A Key to Nematodes Parasitic in Humans

1. Heterogenic. Parasitic form parthenogenetic with direct life cycle. Small buccal capsule without teeth — RHABDITIDA *Strongyloides*

   Not heterogenic. Parasitic forms sexually differentiated — 2
2. Pharynx consisting of a narrow tube running through the centre of a single row of cells — ENOPLIDA (TRICHUROIDEA) *Aonchotheca Calodium Eucoleus Trichuris Trichinella*

   Pharynx muscular and not consisting of intracellular tube — 3
3. Males with copulatory bursa — 4
   Males without copulatory bursa — 5
4. Copulatory bursa muscular and without rays — ENOPLIDA (DIOCTOPHYMATOIDEA) *Dioctophyma Eustrongylides*

   Copulatory bursa cuticular and supported by rays — STRONGYLIDA see subkey below
5. Pharynx dilated posteriorly into a bulb, usually containing a valvular apparatus and often separated from rest of pharynx by constriction. Usually small forms — OXYURIDA *Enterobius*

   Pharynx not dilated posteriorly into a bulb — 6

6. Relatively stout worms. Head with 3 large lips
           ASCARIDIDA
             Ascaris
             Toxocara

   Relatively slender filiform worms. Head with 2
   lateral lips or 4 or 6 small lips or absent.
   Arthropod intermediate hosts   7

7. Usually 2 lateral lips. Chitinous buccal capsule.
   Vulva in middle of body or posterior. Parasites of
   alimentary canal, respiratory system or orbital, nasal or
   oral canal
           SPIRURIDA
           (except FILARIOIDEA
           and DRACUNCULOIDEA)
             Gnathostoma
             Habronema
             Physaloptera
             Thelazia

   Usually without lips. Buccal capsule absent. Vulva in
   pharyngeal region. Parasites of circulatory or lymphatic
   system, serous cavities, muscles or connective tissues   8

8. Females not more than three times longer than males.
   Vulva not atrophied
           SPIRURIDA
           (FILARIOIDEA)
             Filariae

   Females enormously longer than males. Vulva atrophied
   in gravid female
           SPIRURIDA
           (DRACUNCULOIDEA)
             Dracunculus

Subkey to the order Strongylida

(a) Parasites of alimentary canal or rarely in renal tissue   (b)
    Parasites of respiratory system   (d)

(b) Buccal capsule feebly developed or absent.
    Threadlike worms
           TRICHOSTRONGYLOIDEA
             Trichostrongylus

    Buccal capsule well developed   (c)

(c) Buccal capsule with ventral teeth or cutting plates   ANCYLOSTOMATOIDEA
             Ancylostoma
             Necator

    Buccal capsule without teeth, etc. but mouth typically
    with a leaf crown
           STRONGYLOIDEA
           (Family Chabertiidae)
             Oesophagostomum
             Ternidens

(d) Well-developed chitinous buccal capsule. Male often
    attached to female
           STRONGYLOIDEA
           (Family Syngamidae)
             Syngamus

    Rudimentary buccal capsule or absent. Filiform   METASTRONGYLOIDEA
             Parastrongylus

The section on the nematodes has been split into two parts, those that are intestinal and others that are tissue parasites. This has allowed the control of the common intestinal nematodes to be considered together. However, it has resulted in treatment of one of the main zoologically related group of nematodes being divided by the other as below:

Intestinal nematodes | Tissue nematodes
Class Secernentea | Class Adenophorea |
Class Secernentea

Intestinal Nematodes

Geohelminths

This is a group of intestinal nematodes which, while not closely related zoologically, are all soil-transmitted and have great similarities in epidemiology and in methods of control: it includes *Strongyloides*, the hookworms (*Necator* and *Ancylostoma*), *Ascaris* and *Trichuris*.

Order Rhabditida
Family Strongyloididae

Strongyloides stercoralis
(Bavay, 1876) Stiles and Hassall, 1902

SYNONYMS
Anguillula stercoralis, Bavay, 1876 (larvae from faeces); *A. intestinalis,* Bavay, 1877 (parasitic females from intestine); *Pseudorhabditis stercoralis* Perroncito, 1881 (free-living adults).

DISEASE AND POPULAR NAME
Strongyloidiasis or strongyloidosis, anguillosis; Cochin-China diarrhoea. Included as one of the geohelminths.

GEOGRAPHICAL DISTRIBUTION
Strongyloides infection is widely distributed in tropical regions of Africa, Asia and Central and South America (particularly Brazil, Colombia and Guyana); it also occurs in eastern Europe and sporadically in the USA and southern Europe. Distribution is similar to that of hookworms but the prevalence is usually much lower – an estimated 100 million cases worldwide (Grove, 1996).

LOCATION IN HOST
Parthenogenetic females live embedded in the mucosa of the small intestine – the duodenum and the first part of the jejunum in light infections, back to the terminal ileum in heavy infections.

MORPHOLOGY
Parasitic females are small, transparent, filiform nematodes, measuring 2.0–2.7 mm in length by 0.03–0.075 mm in width. The cuticle is finely striated and the tail pointed. The oesophagus occupies the anterior third of the body and joins the midgut, which opens at the ventral anus a short distance from the posterior end. The vulva opens ventrally at the junction of the middle and posterior thirds of the worm. The uteri, oviducts and ovarian tubules are paired, one branch extending forwards from the vulva and the other backwards. About 10–20 eggs are present in the two uteri at one time. The eggs are thin-shelled, transparent and ovoid; they measure 50–60 µm × 30–35 µm when laid. The eggs are partially embryonated and usually hatch in the tissues of the mucosa, so that larvae rather than eggs are passed out in the faeces (Figs 123 and 125).

The females produce eggs parthenogenetically and, although parasitic males similar to free-living ones described below were recorded twice, they have never been seen since.

Strongyloides is also capable of undergoing a complete life cycle in the soil, living as a free-living nematode with a distinct morphology. The free-living female is shorter and stouter than the parasitic form (1.0 mm × 0.06 mm) and has a short rhabditiform oesophagus (muscular and with an enlarged posterior bulb, similar to that of the saprophytic soil nematode *Rhabditis*).

The free-living male measures about 0.7 mm × 0.04 mm and has a pointed tail, curving ventrally, with two spicules and a gubernaculum (this is a chitinous sheath in which the spicules can slide up and down; it is presumed to aid in the transference of

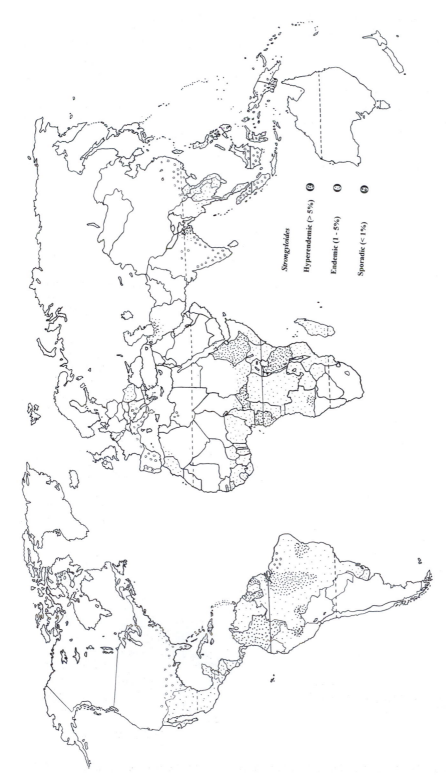

Map 7. Distribution of *Strongyloides stercoralis* (and *S. fuellebornius* in New Guinea).

sperm during copulation and is often of taxonomic importance). The oesophagus is rhabditiform.

LIFE CYCLE (Fig. 52)

Parasitic (= direct) life cycle. Eggs are laid in the mucosa and submucosa of the small intestine. There they hatch as rhabditiform first-stage larvae, which escape into the intestinal lumen and pass out in the faeces, where they are very active. The larvae mea-

sure 250 µm × 20 µm and can be differentiated from those of hookworms by the smaller buccal capsule (Fig. 53). The larvae feed on bacteria in the soil and moult twice to give the infective filariform stage, measuring 550 µm × 20 µm, in the surface layers of the soil. The infective larvae differ from those of hookworms by the lack of a sheath, by the triradiate tip to the tail and in the greater length of the pharynx. They ascend soil particles and damp vegetation

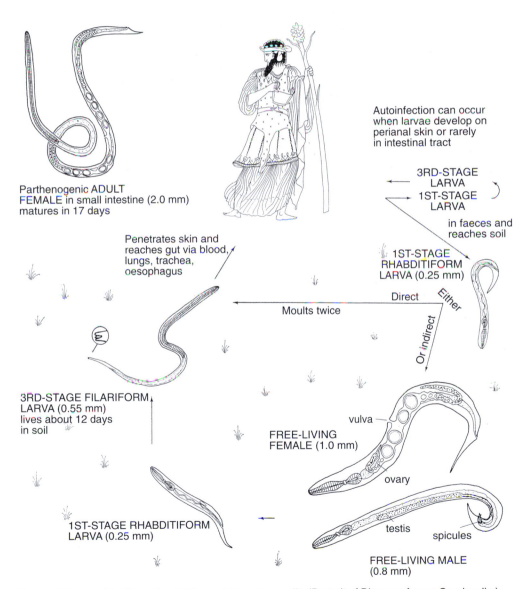

Parthenogenic ADULT FEMALE in small intestine (2.0 mm) matures in 17 days

Autoinfection can occur when larvae develop on perianal skin or rarely in intestinal tract

3RD-STAGE LARVA
1ST-STAGE LARVA

in faeces and reaches soil

Penetrates skin and reaches gut via blood, lungs, trachea, oesophagus

1ST-STAGE RHABDITIFORM LARVA (0.25 mm)

Direct
Either

Moults twice

Or indirect

3RD-STAGE FILARIFORM LARVA (0.55 mm) lives about 12 days in soil

vulva

FREE-LIVING FEMALE (1.0 mm)

ovary

1ST-STAGE RHABDITIFORM LARVA (0.25 mm)

testis   spicules

FREE-LIVING MALE (0.8 mm)

Fig. 52. The possible life cycles of *Strongyloides stercoralis*. (Portrait of Dionysus from a Greek cylix.)

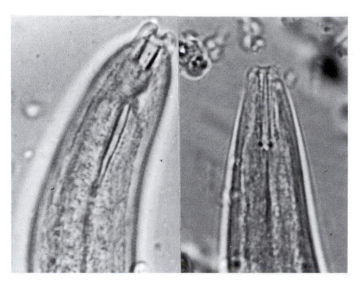

Fig. 53. The anterior ends of the first-stage larva (L_1) of *Strongyloides* (left) and hookworm (right) in soil. The former has a shorter buccal capsule.

in the surface film, often standing on their tails in tufts or aggregates. Under optimum conditions the larvae live in the soil for about 2 weeks but, when they come into contact with the skin, usually of the feet (or more rarely the buccal mucosa), they penetrate and reach the small cutaneous blood-vessels and then the lungs. After penetration of the alveoli, the larvae moult twice and the young adults pass up the bronchi and trachea and then down the oesophagus to reach the small intestine (although it has recently been suggested that they may use other routes). Once there, the female burrows into the mucosal tissues, becomes mature and lays its partheno-genetically produced eggs in the mucosa and crypts about 17 days after penetration.

Very unusually among human helminths is the possibility of replication within the human host. Autoinfection is usually brought about because the rhabditiform larvae in faecal matter are deposited on the perianal skin and develop into filariform larvae, which penetrate through the skin. This accounts for the persistence of strongyloidiasis in patients up to 65 years after they have left an endemic region (most notably in former Second World War prisoners in the Far East, who are still suffering from recurrent larva currens), although the adult worms live for only a few months. In severely ill patients or in chronic carriers, rhabditiform larvae passing down the gut may develop into filariform larvae without reaching the exterior at all, and these then penetrate the intestinal mucosa. Exceptionally, when the patient's resistance is low, all larval stages may be found in many of the visceral organs and rhabditiform and filariform larvae may even appear in the sputum.

Free-living (= indirect or heterogonic) life cycle. A free-living cycle often occurs in warm climates, provided that there is plenty of moisture and nutrients in the soil. The rhabditiform larvae passed out in faeces feed and undergo four moults in the soil to become free-living adult males and females in 24–30 h. The eggs, which develop in the uterus of the free-living female after mating, occupy a large portion of the body and are laid in a partly embryonated state. They hatch in a few hours after completing development and rhabditiform first-stage larvae emerge. These first-stage larvae moult twice and develop into non-feeding, filariform, third-stage larvae in a few days. The infective larvae survive on soil and vegetation in warm moist conditions and penetrate the skin when they come in contact. There is no second free-living cycle.

The factors determining whether direct or indirect development occurs is not well understood but it is believed that the higher the immune status of the host the more likely that larvae passed in the faeces will undergo an indirect cycle. In other species at least there are genetically determined strain differences and environmental factors also help to determine whether males and females or infective larvae develop in soil.

CLINICAL MANIFESTATIONS

There may be pruritic eruption at the site of entry of the larvae ('ground itch') in heavy infections, followed by a cough after a few days.

The majority of cases are of chronic, uncomplicated, strongyloidiasis and are symptomless, with just a few worms present and no alteration to the mucosa. There may, however, be abdominal discomfort, with intermittent gastric pains, accompanied by nausea, diarrhoea, weight loss and a generalized urticaria. Recurrent, linear, rapidly progressive, urticarial weals ('larva currens') can occur on the buttocks, groins or trunk. Lesions in the gluteal region indicate that autoinfection is occurring and are likely to be present in all clinically important cases.

In a proportion of heavily infected cases, more serious clinical disease ensues, characterized by enteritis with malabsorption syndrome and electrolyte imbalance (Plate 12). Such infections in children may have serious consequences, precipitating kwashiorkor and emaciation.

Disseminated (complicated, hyperinfective or overwhelming) strongyloidiasis is always serious and often fatal and can have a variety of manifestations, depending on the intensity of infection and the organs involved. Complications affect particularly the bowel, lungs and central nervous system (CNS) and are often accompanied by secondary bacterial infection. Parasitic ileus (pseudo-obstruction), pneumonitis with pulmonary infiltrates, meningitis, brain abscess and septicaemia are all possible.

Disseminated strongyloidiasis occurs when the body's cell-mediated immune responses are deficient, often in patients with malignant lymphoma or acute leukaemia, on immunosuppressive drugs, after renal transplantation, or suffering from malnutrition. It does not seem to be strongly associated with cases of AIDS, although there is a correlation with HTLV-1 infection and it is possible that *Strongyloides* leads to immunoglobulin E (IgE) deficiency (Phelps and Neva, 1993). Hyperinfection may also be potentiated by a decrease in mobility of the intestine, which allows first-stage larvae to mature into infective forms before being passed out in the faeces. This postulate is supported by the fact that, in cases of hyperinfection, ulcerations caused by infective larvae are always present in the colon as well as the ileum. It has been postulated that hyperinfection is not an immune phenomenon but is caused by corticosteroid therapy stimulating the production of ecdysteroids (moulting hormones) (Genta, 1992). However, hyperinfection occurs in many patients who have not received corticosteroids.

There is evidence that the immunomodulatory effect of many helminths may increase susceptibility to tuberculosis (TB) and AIDS (Borkow and Bentwich, 2000; Bundy *et al.*, 2000).

PATHOGENESIS

This can be divided into three stages.

1. The penetration of the skin by filariform larvae usually causes no symptoms in non-sensitized patients, provided infection is light. Larvae secrete a metalloprotease of molecular mass 40 kDa, which is immunogenic; in heavier infections a rash often appears at the site of entry ('ground itch') and there may be severe pruritus. Where autoinfection is occurring there may also be perianal and perineal ulceration.
2. The larvae that reach the lungs and pass into the alveoli can cause a pneumonitis similar to Loeffler's syndrome in ascariasis (p. 150).
3. The adult females live in the depths of the crypts of the ileum and lay their eggs there. Larvae hatching from deposited eggs burrow through the lumen and cause superficial catarrhal damage to the mucosa, often with excessive production of mucus.

In severe cases of autoinfection, parasites are present in the submucosa, which becomes oedematous. The mucosa becomes flattened and atrophic (Fig. 54), the pathological picture resembling that of tropical sprue or of infection with *Aonchotheca philippinensis* (p. 173). There may be severe ulceration with a non-reversible fibrosis and often a pronounced inflammatory response to secondary bacterial invasion. Larvae in the lymphatics cause a granulomatous lymphangitis; this, coupled with the inflammation, atrophic mucosa and fibrosis, causes a marked congestion and loss in elasticity of the gut. Paralytic ileus can result and there can also be a severe haemorrhagic, ulcerative enterocolitis, with massive invasion of the whole bowel wall by larvae. In cases of complicated disease, larvae can be found in almost any organ, particularly the intestinal lymph nodes, lungs, liver, heart, urinary tract and nervous system.

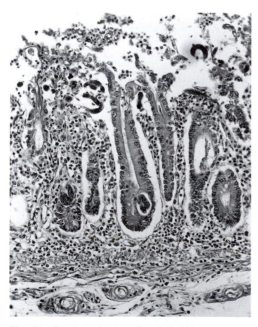

Fig. 54. Section of colon of patient with hyperinfective strongyloidiasis. The section is at the edge of an ulcer and shows inflammation. Adults of *S. stercoralis* are in the crypts and rhabditiform larvae in the lumen.

IMMUNOLOGICAL ASPECTS OF INTESTINAL NEMATODES

Infections with intestinal nematodes generate characteristic patterns of immune responses in their hosts. Typically, infected individuals have elevated levels of IgE, high peripheral eosinophilia and a variety of allergic symptoms, some of which are generalized, others being localized to the tissues invaded. For example, where infection occurs through the skin (e.g. hookworms, *Strongyloides*) there may be dermatitis and pruritus, where parasite development involves the lungs (e.g. *Ascaris*, hookworms) there may be bronchitis or pneumonitis, while invasion of muscles (*Trichinella*) causes myositis. Collectively these symptoms imply that intestinal nematodes generate responses dominated by the T-helper 2 (Th2) subset, and this is in agreement with experimental studies in laboratory rodents. Many species cause forms of intestinal pathology that again can be related to immunological causes, e.g. the protein-losing enteropathy seen in patients infected with *Strongyloides* spp. or *Aonchotheca philippinensis*, and the dysentery syndrome seen in children heavily infected with *Trichuris trichiura*, although the extent to which these are Th2-related is debatable. A major difference between experimental studies and observations on human infections is that, whereas laboratory rodents mount strong protective responses against the majority of species used (e.g. *Nippostrongylus brasiliensis*, *Strongyloides ratti* and *S. venezuelensis*, *Trichinella spiralis*, *Trichuris muris*), evidence for protective responses in humans is very limited. The rapid reacquisition of infection with the common geohelminths after chemotherapy suggests little immunity to reinfection, but, against this, in some species, is evidence of an age-related decline in infection intensity, if not in prevalence (Crompton, 1998; Fig. 55).

Experimental studies suggest that Th2 cells mediate immunity against intestinal nematodes through changes in mucosal structure and function, resulting in an altered parasite environment (Wakelin, 1996). Changes in mucosal architecture (through villous atrophy) and epithelial function, development of mucosal mastocytosis, increased secretion of mucus from

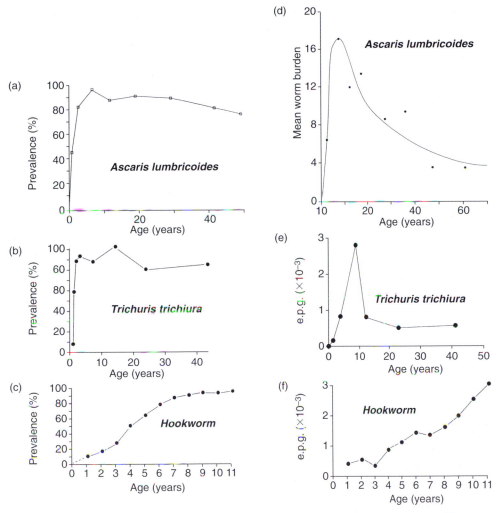

Fig. 55. Left: Graphs showing the relationship between prevalence and age for (a) *Ascaris*, (b) *Trichuris*, (c) hookworms. Each graph is based on a different research study. Right: Graphs showing the relationships between intensity of infection and age for (d) *Ascaris*, (e) *Trichuris*, (f) hookworms. Curve (d) is based on recovery of worms after chemotherapy and (e) and (f) on egg counts. e.p.g., eggs per gram. Each graph is based on a different research study (all graphs from Crompton, 1998).

goblet cells and altered muscular activity have all been implicated. Although infection does elicit Th2-dependent antibodies (e.g. in mice IgA, IgE and IgG1), these are not thought to play a major role. Little or nothing is known of comparable mucosal changes in infected humans and, although antibody responses are made, these are often positively correlated with the duration and intensity of infection, suggesting no role in protection. Arguments have been made, however, for inverse correlations between levels of IgA and level of infection with *Trichuris* and between the levels of IgE and development of *Necator*.

The reasons for the apparent lack of protective immunity against intestinal worms are not fully understood, although many suggestions have been made. In countries where these infections are common, nutritional levels are often low and immunity impaired as a consequence. The pathological consequences of the worm infection may exacerbate nutritional problems, leading to a vicious circle. Infections are sometimes associated with reduced immune responsiveness, and it is clear that worms themselves can interfere with the protective responses of the host in a variety of ways (Prichard, 1993). It is also possible that genetic factors influence the ability to control infections, as has been amply demonstrated in experimental systems (Wakelin, 1994). It is characteristic of infections with intestinal nematodes in populations that their distributions are highly aggregated, i.e. most individuals have low infections while a few are heavily infected (Crompton, 1998). There has been much debate about the cause of such aggregation, with polarized views that it is due primarily to environmental exposure or that it is a consequence of variation in immune responsiveness. It would be unlikely that genetic factors did not influence the ability to respond protectively to intestinal worms, and indeed there have been claims that possession of particular major histocompatibility complex (MHC)-linked genes does correlate with an individual's likely level of infection.

DIAGNOSIS

Clinical. There is no well-defined clinical picture, although watery diarrhoea with mucus, perhaps interrupted by constipation, abdominal pain and with a high eosinophilia, may suggest strongyloidiasis. The lesions in the gluteal region and larva currens are almost pathognomic if present. Imaging techniques can show infiltration in the lungs (Fig. 56).

Parasitological. The presence of rhabditiform first-stage larvae in a fresh faecal sample provides a positive diagnosis (Figs 123 and 125). In an old sample mixed with soil, hookworm larvae could have hatched from eggs and must be differentiated (when living, *Strongyloides* larvae lash like a whip, while hookworm larvae move sinuously like a snake). Also in old faeces (30 h) free-living adults of *Strongyloides* might be found.

To concentrate the larvae, Baermann filtration or formol–ether concentration (p. 263) can be used. In the Baermann technique 10 g (or more) of faeces is spread on a six-

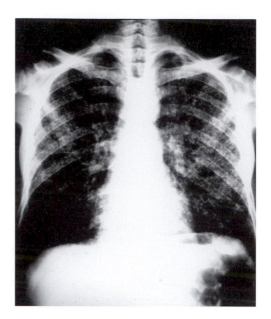

Fig. 56. Radiograph of lungs in a patient with disseminated strongyloidiasis, showing diffuse infiltrations.

layered gauze pad on a coarse sieve with a wooden applicator and placed in a sedimentation flask that has been filled 25 mm below the rim with 0.9–1.2% saline or water at 37°C. Alternatively, a funnel can be used with a length of plastic tubing clamped at the bottom. If the faeces is watery, it can be spread on filter-paper, which is then placed face down on the gauze. After 2 h, 5 ml of the bottom sediment can be removed with a Pasteur pipette and transferred to a 5 cm Petri dish. This is examined under a dissecting microscope for first-stage larvae. If no larvae are found, the flask can be left overnight at room temperature and re-examined; then a drop of iodine can be added and the larvae examined on a microscope slide for generic identification.

There are various culture methods that can be used if no larvae can be found but disease is clinically indicated.

1. The Harada–Mori, filter-paper, test-tube culture and formol–ether concentration methods, which can also be used for hookworms, are given on p. 263.

2. In the agar plate method, 2 g of faeces is placed in the centre of an agar medium in a 9 cm plastic Petri dish, covered and sealed round the edge with adhesive tape, and incubated at room temperature (about 28°C) for 48 h. For greater safety, a double-walled Petri dish (or a smaller dish inside the larger) can be used, the outer area containing 25% glycerine to prevent infective larvae from reaching the edge of the lid. The tracks of larvae can be seen with the naked eye but the dish should also be examined under a compound microscope with a green filter at ×40 magnification. For generic identification, a hole can be made in the agar with hot forceps, 10% formalin added, liquid removed from the bottom with a Pasteur pipette, sedimented and the sediment examined on a microscope slide at high power. This is probably the most sensitive method.

3. In the watch-glass culture method several grams of faeces are spread out on a watch-glass, moistened with water, placed in a Petri dish containing a 2–3 mm layer of water, covered and re-moistened as required. Free-living adults may be seen on the watch-glass after several days or infective larvae after 3 days.

4. A charcoal culture method is also sometimes employed. Five to 10 g of faeces is mixed with activated charcoal in a 10 cm diameter Petri dish, well dampened with distilled water and left covered for 4 days in an incubator at 26–28°C. The infective larvae can be recovered with a soft paint-brush from the condensation drops on the lid. For large quantities of faeces, a sealed jam jar can be used, 5 cm full, and large numbers of larvae will be found in the meniscus around the edge of the mixture when left as before.

5. The entero-test involves swallowing a brushed-nylon thread inside a gelatin capsule and then withdrawing it together with entrapped larvae, fixing in 10% formalin and examining under the microscope. In cases of hyperinfection, larvae may be found in sputum or even urine.

Immunological. These tests cannot usually differentiate between current and past infections. A skin test using extracts of filariform larvae has been in use for 70 years. It measures IgE and is about 80% reliable, although, like other tests, it cross-reacts with filarial infection.

The ELISA is fast and efficient, using stored antigen, and is in routine use in some laboratories (Mangali *et al.*, 1991). The test gives sensitivity and specificity of about 95% when measuring IgG. Specificity of the indirect test can be improved by prior absorption with filarial and hookworm antigens (Conway *et al.*, 1993).

The indirect fluorescent antibody (IFA) test has been used with living larvae as antigen, preabsorbed against other nematodes, and recently a simple gelatine agglutination test has been proposed (Sato *et al.*, 1991).

There is as yet no method for measuring circulating antigens.

TREATMENT

Chemotherapy is principally by benzimidazoles, which appear to act by binding to tubulin and disrupting the assembly of microtubules and by altering transmembrane proton discharge (Grove, 1996).

Thiabendazole. Given orally twice a day for 3–7 days, 25 mg kg^{-1} body weight has a cure rate of about 80%. This is still the drug of choice – unfortunately, since side-effects (nausea, dizziness and anorexia) are common – chemical formula: (2-(4-thiazolyl)-1-*H*-benzimidazole-2-yl)-carbamate,

Mebendazole. If given at 100–200 mg twice daily for 3 days, it is probably effective against adult worms but not against migrating larvae. Treatment for several weeks is more effective, probably because it kills autoinfecting larvae when they develop into adults. Higher dosages may be more effective for cases of disseminated strongyloidiasis – chemical formula: methyl(5-(benzyl)-1-*H*-benzimidazole-2-yl)-carbamate.

Albendazole. When given at 400 mg twice daily for 3 days, it has given variable results in trials, with 50–85% cure rates. Long-term treatment will probably prove to be as effective as mebendazole, perhaps with fewer side-effects and greater action against larvae – chemical formula: methyl-(5-propylthio-1-*H*-benzimidazol-2-yl)-carbamate.

Ivermectin. In clinical trials of uncomplicated cases, this macrocyclic lactone was fairly effective (over 80% cure rate) against adults and larvae at a single dose of 0.2 mg kg^{-1} body weight (Marti *et al.*, 1996). Long-term treatment (0.2 mg kg^{-1} once a week for 4 weeks) with ivermectin may prove to be the best option for complete cure in patients who fail to respond to initial treatment. For disseminated strongyloidiasis, treatment over 3–4 weeks is necessary (Grove, 1996).

It is very difficult to treat cases of disseminated strongyloidiasis with intestinal obstruction, where patients usually need suction and drainage, intravenous fluids and thiabendazole given daily for a week, perhaps rectally, since there is no intravenous formulation. Since patients often die, parenteral ivermectin or use of cyclosporin (3 mg kg^{-1} daily) could be tried as a last resort.

EPIDEMIOLOGY

In many areas strongyloidiasis is coextensive with hookworm infection since the environmental conditions favouring the free-living stages and the mode of infection are similar, but this is not always true. Like hookworm, it is primarily a disease of poverty and insanitary conditions, particularly where there are poor conditions for disposal of human waste and inadequate water supplies. In a study in Bangladesh, occupants of an urban slum community were more likely to be infected if they used communal latrines rather than individual latrines, if they had an earth floor rather than a concrete floor and if they were aged between 7 and 10 (Hall *et al.*, 1994). Both are primarily rural infections, particularly common in coffee, cocoa and banana plantations. Infection is also common in closed communities, such as mental institutions. Infection appears to be acquired progressively between the ages of about 6 and 20 and then prevalence remains constant for the whole of adult life. The larvae of both parasitic and free-living forms are unable to survive temperatures below 8°C or above 40°C for more than a few days. They have little resistance to drying, excessive moisture or marked changes in temperature. Infective larvae live for about 14 days in soil.

Where *Strongyloides* occurs together with hookworms, the former is almost always found to be rarer. This is rather surprising when it is considered that the parasitic females are more prolific than female hookworms and the presence of free-living generations should increase the numbers of larvae in the soil. There are three possible explanations: the first is that the first-stage larvae in the faeces are not as resistant as hookworm eggs; the second that the filariform larvae have shorter longevity; and the third that reported prevalence rates are much too low because of the difficulties of diagnosis.

Infection rates reported recently from surveys in various countries are: Aborigines in Queensland, Australia (large-scale survey) 2%; north-eastern Brazil 5.3% and 9.6%, São Paulo (infants) 2%; Dagestan (large-scale) 1–1.4%; Bihar, India 10%; Jamaica 1%; Laos 19% (10% in under-10s); Bauchi in Nigeria 0.4%; Okinawa (Ryuku Islands) 4–22%; USA (large-scale) 0.2%, Kentucky 0.9%, Tennessee 3%.

PREVENTION AND CONTROL

Personal prevention is aided by the wearing of shoes. Control is principally by the provision of adequate sanitation facilities consequent on a rise in living standards; it is sobering to realize that 2400 million people (45% of the population of the world) still do not have sanitation. In some areas water is recycled from sewage systems and larvae can still survive on the soil or grass, and water thus needs further treatment or storage. Targeted chemotherapy of those groups most at risk may prove to be of use (Conway *et al.*, 1995), but occasional mass chemotherapy is unlikely to be effective. However, the repeated mass chemotherapy campaigns against all geohelminths in general being carried out in many countries may have some effect (see p. 134).

ZOONOTIC ASPECTS

Transmission is almost entirely between humans, although chimpanzees and dogs have been found naturally infected.

Another species, **S. fuelleborni** Linstow, 1905, is a common parasite of monkeys in Africa and Asia and occurs in humans in the forest areas of Central Africa (Cameroon, Central African Republic, Congo, Congo Republic, Ethiopia, Malawi, Ruanda, Togo and Zimbabwe). In these countries it appears to be a natural parasite of humans and in some areas is the predominant species of *Strongyloides*, with an infection rate of 25%.

S. fuelleborni can be differentiated from S. stercoralis as eggs, not larvae, are found in the faeces; these measure on average 53 µm × 35 µm (range 48–61 µm × 30–40 µm) (Fig. 124). The eggs are smaller than hookworm eggs and in a later stage of cleavage. The eggs hatch quickly in faecal samples and in cases of doubt a specific diagnosis can be made by culturing to the free-living adult stage, since these differ from those of S. stercoralis (Grove, 1996). Free-living generations of S. fuelleborni tend to develop under semi-aerobic conditions.

An experimental infection resulted in an intense itching at the site of entry, followed by fever, lymphangitis, lymphadenitis and cough, with an eosinophilia of 48% in the early stages. Abdominal pain occurred after 20 days and eggs appeared in the faeces after 28 days.

What appeared to be a morphologically identical parasite has been reported in the last few years from Papua New Guinea (PNG) and Western New Guinea (Irian Jaya), although there are no non-human primates on this island. In some areas of PNG an almost invariably fatal disease ('swollen belly syndrome') was found in babies 1–6 months old, with swollen abdomen, respiratory distress, enteric protein loss and peripheral oedema. There was no fever but over 100,000 eggs g^{-1} faeces, the eggs often being passed in strings (Ashford *et al.*, 1992).

In other areas there are equally high egg counts but no clinical disease. Clinical disease might be potentiated by prenatal infection from symptomless mothers, followed by a very high exposure to faecal contamination in bags used to carry babies. Treatment with thiabendazole was very effective. The parasite has been designated S. fuelleborni kellyi Viney, Ashford and Barnish, 1991, because of small differences from the African parasite.

There are many species of *Strongyloides* from a wide range of mammals in which the infective, third-stage, larvae can penetrate into the skin of humans but develop no further. They include: S. canis Brumpt, 1922 in dogs, S. cebus Darling, 1911 in monkeys (human case in Panama), S. felis (Chandler, 1925) in cats (Australia), S. myopotami Artigas and Pacheco, 1933 in rodents and carnivores (Brazil), S. papillosus (Wedl, 1956) Ransom, 1911 in sheep, S. planiceps Rogers 1943, in dogs, cats and foxes (Japan), S. procyonis Little, 1965 in carnivores (USA, experimental), S. ransomi Schwarth and Alicata, 1930 in pig and rabbit, S. simiae in primates (Guinea-Bissau, experimental), S. westeri Ihle, 1917 in horse and pig. The free-living males of various species can be differentiated by the structure of the spicules (Grove, 1996).

Halicephalus (= *Micronema*) *deletrix* (Anderson and Bemrick, 1965) is a rhabditiform saprophyte living in soil (family Cephalobidae) but on three occasions it has invaded the brain, liver and heart of humans in the USA through deep lacerations and caused death through meningoencephalitis (Gardiner *et al.*, 1981). It has been found more often in horses (female worms only) in North America and Europe; albendazole with diethylcarbamazine was effective in one cutaneous equine case.

Rhabditids (family Rhabditidae) are small, free-living, saprophytic nematodes that are commonly found in soil and there have been many sporadic reports of infections in humans; adults are usually recovered from faeces and some infections may be spurious. Species reported are: *Cheilobus quadrilabiatus* Cobb, 1924, in faeces of children in Slovakia, *Diploscapter coronata* Cobb, 1913, in the stomach of patients with low gastric acidity in Texas, *Pelodera strongyloides* Schneider, 1866, found under the skin of an infant in Alabama, USA, and of a child in Poland (this is a widespread species often found in the lachrymal fluid of voles), *P. teres* Schneider, 1866, found in faeces, *Rhabditis axei* (Cobbold, 1884) in urine samples in China and Zimbabwe, *R. elongata* Schneider, 1866, found twice in girls in South Korea, *R. inermis* (Schneider, 1860) Dougherty, 1955, in faeces of 17 school-children in Japan, *R. niellyi* Blanchard, 1855, in skin of a patient in France, *R. pellio* (Schneider, 1866) Bütschli, 1873 in the vagina of a girl in Mexico, *R. taurica* Mireckij and Skrajabin, 1965, in the faeces of a child in Russia, *R. terricola* Dujardin, 1845, in the faeces of children in Slovakia and *Rhabditis* sp. in faeces of five children in South Korea.

Order Strongylida

The human hookworms comprise two parasites, *Necator americanus* and *Ancylostoma duodenale.* They both cause similar disease, including anaemia, have similar life histories and require the same control measures. Perhaps because of the movement of peoples, they also have widely overlapping distributions. In addition, there are animal hookworms that are occasionally found in humans, and related nematodes, which in some cases are locally important, adults being found in the intestine or, in the metastrongyles including *Parastrongylus*, the respiratory passages.

Family Ancylostomatidae

Necator americanus
(Stiles, 1902) Stiles, 1906

SYNONYMS
Uncinaria americana Stiles, 1902.

DISEASE AND POPULAR NAME
Ancylostomiasis or ancylostomosis (necatorosis), uncinariasis; New World hookworm infection.

LOCAL NAMES
Chek kaung (Burmese), Au chung (Cantonese), Nsunsuma (Fanti), Aonobyo, Junishichochu, Kochu, Koekabure, Koemake, Sakanoshita or Tsuchikabure (Japanese), Njowni (Luo), Kokki pulu or Koku panuwa (Singalese), Gooryan (Somali), Njuka safura (Swahili), Puchi (Tamil), Pa-yard pak khow (Thai), Sondono (Twi), Aran inu (Yoruba).

GEOGRAPHICAL DISTRIBUTION
Necator was at one time confined almost entirely to the tropics and subtropics but has spread widely and is now the dominant hookworm in Portugal, northern Turkey, the Caspian Sea area of Iran and areas of Japan. It is widespread in Africa south of the Sahara, the Americas (Brazil, Colombia, Venezuela, West Indies, southern USA), where it was probably introduced with the slave trade (although *Ancylostoma* has been reported from pre-Columbian mummies), the Far East (southern and eastern India, Sri Lanka, Malaysia, China, Indochina, Japan, Indonesia, northern Queensland) and the South Pacific. It is absent from most arid zones and temperate climates.

LOCATION IN HOST
Adult worms are present in the second and third portions of the jejunum and rarely in the duodenum with the buccal capsule attached to the mucosa. In heavy infections they may be found as far back as the caecum.

MORPHOLOGY
The adults are cylindrical, greyish-yellow, nematodes tapering anteriorly and slightly curved, with the head bent back dorsally (forming a 'hook').

The cuticle is smooth with fine transverse striations and has lateral cervical papillae just behind the nerve ring, at about the level of the middle of the oesophagus. The large buccal capsule opens slightly dorsally and has a pair of short triangular lancets at the bottom of the cavity (Figs 57 and 58). These aid in attachment of the worm to the mucosa and also in cut-

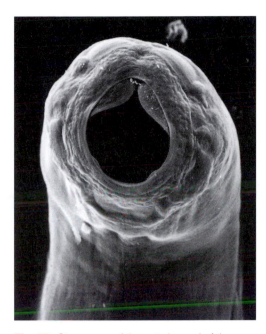

Fig. 57. Stereoscan of the anterior end of the hookworm *N. americanus.*

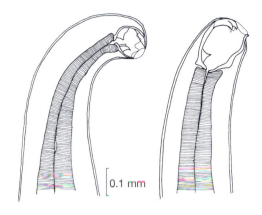

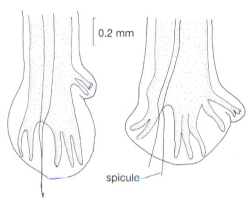

Fig. 58. Anterior end and caudal bursa of male of *N. americanus* (left) and *A. duodenale* (right).

ting off portions for food. A pair of anti-coagulant-secreting glands open into the buccal capsule, producing a histolytic protease with a molecular mass of 37 kDa.

The muscular oesophagus is cylindrical with a slight expansion posteriorly and is about one-sixth of the total length of the worm. The intestine is straight and opens at the posterior end.

The male measures 7–9 mm × 0.3 mm. A single testis lies along the intestine and leads through the seminal vesicle and ejaculatory duct into the cloaca. Immediately noticeable is the broad, membranous, symmetrical, caudal bursa, reinforced by rib-like rays. Within the bursa there are two bristle-like spicules about 2 mm long, which are fused at their distal ends to form a barb. The cloaca opens into the bursa. The shape of the bursa differs in *Necator* and *Ancylostoma* and the two species can also be differentiated by the dorsal ray, which in the former is split to its base (Fig. 58). The female measures 9–11 mm × 0.4 mm. The vulva usually opens just anterior to the middle of the body and from it paired vaginae lead anteriorly and posteri-orly to open into the oviducts, followed by long, slender, coiled ovaries.

LIFE CYCLE (Fig. 59)

The transparent egg is thin-shelled and ovoid, with blunt, rounded ends; it measures 60 (64–76) μm × 40 (36–42) μm. The ovum is unsegmented when discharged by the worm but continues to develop and is usually at the 4- or 8-celled stage when passed in the faeces. It develops quickly and may already be at the morula stage in old faecal samples. On reaching soil the embryo develops into a first-stage larva, which hatches out in 24–48 h. The conditions for maximum rate of development are warmth (+25°C), shade, moisture and a light sandy loam. These larvae are termed

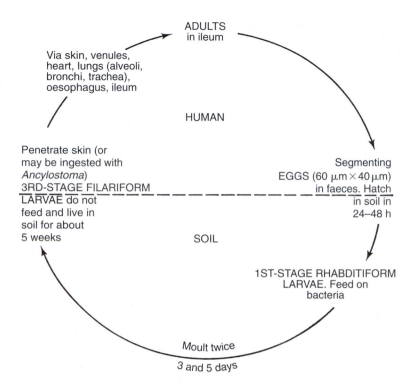

ADULTS
in ileum

Via skin, venules,
heart, lungs (alveoli,
bronchi, trachea),
oesophagus, ileum

HUMAN

Penetrate skin (or
may be ingested with
Ancylostoma)
3RD-STAGE FILARIFORM
LARVAE do not
feed and live in
soil for about
5 weeks

Segmenting
EGGS (60 μm × 40 μm)
in faeces. Hatch
in soil in
24–48 h

SOIL

1ST-STAGE RHABDITIFORM
LARVAE. Feed on
bacteria

Moult twice
3 and 5 days

Fig. 59. Life cycle of human hookworms.

rhabditiform because the structure of the oesophagus (with an anterior portion connected by a thin region to a posterior bulb) resembles that of the free-living nematode *Rhabditis*. They measure 280–300 μm × 17 μm and resemble closely the first-stage larvae of *Strongyloides*, except that hookworm larvae are slightly longer, less pointed posteriorly and have a longer buccal cavity (Fig. 53). The larvae feed on bacteria and organic debris in the soil and moult twice; once on the 3rd day when 400 μm long and again on the 5th day when 500–700 μm long. The third-stage or filariform larvae do not feed and retain the shed cuticle for a time. The mouth becomes closed with a plug and the oesophagus occupies one-third of the length of the body. The larvae are now infective; those of *Necator* and *Ancylostoma* can be differentiated by the apparent space between the oesophagus and intestine in *Necator* and by differences in the structure of the oesophageal spears (Fig. 60 and Table 8).

Hookworm larvae may also need to be differentiated from other nematode larvae in soil or cultured from faeces (Table 9).

The filariform larvae are most numerous in the upper 2 cm of soil, or they may be supported singly or in tufts in the surface film of water on blades of grass. They wave their anterior ends in the air in a questing (nictating) manner. They thrive best in shady, moist open soils covered with vegetation; drying, flooding or direct sunlight are rapidly fatal (Plate 2). Their average life in the tropics is about 2–6 weeks but some larvae may survive under favourable conditions for up to 15 weeks. The optimal temperature range is 28–35°C. They are capable of ascending 60–90 cm of sandy loam but lateral movement is probably limited to about 30 cm (Udonsi and Atata, 1987).

On coming into contact with human skin, the larvae become active and penetrate, usually between the toes or fingers. The penetrating larvae respond to essential fatty acids; they release proteolytic enzymes and secrete eicosanoids, which are immunomodulative. They enter

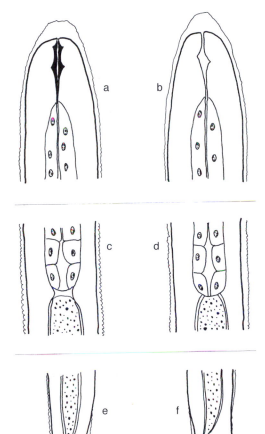

Differential features of
3rd-stage larvae of hookworms

Fig. 60. The third-stage infective larvae (L$_3$s) of *Necator* (left) and *Ancylostoma* (right). (a) and (b) Anterior ends; (c) and (d) junction of oesophagus and intestine; (e) and (f) tail ends.

venules and are carried by the venous circulation to the heart and then to the lungs. The larvae grow in the lungs, penetrate through into the alveoli and ascend the bronchi and trachea. They are then swallowed and reach the small intestine within about 7 days after infection, where they undergo a third moult; this is followed about the 13th day by a fourth moult, by which time they are sexually differentiated. Fertilized females begin egg-laying 4–7 weeks after infection and each produces 2000–11,000 (usually 3000–6000) eggs per 24 h. Each female contains only about 200 eggs at one time, so that the protein turnover involved in egg production is enormous.

The adults can live for 1–14 years but usually for about 4. However, in endemic areas, continuous reinfection and loss occur. This is demonstrated by the fact that in many areas infection rates are much higher after the rainy season (e.g. in western Tanzania there is a variation from 15 to 85%).

CLINICAL MANIFESTATIONS
There is an intense itching and burning at the site of entry. Pruritis may be followed by secondary infection, leading to the condition known as 'ground itch', with papulovesicular dermatitis, subsiding in about a fortnight (Fig. 61).

The larval migration through the lungs can cause a cough due to bronchitis or pneumonitis and patients may pass blood-stained sputum containing eosinophils, but pulmonary manifestations are less marked than with *Ascaris* larvae and these early signs are not usually reported among indigenous populations.

Enteritis, with Charcot–Leyden crystals in the faeces (resulting from breakdown of eosinophils) and a high eosinophilia characterize the early stages of intestinal infection but there is not usually any eosinophilia in the chronic phase.

A variety of gastrointestinal symptoms, such as abdominal pain, diarrhoea, nausea and loss of appetite, have sometimes been attributed to hookworm infection, but the most serious possible effect of an established

Table 8. Differential features of *Necator* and *Ancylostoma*.

	Necator	Ancylostoma
Adults		
Size	♂ 5–9 mm × 0.3 mm ♀ 9–11 mm × 0.35 mm	♂ 8–11 mm × 0.45 mm ♀ 10–13 mm × 0.6 mm
Shape	Head small, bent acutely in opposite direction to general curve	Bow-shaped curve; head in same line as body
Buccal capsule	Almost spherical	Elongated, pear-shaped
Mouth	Guarded by 2 semilunar cuticular cutting plates	Guarded by two pairs of curved teeth
Female		
Tail	No spine	Sharp spine (often lost)
Vulva	anterior to middle	posterior to middle
Male		
Bursa	Narrow, longer than wide	Outspread, wider than long
Dorsal ray	Deeply cleft. Tip of each cleft divided into two	Shallow cleft. Tip of each cleft divided into three
Spicules	Tips usually united and recurved	Tips not united
Eggs	Indistinguishable	
First- and second-stage larvae	Indistinguishable	
Third-stage infective larvae		
Size	Body length 590 µm Overall length 660 µm	Body length 550 µm Overall length 720 µm
Tail	Short and pointed (63 µm)	Long and blunt (85 µm)
Sheath	Marked striations, especially at posterior end	Faint cuticular striations
Head	Pointed	Blunt
Intestine	Apparent gap between intestine and oesophagus	No apparent gap between intestine and oesophagus
Oesophageal spears	Prominent. Anterior and shaped like thistle funnel	Not so prominent. Tips do not diverge

infection is the development of a hypochromic microcytic anaemia, present in about 36 million individuals worldwide. Hookworms are blood feeders and there is a daily loss of about 5 ml of blood in light infections to 100 ml in heavy infections (very roughly equivalent to 2 ml day^{-1} for every 1000 eggs g^{-1} faeces). There may be many symptoms accompanying anaemia, including lassitude, mental apathy, skin pallor, syncope and angina pectoris. In children, stunting of growth is characteristic of severe chronic infections (Fig. 65) and there is evidence that infection also lowers cognitive ability (Sakti *et al.*, 1999).

PATHOGENESIS

In light and moderate infections anaemia is due primarily to insufficient iron intake exacerbated by the presence of the worms but in heavy infections it occurs even when the dietary intake is adequate (Pawlowski *et al.*, 1991). This applies to areas such as western Nigeria, where hookworm anaemia only occurs when many worms are present (i.e. where there are 1000 worms with over 20,000 eggs g^{-1} faeces day^{-1}). On the other hand, in Mauritius, where the average iron intake is only about 5–10 mg day^{-1}, severe anaemia can result from the presence of 100 worms. The time factor must also be considered, as

Table 9. The differentiation of infective filariform larvae found in cultures from human faecal specimens.

	Strongyloides	*Trichostrongylus*	*Ancylostoma*	*Nectator*	*Ternidens*	*Oesophagostomum*
Length (μm) Sheath	500 Absent	750 Present	660 Sheath 720 μm, striations not clear	590 Sheath 660 μm, striations clear at tail end	680 (630–730) Present striated	720–950 Present and
Length of oesophagus as proportion of total body length	$\frac{1}{2}$	$\frac{1}{4}$	$\frac{1}{3}$	$\frac{1}{3}$	$\frac{1}{3}$	$\frac{1}{5}$
Intestine	Straight	Intestinal lumen zigzagged	Anterior end narrower in diameter than oesophageal bulb. No gap between the oesophagus and the intestine	Anterior end as wide as the oesophagus bulb. Gap between the oesophagus and the intestine	Following oesophagus is a pair of sphincter cells. Intestinal lumen somewhat zigzagged	Large triangular cells and lumen zigzagged
Tail	Divided into three at the tip	End of tail knoblike	Blunt	Sharply pointed	Pointed	Sharply pointed
Head Mouth			Blunt Mouth spears not very clear and parallel	Rounded Mouth spears clear and divergent		Rounded Buccal capsule + oesophagus make inverted Y shape

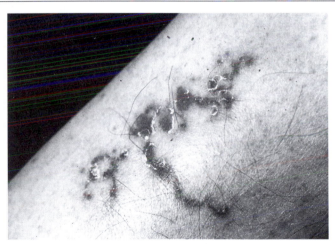

Fig. 61. 'Ground itch' at site of entry of larvae of *Necator* in a sensitized individual. With some non-human species of hookworms, the larvae continue to wander in the skin, causing creeping eruption (also see p. 160).

anaemia will not become apparent until the iron reserves have been completely depleted.

In many areas there is widespread infection but hookworm anaemia is uncommon. This is usually because of an adequate diet, as in Costa Rica or the southern USA but it may also be because other resistance factors limit the numbers of hookworms present, as in India.

Anaemia occurs because the adult worms pass a steady stream of blood through their intestines in order to obtain oxygen for respiration as well as food, with a consequent loss of erythrocytes and protein-containing fluid. The amount of blood passed by an adult *Necator* (0.03–0.05 ml per worm day^{-1}) is less than in an equivalent *Ancylostoma* infection (0.14–0.25 ml per worm day^{-1}) because of its smaller size. Reabsorption of haemoglobin from the intestine occurs, but the amount (about 11%) is less than often assumed in the past; in many areas an adequate diet accompanied by intravenous iron would be more effective in suppressing the clinical signs than anthelminthic treatment.

There is no proof that hookworms depress haemopoiesis but they do appear to decrease erythrocyte life. In addition to anaemia, a characteristic hookworm oedema occurs in heavy infections, resembling the nephrotic syndrome. This is caused by low plasma protein (particularly albumin) but usually only becomes apparent when there is a low iron intake. However, a heavy worm load of about 2000 adults can cause a loss of 4 g of albumin even with an adequate dietary supply of iron.

The extensive damage to the mucosa, including necrosis and haemorrhage, sometimes recorded in cases of hookworm infection is probably due to secondary causes, as is vitamin B$_{12}$ and folic acid deficiency. Similarly, there does not appear to be a direct relationship between hookworm infection and malabsorption (contrast *Strongyloides* (p. 119)).

As with the other geohelminths (Haswell-Elkins *et al.*, 1987a) and the schistosomes, a small minority of infected individuals have high worm burdens with serious disease and are responsible for most of the eggs reaching the environment (Anderson and Schad, 1985).

DIAGNOSIS

Clinical. Chronic anaemia and debility in patients living in an endemic area are suggestive, but may also be caused by malnutrition, malaria, amoebiasis and other helminthiases.

Parasitological. Recovery and recognition of eggs in faecal samples (Fig. 123) are the standard method of diagnosis. The eggs are identical to those of *Ancylostoma* and very similar to those of *Ternidens* and *Oesophagostomum*. Ova must be cultured to the infective larva stage if it is required to differentiate between the two hookworm species (Table 8 and Fig. 59). The Harada–Mori culture method is given on p. 262).

Serological. Not often employed. Complement fixation and indirect haemagglutination tests work well with antigen obtained from adult worms. ELISA and radioimmunological assay (RIA, measuring IgE) both have good specificity when ES antigens are used.

Recently a gene for *Ancylostoma* secreted polypeptide (ASP), a protein produced by infective larvae of *A. caninum*, has been cloned and the amino acid sequence determined. This is very similar to an insect venom that elicits a strong immune response and is being researched as a possible vaccine (Hotez and Prichard, 1995).

TREATMENT

A single course of chemotherapeutic treatment aimed at permanent cure in outpatients living in an endemic area is unlikely to be successful, but it is nevertheless important to reduce the number of worms present below the level causing clinical symptoms. This level will vary in different parts of the world, depending mainly on iron intake and nutritional status. Any drug given should also be supplemented by oral (or intravenous where supervision is not possible) iron therapy. In light infections a single annual treatment is sufficient, but in heavy infections 6- monthly treatment is necessary. The properties of the various drugs are given in Albonico *et al.* (1998).

Albendazole. A single dose of 400 mg for all ages above 2 (60–90% effective) is also active against most other intestinal nematode and cestode infections.

Mebendazole. A single dose of 500 mg for all ages above 2 or 100 mg twice daily for 3 days (20–90% effective) is also effective against other intestinal nematodes.

Levamisole. A single dose of 3 mg kg^{-1} body weight is more effective against *Ancylostoma* than against *Necator* (20–60%).

Pyrantel pamoate. A daily dose of 10 mg kg^{-1} body weight (max. 1 g) for 3 days. More effective against *Ancylostoma* than against *Necator* (20–90%) – chemical formula: (E)-1,4,5,6-tetrahydro-1-methyl-2-(2-(2-thienyl)vinyl]-pyrimidine.

Bitoscanate, bephenium and tetrachlorethylene can no longer be recommended, while ivermectin is not effective.

In a study of 3000 young children in Zanzibar, it was estimated that 1260 cases of moderate and 276 cases of severe anaemia were prevented by treatment with mebendazole, with improved motor development. In children in East Africa learning potential improves for months after treatment, with much higher school attendance (about 100 million children worldwide do not attend school because of soil-transmitted nematode infections).

EPIDEMIOLOGY

It has been estimated that there are from 1050 to 1277 million cases worldwide (about two-thirds due to *Necator*) with 90–130 million suffering morbidity and 65,000 deaths annually, principally from the anaemia. Hookworm infection is essentially a rural disease of poverty and is particularly common in cocoa, coffee and banana plantations, owing to the dense shade and high rainfall (Plate 13). Heavy infections are not found in areas with much less than 100 cm of rain per year and are rare in arid regions.

Recent estimates of infection rates in various regions are: 46% in Cameroon, 6% in peninsular Malaysia, 14–50% in southern Nigeria, 68% in Bobei County in China, 2.5% in Burma (Myanmar), 69% in Indonesia and 54% in Surinam.

Soil type is of great importance to the larvae, which migrate up against the water flow and down again when the top layer of soil is drying. Clay soils are less well aerated and, where there is heavy rainfall, the larvae are not able to survive so well as in sandy soils. This is in contrast to the situation with *Ascaris* and *Trichuris* eggs, which survive better on clay soils, as they dry out less in drought and have better adhesive properties. Larvae are also better able to migrate in well-filled soil that has a crumb structure than in highly compacted soil.

PREVENTION AND CONTROL

Personal prevention is provided by the wearing of shoes.

The control of hookworms has a long history, beginning with the campaign of the Rockefeller Sanitary Commission to eliminate the infection from the southern USA in 1909, followed by the international efforts of the Rockefeller Foundation in 1913. The strategies used then of mass chemotherapy and improvements in sanitation are still appropriate today. Such measures were also very effective in Japan in the 1950s–1980s (from 4.5% with hookworms and 60% with *Ascaris* in 1950 to 0 and 0.01% in 1987).

The newer single-dose, broad-spectrum, anthelminthics are a great advance for mass campaigns against morbidity caused by all the geohelminths, which are under way in many countries, funded by many international and national agencies and by non-governmental organizations (NGOs). For instance, a campaign for annual treatment of all schoolchildren (6–14 years old) in Ghana with albendazole has begun, primarily to reduce disease rather than interrupt transmission, which is not feasible at present. The World Health Organization (WHO) target is that by 2010 regular chemotherapy will be provided for at least 75% of schoolchildren in endemic countries at risk of morbidity (a global school health initiative against both geohelminths and schistosomes is being supported by many international agencies). However, the possibility of resistance to drugs needs to be carefully monitored, particularly because of the sale of substandard products in some countries (Crompton, 2000).

There are three possible strategies for chemotherapy campaigns against all the geohelminths.

1. Universal (= mass) campaigns, in which communities are treated irrespective of infection status, age, sex or social characteristics.
2. Targeted campaigns with group-level application, irrespective of infection status.
3. Selective campaigns with individual application, based on diagnosis of current infection or on level of infection.

The first is feasible if there are sufficient funds; otherwise, the second is most cost-effective, with treatment aimed at high-risk groups, such as school and preschool children and women of childbearing age, while the third is expensive, difficult to implement and likely to be unacceptable to the majority of infected individuals.

Wider utilization of cheap and effective sanitation technologies, such as the ventilated improved pit (VIP) latrine, first introduced in Zimbabwe, or the pour-flush toilet, which provides a water seal and does not require piped water, needs to be encouraged in addition to chemotherapy. Health education and the provision of latrines are also needed to prevent indiscriminate defecation in the fields.

Integrated campaigns, together with immunization or general school health efforts, can often make the most effective use of primary health-care workers.

There are large-scale control campaigns under way in Mexico, Seychelles, South Africa (Natal), Sri Lanka and Zanzibar (Albonico *et al.*, 1998).

ZOONOTIC ASPECTS
Virtually none, although *Necator* is found occasionally in chimpanzees and pigs. Young hamsters can be successfully infected in the laboratory, which is stimulating research into the physiology, pathology and particularly the immunology of

infection, although the fecundity of the parasites is suppressed.

Ancylostoma duodenale
(Dubini, 1843) Creplin, 1845

SYNONYMS
Agchylostoma duodenale Dubini, 1843; *Ankylostomum duodenale*; *Uncinaria duodenalis*.

DISEASE AND POPULAR NAMES
Ancylostomiasis or ancylostomosis, uncinariasis; Old World hookworm infection.

LOCAL NAMES
As for *Necator*.

GEOGRAPHICAL DISTRIBUTION
Ancylostoma extends into more temperate regions than *Necator*. It is present in the North African and European Mediterranean littoral; Asia (northern India, Myanmar, Cambodia, Laos, Vietnam, Malaysia, Indonesia, China, Taiwan, Japan); the South Pacific; and the Americas (particularly Chile, Mexico, Venezuela).

LOCATION IN HOST
As for *Necator*.

MORPHOLOGY
Ancylostoma is a larger and more robust worm than *Necator*. The head is curved dorsally in a smooth curve so that specimens do not have the hook-like appearance characteristic of *Necator*. The large buccal capsule has bilaterally symmetrical curved cutting processes, consisting of two fused teeth, and there is a pair of internal teeth at the bottom of the capsule, with histolytic glands at the base. These aid the attachment of the worm to the mucosa and also assist in cutting off portions for food (Figs. 62 and 63). The features differentiating *Ancylostoma* from *Necator* are shown in Table 8.

The male measures 8–11 mm × 0.4–0.5 mm; the shape and structure of the caudal bursa differs from that of *Necator* (Fig. 58).

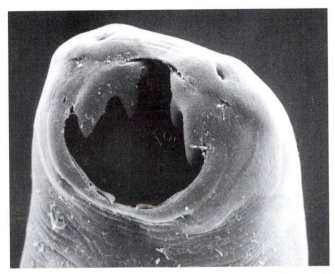

Fig. 62. Stereoscan of anterior end of *A. duodenale* showing two pairs of cutting teeth in mouth capsule.

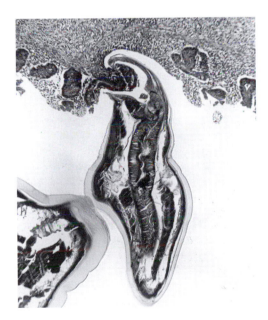

Fig. 63. Section of jejunum with anterior portion of *Ancylostoma* biting off a piece of mucosa.

The female differs principally in having the vulval opening posterior to the middle of the body (Fig. 64).

LIFE CYCLE

The larger females of *Ancylostoma* lay about twice as many eggs (20,000–30,000 per female per 24 h) than those of *Necator*. The eggs of the two genera in faeces are identical and develop in a similar manner in the soil.

In contrast to *Necator*, oral infection with infective third-stage, filariform, larvae, presumably principally on salad vegetables, is thought to be more important than skin penetration. Following oral infection, the larvae travel directly to the intestine without visiting the lungs. They enter the mucosa of the duodenum for 2–3 days before emerging and undergoing the third moult. Adults mature in 4–7 weeks and usually live for about 1 year.

CLINICAL MANIFESTATIONS

If infection is by skin penetration, there can be an itching and burning at the site of entry, followed by a pruritic response. Pulmonary reactions are more pronounced than with *Necator*. In Japan, 'Wakana disease', caused by the migrating larvae, was characterized by dyspnoea, cough, nausea, vomiting and high sputum and blood eosinophilia (up to 90%).

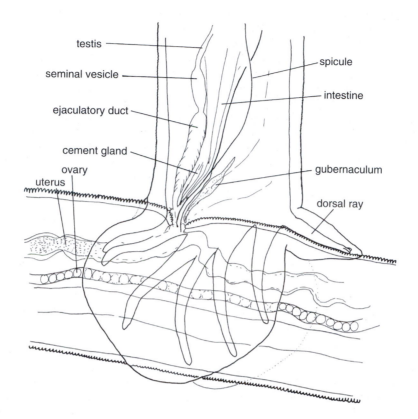

Fig. 64. Vulval region of female of *A. duodenale* and caudal bursa of male showing process of fertilization.

Weakness, anorexia and pica (dirt-eating) are sometimes found in heavy chronic infections.

PATHOGENESIS

This is similar to infection with *Necator* but, because an adult *Ancylostoma* is larger, the anaemia caused by an equivalent number of worms is more severe.

DIAGNOSIS AND TREATMENT

As for *Necator*.

EPIDEMIOLOGY

As for *Necator*. In many areas both types of hookworm are present, possibly in the same patient.

Infection rates recorded recently for various areas where specific identification has been made are: north-eastern Australia in Aboriginals 31–77%, Benin 25–35%, China (Fujien Province) 50%, (Sichuan Province equally with both species) 74%, Egypt 6–8%, Ethiopia 67%, Kenya (preschool children in Kilifi) 29%, southern Nepal 11–79%, Paraguay (school children) 59% with both species.

The ova can develop at a lower temperature (a minimum of 14°C) than those of *Necator*, so that infection is more common in subtropical and temperate climates. The optimum temperature for hatching of eggs is 20–27°C and they fail to develop above 40°C. Infection was formerly common in tin miners in England and in workers building the St Gotthard tunnel between Switzerland and Italy.

PREVENTION AND CONTROL

As for *Necator* except that the thorough washing of salad vegetables is more important than the wearing of adequate footwear.

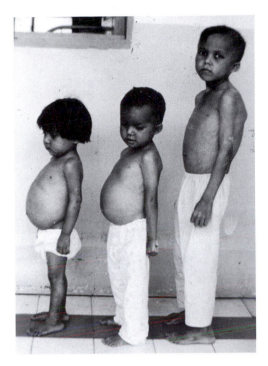

Fig. 65. Severe stunting of growth in children with very heavy hookworm infections. The eldest child is aged 15 with a haemoglobin level of 1.8 g dl^{-1}. Height of windowsill equals 85 cm.

ZOONOTIC ASPECTS
None.

Ancylostoma ceylanicum Looss, 1911, is a parasite of dogs in Asia and South America but also occurs as a human parasite in India and the Philippines. Infection is by the oral route, with a prepatent period of about 25 days. Infections are light and blood loss does not appear to have any clinical significance; the larvae do not cause creeping eruption. Diagnosis is by culturing the larvae to the third stage. Chemotherapy is effective.

Recently, 200 cases of infection with the dog hookworm, ***Ancylostoma caninum***, have been diagnosed in Queensland, Australia, with another 200 probable cases. All were Caucasians and presented with severe abdominal pain, sometimes also with diarrhoea and weight loss, followed by blood eosinophilia (Croese *et al.*, 1994; Prociv and Croese,

1996). In this area this is the leading cause of eosinophilic enteritis and patients may have aphthous ulcers of the terminal ileum, caecum and colon. In 15 cases, adults were seen *in situ* and in nine the typical buccal capsule with three teeth could be recognized in biopsy tissue sections. The adults produced no eggs but were diagnosed by biopsy or by an IgG ELISA. Recently, a Western blot using ES antigens from adult worms to identify IgG4 antibodies to a protein of 68 kDa (Ac68) was found to be more specific and sensitive than the ELISA. However, human species are likely to cross-react and the specific IgE ELISA for *Necator* may be necessary in order to differentiate.

All patients had dogs and walked around the garden in bare feet and it is assumed that infection was contracted from front lawns, which were watered with sprinklers and thus washed dog faeces into the lawn. There were fewer cases in the winter months. The patients were in an affluent area with good hospital facilities for the difficult diagnosis and it is likely that infection with this species also occurs in other parts of the world. One case has been reported from New Orleans, USA, in an 11-year-old girl who had chronic abdominal pain, vomiting, anorexia and weight loss, which resolved after two doses of mebendazole.

Various hookworms of animals very occasionally parasitize humans: *A. japonica* Fukuda and Katsurada 1925, possibly in Japan; *A. malayanum* (Allesandrini, 1905), a natural parasite of bears; *Cyclodontostomum purvisi* Adams, 1933, in Thailand and naturally in the rat; *Necator argentinus* Parodi, 1920 (doubtful); *N. suillus* Ackert and Payne, 1922, once or twice in humans and widespread in pigs. Species causing cutaneous larva migrans (creeping eruption) are considered on p. 160.

Other Strongyles

As well as the hookworms, there are various other bursate intestinal nematodes that can sometimes be recovered from humans. Almost all are principally zoonotic infections, but a few, such as *Trichostrongylus, Ternidens* and *Oesophagostomum*, do have human-to-human transmission in some areas.

Family Trichostrongylidae

Trichostrongylus spp.
Looss, 1905

POPULAR NAME
Wireworms (when in domestic stock).

DISTRIBUTION
Species of *Trichostrongylus* occur locally in humans in Iran (67% in Isfahan), Iraq (up to 10%), Israel, Egypt (11–60%), Ethiopia (23%), Armenia, Japan, Korea (80% in one area), Indonesia and the Cape Verde Islands. Sporadic cases may occur in many areas where people and cattle are in close proximity (e.g. Africa, Australia, India and South America).

LOCATION IN HOST
The adults attach to the wall of the duodenum and jejunum by the anterior end.

MORPHOLOGY
These are small thin strongyle worms (family Trichostrongylidae) measuring 5–10 mm in length; most species are normally parasitic in ruminants. They have no buccal capsule and live with the head embedded in the mucosa of the small intestine. The males have a well-developed copulatory bursa, and the structure of the spicules provides the most useful feature used to differentiate the 11 species (*T. affinis, axei, brevis, calcaratus, capricola, colubriformis, lerouxi, orientalis, probolurus, skrjabini* and *vitrinus*) recovered from humans; in all they are short, equal, stout and spoon-shaped but have small specific differences.

Eggs found in the faeces are similar to those of hookworms but are longer and narrower (75–100 µm × 30–50 µm) with more pointed ends, and they usually contain a segmented ovum at the morula stage when passed in the faeces.

LIFE CYCLE
Eggs passed in the faeces at the morula stage hatch in the soil in about 24 h. The larvae reach the infective third stage in about 3 days. These occasionally penetrate the skin, but in human infections they are almost always ingested. When this happens, the larvae develop into adults in 25 days; in contrast to hookworms, they never undergo a lung migration.

CLINICAL MANIFESTATIONS AND PATHOGENESIS
Infection is usually light and causes no clinical symptoms. In heavier infections (a few hundred worms) there may be abdominal pain, diarrhoea and a slight anaemia, accompanied by a mild eosinophilia (under 10%).

The head of the adult worm produces traumatic damage to the mucosa, with inflammation at the site of attachment. The worms may also suck blood but the amount is not sufficient to cause anaemia.

DIAGNOSIS
This is by recognition of eggs in the faeces (Fig. 124), which gives identification to the generic level.

The larvae can also be cultured, using the techniques for hookworms (p. 262). The infective third-stage larvae must be differentiated from those of hookworms and *Strongyloides* (Table 9). The species of trichostrongyle involved can only be determined if adults are obtained after chemotherapy, and veterinary textbooks should be consulted.

TREATMENT
All the drugs used for hookworms work well against trichostrongyles, which are usually easier to eliminate. Mebendazole has been used successfully at 100 mg twice daily for 3 days for adults.

EPIDEMIOLOGY, PREVENTION AND CONTROL
Larvae are usually ingested on contaminated vegetables and these should be

thoroughly washed or cooked. The eggs and infective larvae are both very resistant to desiccation, which makes control difficult. In areas of Iran and Iraq cattle are kept in the backyards of houses (Plate 14) and a particularly heavy build-up of larvae occurs after the rainy season.

It was reported in 1953 that there were 48 million human cases worldwide; it is not known if prevalence is now much lower.

ZOONOTIC ASPECTS
In many areas infection is contracted from livestock, although with *T. orientalis* from sheep and camels, which is the most common species in humans in China, Japan, Iran, Iraq, Korea and Taiwan, there is probably a human cycle involved.

Other trichostrongylids that are common parasites of domestic stock in many areas of the world, such as *Haemonchus contortus*, *Marshallagia marshalli*, *Mecistocirrus digitatus*, *Nematodirus abnormalis*, *Ostertagia circumcincta* and *O. ostertagi*, may occasionally occur in humans, particularly in Iran and Azerbaidjan. For further details of these parasites, textbooks of veterinary medicine should be consulted (see General References, p. 282).

Family Chabertiidae

Ternidens deminutus
Railliet and Henry, 1909

SYNONYMS
Triodontophorus deminutus Railliet and Henry, 1905.

DISEASE AND POPULAR NAME
Ternidens infection (ternidensiasis or ternidensosis), false hookworm infection.

GEOGRAPHICAL DISTRIBUTION
Comoros Islands, Congo Republic, Mauritius, southern Tanzania and Zimbabwe (up to 87% in one area).

LOCATION IN HOST
Adults occur in the colon and occasionally the ileum, with the anterior end attached.

MORPHOLOGY
The adults superficially resemble hookworms but are rather larger. The subglobose buccal capsule of *Ternidens* is directed anteriorly and has forked teeth in its depths. The mouth is surrounded by a double 'leaf crown' or corona radiata of cuticular bristles.

Females measure 12–16 mm × 0.65–0.75 mm. The vulva opens just in front of the anus. Males measure 9.5 mm × 0.55 mm and have a caudal bursa with the rays arranged in a characteristic pattern. The spicules are long and equal, measuring about 0.9 mm in length.

LIFE CYCLE
Eggs measure 81 (70–94) µm × 52 (47–55) µm. They pass out in the faeces, usually in the 8-celled stage, and develop into rhabditiform larvae in about 30 h. The larvae feed on bacteria and moult twice (once on the 6th day and again in 8–10 days at 29°C). The third-stage larva retains the cast cuticle as a sheath, but it is not known how transmission to humans occurs. All attempted experimental infections either by mouth or by skin penetration have failed. It is possible that an invertebrate intermediate host, such as the termite, is required (Goldsmid, 1991).

CLINICAL MANIFESTATIONS
The great majority of cases have a light worm load and appear to be symptomless, although little is known of the effects of the parasites and they could be involved in the formation of intestinal nodules.

PATHOGENESIS
The parasites feed on blood and probably cause ulceration of the mucosa. While the loss of blood from the large bowel could be more serious than that caused by hookworms in the jejunum, as no reabsorption occurs, anaemia has not been reported. This might be because usually only a few worms are present.

In experimental studies in rhesus monkeys, adults eventually become encapsulated in nodules, but it is not known if a similar effect occurs in humans.

DIAGNOSIS AND TREATMENT

Diagnosis is by recognition of the eggs in faeces (Fig. 124); concentration methods can be used if necessary. The eggs must be differentiated from those of hookworms, which can be done with difficulty by the larger size and particularly by the larger volume occupied by the dividing ovum. For more positive identification the larvae can be cultivated to the infective third stage (p. 262 and Table 9). These have characteristic paired sphincter cells at the junction of the oesophagus and intestine. *Ternidens* is still frequently misdiagnosed as hookworm.

Chemotherapy is the same as for hookworm; albendazole at 400 mg was successful in a trial in children (Bradley, 1990).

EPIDEMIOLOGY AND ZOONOTIC ASPECTS

Ternidens is a very common parasite of monkeys in tropical areas of Africa and Asia (China, Indonesia, Malaysia, southern India and Vietnam) and these probably act as reservoir hosts. It is not known why human infection is restricted to areas of Africa, where it may be very common, but this is presumably related to its (unknown) mode of transmission. One case has been diagnosed from Surinam.

Oesophagostomum bifurcum
(Creplin, 1849)

DISEASE AND POPULAR NAME

Oesophagostomiasis or oesophagostomosis; nodular worm (for species in veterinary practice).

GEOGRAPHICAL DISTRIBUTION

Oesophagostomum bifurcum is a strongylid nematode (family Chabertiidae) and has been reported many times from humans in West Africa and also from East Africa and Asia. It is a common parasite of monkeys, while some other species may be found in ruminants and pigs. *O. aculeatum* (Linstow, 1879) has been reported once each from a human in Brunei and Indonesia (Ross *et al.*, 1989), *Oesophagostomum* sp. from the peritoneal cavity of a patient in Malaysia and *O. stephanostomum* Railliet and Henry, 1909, very rarely from Côte d'Ivoire, with a case from Brazil and probably another from Surinam.

LOCATION IN HOST

Adults in nodules in the wall of the colon and caecum.

MORPHOLOGY

Species of *Oesophagostomum* resemble hookworms in shape and size but have a buccal capsule that opens forwards, with a cuticular 'leaf crown' surrounding the mouth opening, and a cylindrical rather than globose buccal capsule. The caudal bursa of the male is symmetrical and the long spicules are equal. Each female has been estimated to produce about 5000 eggs 24 h^{-1}.

LIFE CYCLE

The eggs closely resemble those of hookworms, measuring 58–69 μm × 39–47 μm. Larvae hatch in 2 days at 30°C and develop in the soil into third-stage infective larvae in 5–7 days. These are ingested, invade the wall of the colon and caecum and become encapsulated. A nodule forms, measuring about 1.5 cm in diameter, with a fibrous tissue wall and having a living worm in the centre of an unruptured abscess (Fig. 66). When the worms mature, they break out of the nodule in about 6–7 days and sometimes become attached to the caecal wall. Shrunken third-stage larvae inside the sheath can survive for a considerable period in the environment under desiccated conditions.

CLINICAL MANIFESTATIONS AND PATHOGENESIS

Some worms apparently mate in the lumen of the colon and cause no symptoms. However, others may stay in small nodules in the intestinal wall or penetrate through into the abdominal cavity, where they can cause significant pathology. There can be

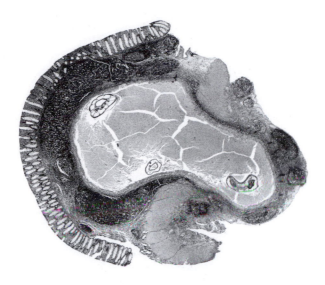

Fig. 66. Nodular lesion caused by *O. bifurcum* presenting as a para-umbilical mass in an 8-year-old girl in Nigeria. At laparotomy the mass was found adhering to muscles and fascia of the anterior abdominal wall of the ascending colon (magnification × 11). Sections of the nematodes can be seen.

dozens of nodules, each 2–3 cm in diameter. The wall of the colon becomes grossly thickened, although the mucosa and serosa remain intact. There is no definite cyst wall but there is a layer of macrophages, epithelial cells and fibroblasts, and often many plasma cells and eosinophils. Nodules contain thick pus or caseous material. In the majority of cases the infection is self-limiting and eventually resolves without treatment.

In northern Ghana and Togo and probably southern Burkina Faso, infected individuals often have an epigastric or periumbilical swelling recognized by local people and known as a 'tumeur de Dapaong' (Plate 15). These may be accompanied by considerable pain, and abdominal occlusion or the presence of the abscesses may require surgical intervention. Many cases are in children, most about 10 years old. The wall of the colon is often oedematous and the whole of the bowel loop becomes hardened and surrounded by adhesions. There may also be involvement of the liver, and worms in the abdominal cavity can cause peritonitis

(Polderman *et al.*, 1991, 1999; Polderman and Blotkamp, 1995). Nodules sometimes calcify and then show up on X-ray. In a case of infection in Brunei, probably caused by *O. aculeatum*, a single worm was removed from a painless lump on the back measuring 3 cm and containing thick brown pus. Infection may have been contracted by direct penetration (Ross *et al.*, 1989).

DIAGNOSIS
Clinical diagnosis is often difficult and oesophagostomiasis has often been mistaken for other conditions, such as carcinoma, appendicitis or amoebiasis; laparotomy will provide a positive diagnosis and ultrasound can be useful.

In order to differentiate the eggs in faeces from those of hookworms, the larvae have to be cultivated to the third stage (Table 9). An activated charcoal/faeces filter-paper technique for 5–7 days works well (p. 123). The larvae measure 720–950 μm and have a cuticle with prominent striations, 28–32 (or sometimes 20) large, characteristic triangular-shaped intestinal cells and a buccal capsule that differs from that of hookworm larvae (Blotkamp *et al.*, 1993; Pit *et al.*, 1999).

An ELISA based on detection of specific IgG4 in sera had a specificity of over 95% in one study and may prove useful in differentiating *Oesophagostomum* from hookworm in epidemiological studies (Polderman *et al.*, 1993).

TREATMENT

Surgery to resect the infected portion of the colon is sometimes necessary.

Albendazole (400 mg or better 10 mg kg^{-1} body weight daily for 5 days) and pyrantel pamoate (two doses of 10 mg kg^{-1}) are both effective but thiabendazole and levamisole are not.

EPIDEMIOLOGY AND CONTROL

It is likely that infection with *O. bifurcum* in northern Ghana and Togo and maybe Uganda now involves human-to-human transmission and monkey reservoirs are no longer necessary. In the focus identified in West Africa it is estimated that there are about a quarter of a million cases and in some villages in rural areas there are infection rates of 30–60%, although infections are rarely found in young children (Polderman *et al.*, 1991, 1999; Polderman and Blotkamp, 1995). Transmission is limited to the rainy season, but it is not clear exactly how humans become infected. Another species, *O. apiostomum* (Willach, 1891) Railliet and Henry, 1905, a parasite of monkeys in West Africa, has been reported from the colon of a patient in Togo, but specific identification of human cases is difficult unless adults are expelled.

Infections are easier to treat than hookworm infections and should be much reduced by any hookworm control campaign.

Family Syngamidae

Mammomonogamus laryngeus
(Railliet, 1899) Ryzhikov, 1948

SYNONYMS

Syngamus laryngeus Railliet, 1899. *Syngamus kingi* Leiper, 1913. The genus name *Syngamus* is now used only for the species in birds, such as *S. trachea* causing 'gapeworm' in poultry, although *S. laryngeus* may still be found in some textbooks.

DISEASE NAME

Mammomonogamiasis or mammomonogamosis.

GEOGRAPHICAL DISTRIBUTION

There have been over 90 reported cases from humans, the majority in South America (25 from Brazil), with a few cases in North America, the West Indies and China and single cases from Australia, Korea, the Philippines and Malaysia (or possibly Thailand).

LOCATION OF ADULTS

Adults inhabit the air passages of the upper respiratory tract, particularly the larynx or pharynx.

MORPHOLOGY AND LIFE CYCLE

The male worm (4 mm × 0.35 mm) is much smaller than the female (20 mm × 0.5 mm) and the two are joined in permanent copulation, giving a characteristic Y shape (family Syngamidae). The buccal capsule of both sexes is well developed and globular. It is used to attach the worms to the air passages, where they suck blood. The copulatory bursa and supporting rays of the male have characteristic structures that are of specific importance.

The eggs measure 85–90 µm × 50 µm and have a sculptured appearance. Infective third-stage larvae develop from eggs in 9–15 days at 26–30°C and are probably ingested on salad vegetables. Larvae are believed to reach the trachea via the bloodstream and lungs.

CLINICAL MANIFESTATIONS AND PATHOGENESIS

There is an incubation period of 25–40 days. Worms are found in the trachea, larynx and sometimes the smaller bronchi and produce headache, nausea, irritation and a severe dry cough. There may also be blood in the sputum (haemoptysis). An eosinophilia of 23% has been reported.

DIAGNOSIS AND TREATMENT

Adults can usually be seen in the larynx and pharynx and eggs may be found in the sputum. Adults are sometimes expelled after coughing and a recent Thai patient who had worked in Malaysia coughed up 96 worms.

Benzimidazoles, such as albendazole or mebendazole would probably be effective. Treatment with thiabendazole was effective in one case.

ZOONOTIC ASPECTS

This is entirely a zoonotic infection. Natural hosts are cattle, water-buffaloes, goats and, in Thailand, wild felids. A single human case of infection with *M. nasicola* (Buckley, 1934), a similar species found in a wide range of herbivores, has been reported.

Family Angiostrongylidae

Parastrongylus cantonensis
(Chen, 1935) Chabaud, 1972

SYNONYMS

Pulmonema cantonensis Chen, 1935; *Angiostrongylus cantonensis* Dougherty, 1946.

DISEASE

Parastrongyliasis or parastrongylosis, angiostrongyliasis. A cause of eosinophilic meningitis.

GEOGRAPHICAL DISTRIBUTION

This is entirely a zoonosis, occasional cases occurring in Indonesia, Laos, Malaysia, many Pacific islands, the Philippines, Taiwan, Thailand and Vietnam. In recent years it has also been reported from humans in Australia, China, Côte d'Ivoire, Cuba, Dominican Republic, India, Japan, Mauritius, Puerto Rico, Reunion and the USA and the infection appears to be spreading.

LOCATION IN HOST

P. cantonensis does not usually develop to maturity in humans, the third-stage larvae migrating to the brain, CNS or eyes.

MORPHOLOGY

The third-stage larva measures 0.46–0.5 mm × 26 µm when ingested. It has small lateral alae and characteristic chitinous rods in the buccal cavity.

The adult worms are normally found in the main branches of the pulmonary artery of rats, but not in humans. They are slender strongyloid nematodes (superfamily Metastrongyloidea; many species in livestock are known as lungworms), with a small buccal capsule containing two lateral triangular teeth. Females measure 22–34 mm × 0.34–0.56 mm. The vulva opens near the anus and the red, blood-filled gut and white uterus give a characteristic 'barber's pole' effect. The male measures 20–25 mm × 0.32–0.42 mm and has a well-developed caudal bursa, with subequal spicules (1.02–1.25 mm long).

LIFE CYCLE

In rats, the eggs hatch in the lungs and first-stage larvae are passed out in the faeces; they can survive up to 2 weeks in water. For further development the larvae need to be ingested by or to penetrate into snails or slugs. They moult twice in the muscles and the infective larvae remain coiled up in the mantle. They are infective in 2–3 weeks at 26°C. When an infected mollusc is eaten by another rat, the larvae penetrate the intestinal wall and are carried by the circulatory system via liver, heart and lungs to the main arterial circulation. They then reach the CNS and congregate in the spinal cord, medulla, cerebellum and diencephalon. After moulting, the fourth-stage larvae migrate into the subarachnoid space and 26–33 days after infection they reach the pulmonary arteries. Here they become sexually mature in another 7 days.

In humans the third-stage larvae ingested in snails or slugs can migrate via the liver, heart and lungs to reach the CNS.

CLINICAL MANIFESTATIONS

There is an incubation period of 12–36 days before symptoms of severe headache, back and neck stiffness, extreme tiredness, photophobia, nausea, vomiting and vertigo occur. There is a generalized hyperaesthesia of the skin, with signs of paralysis of one or more nerves and eye muscles and facial paraesthesia (burning, tingling, etc.). The symptoms usually last for about 2 weeks but may be prolonged.

Mortality due to the disease is generally low (although in Thailand a mortality rate of 1.2% has been reported) and most cases are self-limiting, with recovery occurring in about 4 weeks.

PATHOGENESIS

There are two distinct forms of the disease; more typical is the cerebral form, with a meningitic syndrome, but there is also a much rarer ocular form, with acute inflammation of the eye but no signs of meningitis (Wariyapola *et al.*, 1998).

Most of the knowledge of the pathology of the disease has been obtained from experimental infections in animals. However, in autopsy cases, worms have been found in the brain, with inflammation spreading along the perivascular spaces into the brain substance. The inflammatory reaction in the brain and meninges is localized, particularly in the vicinity of the parasites under the arachnoid (Fig. 67). Eosinophils, Charcot–Leyden crystals and giant cells are apparent histologically. Dead larvae are found inside

granulomatous lesions with necrotic debris in the cerebellum, pons and medulla, death in these cases probably being due to impairment of the bulbar functions.

Eosinophilia is common in this infection and there is a raised cell count in the cerebrospinal fluid (in one fatal case there were 880 cells mm^{-3}, of which 92% were eosinophils). In experimental animals an inflammatory reaction develops after a few weeks, with leucocytic infiltration and a preponderance of eosinophils in the meninges and the parenchyma of the CNS. The severity of the disease is related to the number of third-stage larvae that reach the CNS, most of the pathology being caused by the dead worms.

DIAGNOSIS

Clinical diagnosis is usually possible, particularly if there is evidence of raw snails having been eaten. Particularly important is the eosinophilic pleocytosis of the cerebrospinal fluid (at least 25% eosinophils) with Charcot–Leyden crystals; foreign-body giant cells and sometimes larval worms can also be seen in a lumbar puncture (about 10% of patients).

The meningitis must be differentiated from that caused by a cerebral tumour or

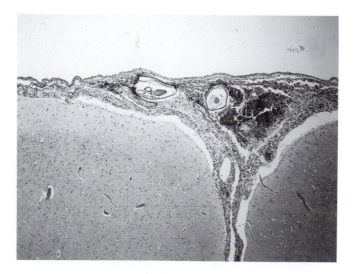

Fig. 67. Larvae of *P. cantonensis* migrating through the meninges of the central nervous system, exciting meningeal infiltration, eosinophilic pleocytosis in the cerebrospinal fluid and sometimes subarachnoidal haemorrhage (magnification × 50).

haemorrhage or from the presence of other helminths, such as *T. solium* cysticerci and *Gnathostoma*, or possibly *Paragonimus*, *Schistosoma* eggs, *Echinococcus*, *Trichinella* and *Toxocara*. Isolated instances of eosinophilic meningitis have been reported from parts of the world where *P. cantonensis* is not known to occur and may be due to other helminths, although this is clearly a helminth that is being carried to new parts of the world inside the rat hosts (Cross, 1987; Kliks and Palumbo, 1992).

Recently there has been a good deal of work on serodiagnostic tests. Two monoclonal antibodies (AcJ1 and AcJ20) are able to recognize the epitope on an antigen with a molecular mass of 204 kDa. A double-antibody sandwich ELISA showed good specificity with sera, but not with CNS fluid (Chye *et al.*, 1997), and an immunoblot technique is promising.

Larvae have been recovered from the eye on three occasions (a recent case in Sri Lanka may have been of a new species).

TREATMENT
It is not certain that chemotherapy is advisable, as live worms cause far less tissue reaction than dead ones and the infection is usually self-limiting.

EPIDEMIOLOGY
Human infection usually occurs from eating the giant African land snail (*Achatina fulica*), which is popular among people of Chinese descent and has been introduced by them to Hawaii and other Pacific islands. Another snail, *Pila*, is similarly eaten in Thailand, as are freshwater prawns in Tahiti. In addition, small slugs (e.g. *Veronicella*), snails and planarians may be ingested inadvertently in salads. It is possible that larvae escape from the invertebrates in faeces or slime and are ingested on vegetables or fruit. At least six species of terrestrial snails, nine species of aquatic snails and five species of slugs, freshwater prawns, frogs and toads have been found naturally infected, and many other invertebrates and probably fish can serve as paratenic hosts. In some Asian countries some of these hosts are ingested for medicinal purposes.

The natural hosts are many species of rodents, for human infections principally *Rattus norvegicus* and *R. rattus* (now commonly infected in ports such as Alexandria, New Orleans and Port Harcourt, Nigeria, although human infection has not yet been proved). The bandicoot rat is another natural host.

Parastrongylus mackerrasae possibly causes eosinophilic meningitis in Australia and *P. malaysiensis* in South-East Asia (Prociv *et al.*, 2000). Another species, *P. vasorum*, which occurs in dogs and foxes in Europe and South America, does not have a neurotropic cycle.

Parastrongylus costaricensis
(Morera and Céspedes, 1971) Ubelaker, 1986

SYNONYM AND DISEASE
Angiostrongylus costaricensis Morera and Céspedes, 1971; *Morerastrongylus costaricensis* Chabaud, 1972. Abdominal parastrongyliasis or parastrongylosis (or abdominal angiostrongyliasis).

GEOGRAPHICAL DISTRIBUTION
This parasite was discovered by Morera and Céspedes in the mesenteric arteries of patients in Costa Rica in 1971. In the following 30 years it has been found in humans in Argentina, Brazil, Colombia, Costa Rica, Dominican Republic, Ecuador, El Salvador, Guadeloupe, Guatemala, Honduras, Japan, Martinique, Nicaragua, Panama, Peru, the USA and Venezuela, with a possible case in Congo Republic (Zaire).

LOCATION IN HOST
Adult worms that lay eggs but do not produce larvae are found in the ileocaecal branches of the anterior mesenteric artery or occasionally in the liver or testicles. Full development occurs in the natural host, the cotton rat, *Sigmodon hispidus*.

MORPHOLOGY
Adult males measure 17.4–22.2 mm × 0.28–0.31 mm. The caudal bursa is well

developed and symmetrical with six papillae and equal spicules. Females measure 28.2–42.0 mm $\times$ 0.32–0.35 mm, with the vulval opening about 0.26 mm from the tip of the tail. Both sexes lack a buccal capsule.

LIFE CYCLE

Twelve species of rodents can act as final hosts, as well as marmosets, dogs and the coatimundi. First-stage larvae (L_1s) in the faeces of these hosts enter slugs as intermediate hosts, where they develop into the infective third stage (L_3) and are often excreted into the mucus left on vegetation. In Central America the veronicellid slug, *Vaginulus plebeius,* which is common up to an altitude of 2000 m, is commonly infected (50% overall in Costa Rica) sometimes with large numbers of larvae (Morera, 1994). When these slugs are ingested by cotton rats or other natural hosts, the L_3s penetrate the intestinal wall within 4 h and migrate to the lymphatics of the intestinal wall and mesentery. Following a further two moults, the young adults (females measuring 28–44 mm and males 20 mm in length) migrate to the mesenteric arteries after 10 days. They mature and release eggs by 18 days. The eggs are deposited in the intestinal wall, where they hatch, and the L_1s are excreted in the faeces by 24 days postinfection. Humans become infected by ingesting infected slugs, either intentionally, in the case of young children, or accidentally, on salad vegetables. The L_1s in mucus can also be ingested from food or from the hands of children after playing with slugs.

CLINICAL MANIFESTATIONS AND PATHOGENESIS

Infection is found predominantly in children, but all ages can be susceptible. If worms are present in the tissues of the caecal region, there is usually pain in the right flank and iliac fossa. There may be fever, often accompanied by anorexia and vomiting and constipation or diarrhoea in children. In many patients a tumour-like mass can be palpated in the lower right quadrant (although this procedure may be painful), and this may be mistaken for a malignant tumour. There is usually some degree of leucocytosis, with 20–50% eosinophilia. In children, symptoms may mimic appendicitis, Crohn's disease or Meckel's diverticulum. Some cases have bright red blood in the faeces.

The adult worms and eggs in the arteries provoke damage to the endothelium, causing thrombosis and necrosis of tissues, and the eggs cause inflammatory reactions in the small vessels. The whole wall of the intestine can become thickened and hardened, with yellowish granulatomous areas of inflammation (Fig. 68). In lighter infections only the appendix is damaged but in heavy infections the terminal ileum, caecum and ascending colon may have to be excised.

If the liver is infected, there is likely to be pain in the upper right quadrant, with some degree of hepatomegaly. Palpation is painful and there are enzyme abnormalities and a high eosinophilia; the syndrome resembles visceral larva migrans (p. 157). The presence of adult worms in the spermatic cords of males can result in acute pain from obstruction by adult worms, leading to haemorrhagic necrosis of the testicular parenchyma.

Even without treatment, recovery usually takes place in a few weeks to many months.

DIAGNOSIS

Symptoms in children of an appendicitis-like illness with a high eosinophilia are suggestive. Clinical diagnosis can be greatly aided by X-ray. Contrast medium shows filling defects in the terminal ileum, caecum and ascending colon, with irritability and thickening of the wall. There is also a sudden contraction of the caecum observed by fluoroscopy after a barium enema, typical of chronic granulomatous inflammatory reactions and found also in tuberculosis and amoebic abscesses. Newer imaging techniques would probably be even more useful. Parasitological diagnosis is only possible following biopsy or resective surgery since L_1s are not produced in the faeces.

Serological diagnosis is thus very important. There is a latex agglutination test and an ELISA, both of which are sensitive and specific, and immunoelectrophoresis or Ouchterlony immunodiffusion can also be employed.

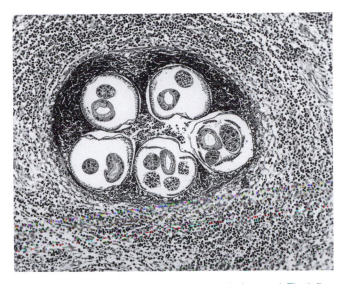

Fig. 68. Cross-sections of five adult *P. costaricensis* in a mesenteric vessel. The inflammatory exudate and eosinophils surrounding them are undergoing necrosis (perhaps following the death of the worms), suggesting both immediate and delayed hypersensitivity responses.

TREATMENT

Surgery is the most common form of treatment, but with more experience many cases have been found to resolve in time without it, and conservative palliative treatment can be employed unless there is an acute flare-up.

Chemotherapy with thiabendazole, albendazole and diethylcarbamazine has been tried and may have some effect but there is evidence from experimental infections in rats that it causes the parasites to wander erratically and cause further lesions.

EPIDEMIOLOGY

This infection is widespread in rodents in the Americas and the numbers of human cases is rising in many countries, probably because it is being increasingly recognized as a public health problem rather than a rare and curious infection. Most cases have been reported from Costa Rica, more than 650 in 1993 in a population of 3 million (Morera, 1994). Almost all of these are in children, and boys are twice as likely to be infected as girls; both are more likely to be infected in the wet season. In Costa Rica, 43% of cotton rats were found to be infected.

Metastrongylus elongatus Railliet and Henry, 1911 (Family Metastrongylidae), a parasite of pigs with earthworms as intermediate hosts, has been recovered once from the human respiratory tract.

Order Ascaridida

Family Ascarididae

Ascaris lumbricoides
Linnaeus, 1758

DISEASE AND POPULAR NAMES

Ascariasis or ascariosis; roundworm infection. One of the geohelminth infections.

LOCAL NAMES

Dedan (Arabic), Cacing (Bahasa Malay), Than kaung (Burmese), San'chik (Cantonese), Nsunsuma (Fanti), Agan afo (Ibo), Kaichu (Japanese), Njowni (Luo), Wata panuwa (Singalese), Gooryan (Somali), Lumbris (Spanish), Safura njoka (Swahili), Nakupoochi (Tamil), Pa-yard sai-doen (Thai), Aràn inú (Yoruba).

GEOGRAPHICAL DISTRIBUTION

Cosmopolitan. *Ascaris* infection is common in both temperate and tropical countries where there are both adequate moisture and low standards of hygiene and sanitation. It is one of the most common human helminths with an estimated 1400 million infected persons in the world (23% of the world population), with about 60,000–100,000 deaths annually.

LOCATION IN HOST

Adults are normally found in the lumen of the small intestine but do not attach to the mucosa.

MORPHOLOGY

These are large, stout nematodes, tapering at both ends. The females (200–400 mm × 3–6 mm) are slightly larger than the males (150–300 mm × 2–4 mm) but may show great variation in size, depending on age and worm load. The mouth opens terminally and has three lips, each of which has a pair of sensory papillae on its lateral margin, and rows of small denticles or teeth. The principal structural protein of the cuticle is collagen, stabilized by disulphide bonds.

In the female the paired, tortuous, tubular ovaries, oviducts, seminal receptacles and uteri lead into a vagina, which opens by a small vulva on the ventral surface about a third of the body length from the anterior end. The average daily output of eggs is about 200,000 per female and each may lay a total of 25 million during her lifetime. The posterior end of the male is curved ventrally and there are two almost equal copulatory spicules (measuring 2.0–3.5 mm) and numerous preanal and postanal papillae. There is no gubernaculum.

The eggs are broadly ovoid and measure 45–70 µm × 35–50 µm. The shell is thick and transparent and usually has a coarsely mammilated outer albuminous coat, stained light brown with bile pigments (Fig. 69). The ova are unsegmented when passed in the faeces. Occasionally eggs are passed without the outer coat and a proportion of eggs (about 15%) are infertile; these are longer and narrower (90 µm × 40 µm), with a thin shell, more irregular outer covering and disorganized contents (Fig. 69). They occur either because the rapid production of eggs allows some to pass through unfertilized or because only female worms are present.

LIFE CYCLE (Fig. 70)

The unsegmented, fertilized, ova, passed in the faeces, take 10–15 days to develop to the infective stage at 20–30°C in moist soil

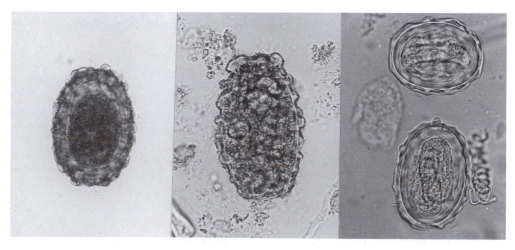

Fig. 69. Egg of *Ascaris*. Left: Fertile unembryonated egg as seen in faeces. Centre: Infertile egg from faeces. Right: Second-stage infective larva in egg after at least 10–15 days' development in soil (original magnification × 350).

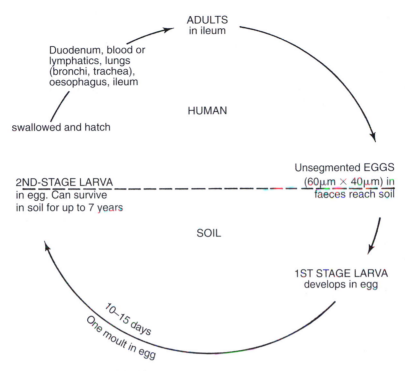

ADULTS
in ileum

Duodenum, blood or
lymphatics, lungs
(bronchi, trachea),
oesophagus, ileum

HUMAN

swallowed and hatch

Unsegmented EGGS
(60μm × 40μm) in
faeces reach soil

2ND-STAGE LARVA
in egg. Can survive
in soil for up to 7 years

SOIL

1ST STAGE LARVA
develops in egg

10–15 days
One moult in egg

Fig. 70. Life cycle of *Ascaris lumbricoides*.

or water. The first-stage larva inside the egg moults after about a week and it is the egg containing the second-stage larva that is infective (Fig. 69). In moist loose soil with moderate shade, infective eggs may survive for up to 7 years (Plate 2).

When the infective eggs are ingested, the larvae hatch in the duodenum. The eggshell is dissolved when there is a temperature of 37°C, high CO_2 concentration, low oxidation-reduction potential and a pH of around 7.0. The second-stage larvae measure 0.2–0.3 mm × 0.014 mm and have a rhabditiform oesophagus extending back about a quarter of the length of the body. They penetrate the mucosa and are carried in the lymphatics or veins through the liver and heart to reach the lungs in 3 days. With *A. suum* in pigs, at least, the larvae penetrate the colon and caecum, not the ileum, and reach the liver in 6 h causing lesions (Murrell *et al.*, 1997). The larvae moult twice in the lungs (at 5–6 days and 10 days) and then penetrate the alveolae, ascend the trachea and pass down the

oesophagus to reach the ileum. They develop into adult males and females in about 65 days and live for 1–2 years.

CLINICAL MANIFESTATIONS
Although the majority of infections are apparently symptomless (about 85%), the presence of even a few worms can be potentially dangerous and there are still over 200 million cases showing morbidity.

The first clinical signs and symptoms are a pneumonitis with cough, dyspnoea, substernal pain, fever and sometimes a blood-stained sputum (which may contain larvae). These symptoms begin 5 to 6 days after infection and usually last 10–12 days. This is known as Loeffler's syndrome and the X-ray findings often show dense pulmonary infiltrations, resembling acute tuberculosis. There is moderate eosinophilia (which increases to a maximum of 40% 3 weeks after infection).

The severity of symptoms depends both on the number of eggs ingested and on the previous infection history; hypersensitive individuals may have severe symptoms, with perhaps urticaria and asthma from the presence of only a few larvae. The relationship between pneumonitis and ascariasis was well shown by a study in Saudi Arabia, where there is a short transmission season in spring when infection can occur. In young adults (and probably children) Loeffler's syndrome occurs at this time of year, with eggs appearing in the faeces 2–3 months later. However, in Colombia, where there is constant transmission, this syndrome does not occur.

The second phase of clinical disease is due to the presence of the adult worms in the intestinal lumen (Fig. 71). The usual symptoms of heavy infections are digestive disorders, nausea, vomiting and colic and, in children, restless sleep and tooth grinding.

Intestinal obstruction is a serious complication of *Ascaris* infection, which usually occurs in children, often as young as 2 (Plate 16). Mortality in such cases admitted to hospital is about 9%. Because of the danger of causing obstruction, it is advisable in an endemic area to examine the faeces, followed by appropriate treatment if necessary, before carrying out an intestinal operation or before giving chemotherapy for other parasites, which may irritate *Ascaris*. The symptoms of intestinal obstruction are recurrent abdominal pain, loss of appetite, nausea and vomiting.

Adult worms causing obstruction can often be seen outlined as a shadow on X-rays after a barium meal. In many areas this is the commonest cause of intestinal obstruction in children. Occasionally worms may cause peritonitis or may wander in the appendix and possibly give rise to appendicitis (but see p. 163).

Adult *Ascaris* appear to be particularly prone to a 'wanderlust', perhaps an attempt to repeat the migrations of their youth when the larvae were only 0.3 mm long (Plate 17). They may migrate up the bile-duct or even up the pancreatic ducts. In children this causes severe colicky pain in almost all patients, with nausea and vomiting. After a few days fever develops, accompanied by a slight jaundice. Complications include ascending cholangitis (in about 15% of cases), obstructive jaundice (1%), acute pancreatitis (4%), and occasionally multiple liver abscesses. Such worms can be removed endoscopically. In China ascariasis has been estimated to account for about 13% of all cases of biliary obstruction (Zhou Xianmin *et al.*, 1999).

Sometimes adults may develop in ectopic sites such as the abdominal cavity and infrequently worms pass out through various orifices – mouth, nose, lachrymal duct, urethra, vagina – much to the consternation of the infected person.

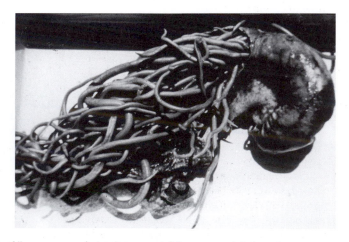

Fig. 71. Portion of ileum removed at autopsy containing many adult *Ascaris*.

Surgical complications are more common in areas where patients have greater worm loads, which in turn are found where the intensity of transmission and prevalence are high.

The amount of host food material removed by *Ascaris* is not negligible and this, together with concomitant anorexia and malabsorption, probably potentiates kwashiorkor in areas where protein intake is only just adequate. Parasitism is often so widespread in many developing countries that the effect on the nutrition of already malnourished children should not be underestimated. It has been estimated that a child who has 26 worms may lose one-tenth of its total daily intake of protein. There is also some evidence that ascariasis in children can contribute to vitamin A and C deficiency. The most important effect of disease in children aged 2–10 is its effect on height and weight, development and probably cognitive ability (Crompton *et al.*, 1989; Thien Hlang, 1993; Crompton, 2000).

PATHOGENESIS

The larvae cause lesions in the liver, spleen and lymph nodes. Sometimes necrotic foci are also found, encapsulated larvae causing a granulomatous reaction. In the lungs they cause petechiae and in severe reactions there is also ulceration of the bronchial mucosa and abundant mucus. Charcot–Leyden crystals may be present from the breakdown of eosinophils.

High IgE production may function to protect both the host and the parasite. *Ascaris* induces a Th2 cell-mediated response, producing interleukin 4 (IL-4) and resulting in production of IgE. It is possible that the parasite also produces an IL-4-type molecule that stimulates the host to produce non-specific superfluous IgE, thus swamping the immune response (Prichard, 1993). Attempts to demonstrate that immune responses can explain the clear predisposition to infection have not been successful (see Crompton, 2000). The immunology of intestinal nematodes is discussed on p. 120.

DIAGNOSIS

Clinical. The pneumonitis caused by the migrating larvae is often not diagnosed, but the accompanying high eosinophilia is suggestive. The adult worms can sometimes be seen as clear spaces on X-rays after a barium meal (the gut of the worms may show as a thin central line of contrast medium) or on a computer-assisted tomography (CT) scan. Ultrasound is particularly useful for worms in the biliary or pancreatic ducts, showing up as long, narrow, moving images maybe with two inner parallel lines. Endoscopy is also useful.

Parasitological. Eggs are usually plentiful in the faeces, although infertile eggs may not be recognized. Direct faecal smears, using about 2 mg of faeces, are usually adequate, while the Kato–Katz thick-smear technique (p. 257) works well. Concentration methods using sedimentation or brine flotation may be used but are not really necessary. Unlike most other nematodes, the number of eggs in the faeces often gives a good indication of the number of adults present (although a few parasites produce proportionally more eggs and very many parasites too few). However, since there are marked variations in fecundity in different countries, the WHO threshold of 50,000 eggs g^{-1} faeces indicating a heavy infection needing regular re-treatment may not be universally applicable (Hall and Holland, 2000).

Immunodiagnosis. All immunodiagnostic tests are very non-specific and none are used in practice. A 25 kDa antigen from the body fluids of larvae and adults of *A. lumbricoides* and the pig ascarid *A. suum* (ABA-1) is highly allergenic against mast cells *in vitro* and could possibly provide the basis for a test, at least at the community level – preferably if it could utilize saliva. It is possible to identify *Ascaris* metabolites in urine but this is not so far a practical test.

TREATMENT

Clinical. Intestinal obstruction in children can usually be treated conservatively with intravenous fluids, but acute infections may require surgical removal. Biliary obstruction, which is more common in adults than in children, can sometimes be treated by using retrograde endoscopy.

Chemotherapy

- Albendazole
  This is 100% effective at a single oral standard dosage of 400 mg for all individuals except pregnant women and the under-5s and will have action against all the geohelminths.

- Mebendazole
  This can similarly be used at a standard single oral dose of 400 mg for all geohelminths although best against *Ascaris* (100%).

- Pyrantel pamoate (= embonate)
  This is given as a single oral dose at 5–10 mg kg^{-1} body weight. It is not effective against *Strongyloides* and *Trichuris* (0–20% cure rate) and only partially against hookworms (20–90%); possibly it may also encourage obstruction by paralysed worms.

- Levamisole
  When given at 150–250 mg (2.5–5 mg kg^{-1}) it is completely effective (paralysing *Ascaris*) but less so against other intestinal nematodes.

EPIDEMIOLOGY

Ascariasis is prevalent in most tropical countries, with estimated infections of: China 523–539 million, Côte d'Ivoire 17% and Kenya 38%. Infection rates are often high in urban (particularly slum) areas: 25% in Brazil (Rio de Janeiro), 47% in Egypt (Alexandria), 35% in India (Hyderabad), 64% in Malaysia (Kuala Lumpur), 55% in Mexico (Coatzacoalcos), 68% in Nigeria (Lagos), 80% in the Philippines (Manila) and 43% in Sierra Leone (Freetown).

The adults are not usually very long-lived and there is often an annual cycle of infection. Evidence from people who move to a non-endemic area shows that eggs cease to be passed in under 18 months. Eggs may continue to be passed in the faeces up to 7 days after the adults have been expelled. Males are expelled first, so that in long-established infections without reinfection there is a preponderance of females.

The use of human faeces as a fertilizer ('night-soil') is common in some parts of the world and can result in eggs getting on to salad vegetables. In China and other areas raw faeces is now being stored. Over 90% of ova are killed by storage for 15 days at 29°C or 6 days at 33°C; but for complete destruction 40 days at 30°C is required (Muller, 1983).

Untreated sewage is sometimes discharged into rivers and lakes, which represents a clear health hazard. Even more common is discharge into the sea and eggs are able to continue development in sea water, as is said to occur in coastal villages of Samoa.

Properly designed modern sewage treatment plants will remove or destroy all *Ascaris* eggs, the bacterial bed treatment not being so effective as the activated sludge process or sand filtration. However, eggs need to be retained for 10–12 months in septic tanks and cesspits before they are all destroyed. Eggs will not embryonate below 18°C but can survive for many weeks at much lower temperatures and continue development when the temperature is raised. In experiments in Russia eggs have survived in soil for 7 years, but in most natural habitats they will be destroyed by sunlight, fungi or acarines in 2–6 months and in temperate climates they survive for shorter periods in summer.

The soil type is important in transmission; clay soils favour survival of eggs, since they retain water better. Complete lack of aeration is not lethal, ova remaining viable for months without oxygen, although their development is interrupted (Mizgajska, 1993).

PREVENTION AND CONTROL

Where there is a marked rise in standards of sanitation over a large area, *Ascaris* infection falls quickly, usually within a year. At the personal level, thorough washing and preferably cooking of vegetables and supervision of children's play areas are important. However, it is difficult to prevent infection and reinfection in young children, particularly where pica (geophagia) is common (Geissler *et al.*, 1998). Mass chemotherapy campaigns for all geo-helminths are discussed on p. 133.

ZOONOTIC ASPECTS

The relationship of human *A. lumbricoides* to the very common parasite of the pig still remains unresolved. Slight morphological differences have been described, such as the labial denticles being concave in the former and straight-sided in the latter, but these have been challenged by other workers (Gibson, 1983). Cross-infection can undoubtedly occur but in Guatemala, for instance, there appears to be little gene flow between infections of humans and of pigs, which is encouraging for control campaigns. In North America, however, a non-endemic region, molecular evidence indicates that most human cases are of pig origin (Anderson and Jaenike, 1997). There also appear to be genetic differences between the two forms (Xingquan *et al.*, 1999) and pig parasites are usually regarded as a separate species, *A. suum* Goeze, 1782. It is probable that human infections originally came when pigs were first domesticated in neolithic times, possibly in China (Peng Weidong *et al.*, 1998; Crompton, 2000); infections of *A. lumbricoides* in other primates appear to have been contracted from humans (cases of 'nosozootic' infections).

Lagochilascaris minor
Leiper, 1909

There have been occasional human cases recorded from Bolivia, Brazil, Costa Rica, Ecuador, Mexico, Surinam, Trinidad and Venezuela.

In humans the first sign of infection is a pustule, usually on the neck, which grows in size to give a large swelling. After the skin breaks, living adults, larvae and eggs are expelled at intervals in the pus. Eggs are continually developing into larvae and then adults in the tissues at the base of abscesses, so that repeated life cycles occur (de Aguilar Nasumento *et al.*, 1993). In the mastoid region, temporal bone can be invaded, with numerous mastoid sinuses and perhaps involvement of the CNS. In one woman worms emerged into the mouth and in a young girl a worm was recovered from a tooth abscess. The zone of induration grows deeper and sinus tracts develop, the openings oozing pus. Eventually a chronic granulomatous inflammation ensues, which can last for months. Some cases are fatal, including one with worms in the lungs.

The natural definitive hosts are unknown but are probably carnivores or opossums. Cats have been found naturally infected in Argentina and Brazil and, in cats experimentally infected with cysts from mice containing third-stage infective larvae, the larvae excysted in the stomach and penetrated the oesophagus, trachea, pharynx and cervical lymph nodes, developing to adults in 9–20 days postinfection. However, the worms did not produce eggs, although they did in animals fed infected mice. In mice infected orally with ova from humans, the first-stage larvae hatched in the gut, penetrated the wall and migrated to the liver, lungs, skeletal muscles and subcutaneous tissues, where they encysted as third-stage larvae. How humans become infected is not known, although presumably it is either from ingestion of wild animals containing cysts or from ingestion of eggs in the environment.

Long-term treatment with levamisole and thiabendazole has not been effective, but albendazole (200–400 mg each day for 5 days) and perhaps mebendazole (200 mg each day) have some (although perhaps a temporary) effect. Ivermectin (300 µg kg^{-1} daily for 4 weeks) has resulted in long-term cure in single cases in Ecuador and Brazil.

Baylisascaris procyonis
(Stefanski and Zarnowski, 1951)

This is a common parasite of racoons in the USA. In humans and small rodents, such as squirrels, or porcupines, rabbits, birds and dogs, it causes a form of visceral, neural or ocular larva migrans. There are about a dozen species of *Baylisascaris* from carnivores and the full life cycle is known only for a species in badgers, which requires an intermediate host. It is likely that racoons ingest small mammals and birds with granulomas containing larvae in the somatic and particularly CNS tissues (although eggs can also be infective); the worms then develop into adults in the intestinal lumen and eggs are evacuated in the faeces, with second-stage larvae developing inside them in soil. They are then infective to the mammalian and bird intermediate hosts, where development to the third stage takes about 2 weeks.

In a fatal case in a 10-year-old boy, the larvae evoked a sessile polyploid mass in the left ventricular myocardium, protruding into the ventricular lumen (Boschetti and Kasznica, 1995). In other cases, with larvae in the brain, a sometimes fatal eosinophilic meningoencephalitis ensues (Plate 18). In an infant who recovered after treatment with a single dose of ivermectin and multiple doses of thiabendazole and prednisolone, there was permanent neurological damage (Cunningham *et al.*, 1994). Other cases in adults have resulted in larvae in one eye causing a diffuse neuroretinitis. In most cases diagnosis is based solely on ELISA or immunoblot techniques although L_3 larvae have been found in usually granulomatous biopsy specimens. Larvae measure 930–1300 µm $\times$ 50–65 µm and have well-developed lateral alae. Neurological cases present with extreme lethargy, with 30–40% eosinophilia (Kazacos, 1983).

The adult worms resemble those of *Ascaris* in size but have cervical alae and an area rugosa, while the eggs are pitted. The larvae inside eggs can survive for long periods in soil, and infection is widespread in racoons throughout North America; similar species parasitize skunks, martens and bears.

Parascaris equorum (Goeze, 1782) Yorke and Maplestone, 1926, is a widespread parasite of horses and other equines that has caused occasional cases of human visceral larva migrans and pneumonitis from inges-tion of eggs in the environment. A biological quirk, shared with *A. suum,* is that nuclear DNA is greatly reduced in all somatic cells but not in germ cells.

Family Anisakidae

Anisakis and other anisakids

DISEASE AND POPULAR NAMES
Anisakiasis or anisakidosis; herring-worm disease, cod-worm disease (from *Pseudoterranova*).

GEOGRAPHICAL DISTRIBUTION
Anisakis simplex (Rudolphi, 1809), synonym *A. marina*, is a natural parasite of marine fish-eating mammals. Human cases occur where fish are eaten raw and was first recognized in The Netherlands in 1960. Cases (almost 34,000 in total) have been reported from Japan (over 16,000), Korea (196 up to 1992), Canada, France, Germany, Italy, The Netherlands, Russia, Spain, the UK and the USA.

LOCATION IN HOST
Larvae are found in abscesses in the wall of the intestinal tract, usually the stomach in Japan but also the small intestine and colon.

MORPHOLOGY AND LIFE CYCLE
L_3s in humans measure about 29 mm $\times$ 0.45 mm, with the typical ascarid three lips and a dorsal boring tooth at the anterior end. The tail is short and rounded, with a small projection at the end. Occasionally larvae in humans develop to the fourth stage but never to adults.

Thin-shelled eggs (50 µm $\times$ 40 µm) are discharged in the faeces by the adults, which inhabit the stomach of marine mammals. Larvae develop inside the egg and moult once to give the L_2. The sheathed larvae hatch and can live in sea water for many weeks. If ingested by planktonic euphausid crustaceans (krill), the larvae penetrate the gut wall and develop to the L_3 stage. When krill is ingested by many (164) species of fish, such as herring, mackerel, cod and salmon, or by squid, the larvae encyst in the muscles or viscera. These act as paratenic hosts, since the larvae do not develop further, but if they are eaten by any of many species of marine mammals (26 cetacean and 12 species of pinniped) the contained larvae develop into adults in the stomach.

CLINICAL MANIFESTATIONS AND PATHOGENESIS

If the parasite is in the stomach, the most common symptoms are nausea, vomiting and epigastric pain, simulating a peptic ulcer or a tumour, beginning 1–12 h after ingestion of infected fish (Plate 19). Sometimes there may be symptoms of acute chest pain. The parasites can elicit severe IgE-mediated hypersensitivity, which might require emergency treatment. There is sometimes urticaria, angioedema and even anaphylaxis. If abscesses are present in the intestine or colon, there is likely to be lower abdominal pain, but sometimes it can resemble acute appendicitis (Plate 20). This develops after about 2 days and lasts for a further few days before ileus or perhaps ascites results. Gastric cancer is much more common in Japan than in any other country and the presence of *Anisakis* larvae has been suggested as a cofactor (Petithory *et al.*, 1990). Occasionally worms may penetrate through to the abdominal cavity and in one patient a larva was discovered in the liver.

In the early stages there is an abscess infiltrated by neutrophils and later an eosinophilic granulomatous reaction. The affected portion of the intestinal tract becomes oedematous (up to 1.5 cm thick), with ulcerations and petechial haemorrhages in the mucosa, each containing a larval worm. Dead worms become surrounded by foreign-body giant cells. Submucosal lesions of the ileum or colon also have larvae in them, surrounded by an area of necrosis.

DIAGNOSIS AND TREATMENT

Clinical and parasitological. Endoscopy can be very useful for viewing the stomach abscess, which is oedematous, and there may be severe erosive gastritis, hyperaemia and bleeding. There are usually only one to nine worms, but in one patient 56 worms were removed (Kagei and Isogaki, 1992). Contrast X-rays can reveal filling defects and oedematous, obstructed, areas in the stomach wall (Ishikura *et al.*, 1992).

Immunodiagnosis. Various monoclonal antibodies have been discovered that recognize specific epitopes from *A. simplex* larvae. One (An2) recognizes epitopes from intestinal cells and ES products and has been used in a micro-ELISA. Another IgG1κ antibody (UA3) of 139 kDa is more specific, but both only detect the presence of the worms about 4 weeks after infection. An immunoblot technique with larval whole-body antigen to detect IgE is positive after a few days (Garcia *et al.*, 1997). An antigenic β-galactosidase helminth-derived recombinant fusion protein (FP) obtained by recombinant DNA techniques and used in an ELISA is stated to be completely specific, in contrast to soluble antigens (Sugane *et al.*, 1992).

The most effective method of treatment for gastric worms is by endoscopy and removal of the larval worms using biopsy forceps; symptoms clear up within hours of removal.

EPIDEMIOLOGY AND PREVENTION

With the ability to easily remove larval worms, it is becoming increasingly evident that other anisakids may be involved, as well as *Anisakis simplex*. There is *A. physetis* Baylis, 1923 (previously known as *Anisakis* type II larvae), *Pseudoterranova decipiens* (Krabbe, 1878) in Japan and North America, *Contracaecum osculatum* (Rudolphi, 1802) and *Hysterothylacium* (syn. *C.*) *aduncum* (Rudolphi, 1802). Larvae of all are found in marine fish; *C. osculatum* caused an infection in Spain from eating sardines and *H. aduncum*, with adults in piscivorous fish, not mammals, was reported from Chile. All cause similar lesions in the gastric and possibly the intestinal wall. A fourth-stage larva of *P. decipiens* that had been removed measured 29.7 mm × 0.94 mm (Sohn and Seol, 1994) and an adult worm (reported once only) 33 mm × 1.0 mm. This is a natural parasite of seals and requires two crustacean intermediate hosts (a copepod and an amphipod).

The various larvae can be distinguished. Those of *Anisakis* have no lateral alae and in section have characteristic Y-shaped lateral cords. *A. simplex* larvae measure on average 28.4 mm × 0.45 mm and have a short tail with a terminal spine, while those of *A. physetis* measure 27.8 mm × 0.61 mm and have a long tail without a terminal spine. Larvae of *Pseudoterranova decipiens* measure 32.6 mm × 0.8 mm and have a short tail with a spine and the proventricular–caecal junction is not straight but diagonal.

A high proportion of food fish may be infected with anisakid larvae, up to 90% in herring and cod. Fish should be gutted as soon as caught, since larvae are thought to move into the tissues after death, and deep-freezing (−20°C) will kill the larvae. Raw (green) herrings are popular in The Netherlands but infection appears to have vanished, since all fish sold must now be deep frozen first. Thorough cooking will also kill the larvae, but raw fish are eaten in some countries, particularly Japan, where 'sashimi' is popular. Also, it has been reported recently that cases of severe allergic symptoms, such as urticaria, dyspnoea and even anaphylaxis, have occurred in patients after eating thoroughly cooked fish and it is probable that the individuals had become sensitized by previous infection with live larvae.

Infection can be divided into two categories:

1. Visceral larval migrans results when ingestion of eggs or larvae leads to the presence of wandering larvae in the deep organs. Potentially, this group constitutes the most serious danger to humans. Species that may be involved include the larvae of *Toxocara canis*, *T. cati*, *Lagochilascaris major*, *Parascaris equorum*, *Gnathostoma spinigerum* and other spirurids, *Parastrongylus cantonensis*, *P. costaricensis*, *Anatrichosoma cutaneum*, *Alaria* spp. and *Spirometra* spp. This definition does not strictly include *Ascaris suum* and *Calodium hepaticum*, which reach maturity in the human body, *Baylisascaris procyonis*, which develops in humans as in its usual intermediate hosts, or *Anisakis simplex*, which develops normally in humans until it dies in the tissues, although these species are often included.

2. Cutaneous larva migrans is caused by skin-penetrating larvae that continue to wander in the superficial layers of the body. Larvae that may be responsible include hookworms, *Strongyloides*, *Gnathostoma hispidum*, fly larvae and spargana of *Spirometra* spp. Some animal schistosomes, including zoophilic strains of *Schistosoma japonicum*, *Heterobilharzia* and *Orientobilharzia* and bird parasites, such as *Australobilharzia*, *Bilharziella*, *Gigantobilharzia*, *Microbilharzia*, *Schistosomatium* and *Trichobilharzia*, cause 'swimmers' itch' at the site of penetration but without wandering in the superficial layers.

Larva Migrans

This is a term used to describe human infection with helminth larvae that do not grow to maturity but wander in the body, sometimes with serious results. The condition is caused by natural parasites of animals, with humans acting as abnormal paratenic hosts, in which the parasites do not develop but are not destroyed, and may also result from invasion by larvae belonging to zoophilic strains of species normally found in humans.

Visceral larva migrans

Only the dog and cat ascarids will be considered in this section, the other possible causative agents being considered in their appropriate sections.

Toxocara and *Toxascaris*

DISEASE AND POPULAR NAME
Toxocariasis or toxocarosis; 'arrowhead worms'. Most important cause of visceral larva migrans (VLM).

Toxocara canis (Werner, 1782) Johnston, 1916, is a very common ascarid nematode of dogs in many parts of the world. ***T. cati*** (synonym *T. mystax*) (Schrank, 1788) Brumpt, 1927, is found in cats and foxes and ***Toxascaris leonina*** (von Linstow, 1902) Leiper, 1907, in dogs, cats and many wild carnivores. Each of these parasites is more common in young animals during the first few months of life.

MORPHOLOGY

The adults are smaller than those of *Ascaris* and have characteristic cervical alae or wings (Table 10).

LIFE CYCLE

The egg is unsegmented when passed, but in soil the ovum inside embryonates to give the infective second-stage larva in 9 days at 26–30°C and 11–18 days at 20°C with a relative humidity above 85%.

The natural hosts are usually infected before birth by the mother ingesting eggs containing second-stage larvae. The hatched larvae penetrate the gut wall and then undergo a 'somatic' migration, reaching the lungs, liver and kidneys and, in pregnant females, penetrating through the placenta to infect the fetus. Young puppies or kittens may also be infected with larvae through the milk or by ingesting eggs, when a 'tracheal' type of migration similar to that of *Ascaris* results. Adult females in the ileum produce eggs in the faeces after 4–5 weeks.

Eggs hatch as second-stage larvae in mice (or in the case of *Toxocara cati* or *Toxascaris leonina* in invertebrates such as cockroaches and earthworms also) and these act as paratenic hosts, the larvae invading many tissues and becoming encapsulated after 12 days. Further development occurs if those are eaten by the definitive hosts.

In humans the eggs are ingested and the second-stage larvae hatch out in the intestine and undergo a similar 'somatic' migration but do not develop further. They measure 350–530 µm and are considerably thinner than the larvae of *Ascaris* and this may explain why they are not filtered out in the liver and lungs.

CLINICAL MANIFESTATIONS AND PATHOGENESIS

Disease occurs mainly in young children (typically 1–4 years old) who have had close contact with infected household pets or have been exposed to eggs in the environment and is due mainly to *T. canis*. In over 80% of cases there is a marked eosinophilia (over 50% with 20,000 eosinophils mm^{-3}) and hepatomegaly. In over 50% of cases, pulmonary symptoms,

Table 10. Differentiation of the dog and cat ascarids.

Toxocara canis	Toxocara cati	Toxascaris leonina

Length:
  Females 6–18 cm
  Males 4–10 cm
	Length:
	  Females 4–12 cm
	  Males 3–6 cm
		Length:
		  Females 4–10 cm
		  Males 3–7 cm

Head bent ventrally	Head bent ventrally	Head straight
Cervical alae elliptical	Cervical alae broad and end abruptly posteriorly	Cervical alae elliptical
Oesophagus with a posterior muscular bulb	Oesophagus with a posterior muscular bulb	Oesophagus with no posterior bulb
Tail of male with digitiform appendage and caudal alae	Tail of male with digitiform appendage and caudal alae	Tail of male conical with no caudal alae
Eggshell pitted (75–85 µm)	Eggshell pitted (65–70 µm)	Eggshell smooth (75–85 µm)
Specific to dog	Specific to cat	Found in dog or cat

such as coughing and wheezing with dyspnoea and fever (Loeffler's syndrome), lasting up to 3 weeks, are found and there may be acute bronchitis with pneumonia. Chest X-rays often show bilateral infiltrates. These are followed by gastrointestinal disturbances, with larvae present in the liver and maybe the brain as well as the lungs, causing eosinophilic granulomas. Hepatomegaly and eosinophilia can last for many months. Larvae in the brain can cause convulsions or hemiplegia (Plate 21). There is the possibility that *Toxocara* larvae are responsible for carrying viral (including poliomyelitis and Japanese B encephalitis), bacterial and protozoal pathogens into the brain and other organs. Very rarely there can be myelitis.

Another form of the disease, which usually occurs in older children or adults when larvae invade the eye but do not cause the typical visceral symptoms, can be termed ocular larva migrans (OLM). The larvae cause unilateral chronic granulomatous endophthalmitis (in 60% of cases) or peripheral retinitis (in 10% of cases). These granulomata cause distortion or even detachment of the retina, and blindness is common (Gillespie, 1993; Gillespie *et al.*, 1993). There can also be papillitis, leading to glaucoma. One danger is that the lesion will be mistaken for a retinoblastoma and the eye hurriedly removed. However, the eye lesions in toxocariasis are raised and always unilateral (Fig. 72).

A few human infections with adult *T.*

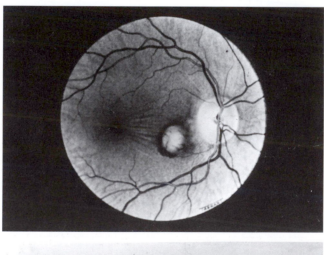

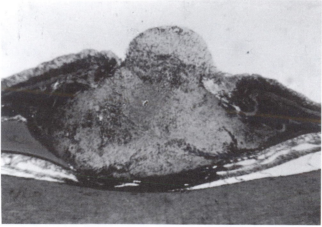

Fig. 72. Top: Ophthalmoscope view of the retina with raised area near the optic disc (haemorrhage on left). Bottom: Section of granulomatous lesion of retina, with a larva in the centre of fibrinoid necrosis.

canis and *T. cati* have been recorded, possibly from ingestion of larvae in an invertebrate intermediate host.

Histopathology. In experimental animals, petechial haemorrhages occur in the liver when the larvae leave the sinusoids and burrow through the tissues, leaving necrotic trails behind. These are inflammatory at first but then become granulomatous, containing eosinophils, lymphocytes, fibroblasts, epitheloid cells and giant cells. The live larvae become encapsulated and can sometimes live for months or even years but usually soon die. Similar lesions occur in the lung and there can also be myocardial or CNS involvement. In experimentally infected mice, larvae of *T. canis* entered the brain in all cases and the eye in 5%, while those of *T. cati* migrated to the brain in 8% of cases but never to the eye.

The migrating larvae evoke both delayed-type and immediate-type hypersensitivity reactions. The levels of both IgG and IgM are raised greatly but much is nonspecific. There is a carbohydrate (trisaccharide) cuticular-associated epitope that is immunogenic (Kayes, 1997).

DIAGNOSIS

Clinical. Hepatomegaly with eosinophilia is suggestive, as is elevated gammaglobulin and isohaemoagglutinin titres. Ultrasonography and magnetic resonance imaging (MRI) show hepatic granulomas as characteristic multiple hypoechoic nodular lesions.

Parasitological. Liver biopsies may show granulomatous lesions but it is rare to find a portion of a larva in tissue sections. The second-stage larva measures 350–450 µm × 18–21 µm and, if one is seen, can be differentiated from an *Ascaris* larva in sections by its smaller diameter.

Immunodiagnosis. ELISA, using antigens from second-stage larvae or their ES products, has about 90% specificity and 80% sensitivity. Low-molecular mass (26.9 to 38.9 kDa) polypeptides from L_2s recog-

nized by infected sera show a very high specificity in an SDS-PAGE or enzyme immunotransfer blot assay.

TREATMENT

Albendazole (400 mg or 10–15 mg kg^{-1} day^{-1} for 10–21 days) or mebendazole (100 mg daily for 10–21 days) have been successfully used in recent trials. Diethylcarbamazine can no longer be recommended, although thiabendazole is still used. The majority of cases resolve in a few months even without treatment, although corticosteroids (e.g. 30 mg of prednisone day^{-1} for 21 days) can be given to reduce inflammation and relieve symptoms in severe cases.

EPIDEMIOLOGY, PREVENTION AND CONTROL

Infection is very common in dogs and cats in most parts of the world, e.g. Chile (19% *T. canis*, 65% *T. cati*), Slovakia (70% *T. cati*). Many children also react positively in serological tests, e.g. 33% in Corunna, Spain, 35% in Malaysia. It is clear that the great majority of children exposed do not suffer clinical disease (Gillespie, 1988).

Puppies and kittens should always be dewormed as a routine. There are often many infective eggs around houses from the faeces of household pets and measures should be taken to prevent indiscriminate defecation and also to prevent young children from playing in and ingesting contaminated soil (pica). In many developed countries children's play sandpits are now protected with a fence.

Toxocara pteropodis Baylis, 1926, is a parasite of fruit bats on the Pacific islands comprising Vanuatu. It has been suggested as the cause of a disease outbreak known as Palm Island mystery disease with hepatitis-like symptoms, but this may have been due to poisoning (Prociv, 1989).

Cutaneous larva migrans or 'creeping eruption'

Of the various possible causes of this condition, *Spirometra* is considered on page

70, *Strongyloides* on page 115, *Gnathostoma* on page 184 and fly larvae on page 241, and only the animal hookworms are considered here.

Ancylostoma braziliense Gomez de Faira, 1910, is a hookworm of dogs and cats in many tropical regions of the Americas. The buccal capsule has a smaller aperture than that of *A. duodenale* and has a small inner tooth and a large outer one. When the infective filariform larvae penetrate the skin of humans, they follow a tortuous path under the skin, progressing at 2–5 cm day^{-1}. An erythematous inflammatory reaction follows the tunnel made by the larvae between the germinal layer of the epidermis and the dermis. The tunnel fills with serum and the surrounding oedematous tissues contain many polymorphs and eosinophils. The larval movement results in intense itching and pruritus, and often secondary bacterial infection is caused by scratching; the larvae die after a few weeks, even without treatment, and the symptoms subside (Jelinek *et al.*, 1994). Other species of animal hookworms, such as *A. caninum*, *A. tubaeforme*, *Bunostomum phlebotomum* or *Uncinaria stenocephala* may also be responsible. The condition is similar to the 'ground itch' that sometimes follows penetration by the larvae of human species of hookworms and by *Strongyloides stercoralis*, but lasts longer. Local treatment with an ethyl chloride spray or topical application of thiabendazole is effective.

A. caninum (Ercolani, 1859) is a common and important parasite of dogs and cats in most tropical and semi-tropical parts of the world and the larvae can be a cause of folliculitis; development to adults in humans is discussed on p. 138, together with *A. ceylanicum*, which is morphologically very similar to *A. braziliense* and is found in dogs in Asia and South America, but does not appear to cause creeping eruption.

A. tubaeforme (Zeder, 1800) is a cosmopolitan parasite of the cat, **Uncinaria stenocephala** (Railliet, 1884), a similar parasite to *Necator*, is found in the dog, cat

and fox in Europe and North America and **Bunostomum phlebotomum** (Railliet, 1900) is a widely distributed parasite of cattle.

Order Oxyurida

Family Oxyuridae

Enterobius vermicularis
(Linnaeus, 1758) Leach, 1853

SYNONYMS
Ascaris vermicularis L., 1758; *Oxyuris vermicularis* Lamark, 1816.

DISEASE AND POPULAR NAMES
Enterobiasis or enterobiosis, oxyuriasis; pinworm, seatworm or threadworm infection.

Local names

Deedan dabousia (Arabic), Cacing kerawit (Bahasa Malay), Toke kaung (Burmese), Kira panuwa (Singalese), Njoka safura (Swahili), Keeri pulu (Tamil), Pa-yard senderi or Kem-mood (Thai), Nnoko-boa (Twi).

GEOGRAPHICAL DISTRIBUTION
Taking into account the difficulty of diagnosis, enterobiasis is undoubtedly one of the most common human helminth infections worldwide, certainly in temperate climates, with an estimate of 1000 million cases worldwide (Cook, 1994). In general, infection is less common in tropical and less developed countries, presumably because of the fewer clothes worn.

LOCATION IN HOST
The adults are located in the lumen of the caecum and appendix, sometimes with the anterior end attached to the mucosa. In heavy infections they may also be present in the ascending colon and ileum.

MORPHOLOGY
Pinworms are small cylindrical nematodes, pointed at either end. They have three lips around the mouth but no buccal capsule.

The oesophagus is muscular and has a posterior bulb characteristic of the order Oxyurida. The cuticle has cervical alae continued as lateral projections, which enable *Enterobius* to be easily recognized in sections of appendix, etc. (Figs 51 and 73). The female measures 8–13 mm × 0.3–0.5 mm and has a long pointed tail (about one-third of the total length). The vulva opens midventrally almost a third of the way down the body. The paired uteri are usually filled with thousands of eggs and the whole body becomes distended. The male is much smaller, measuring 2–5 mm × 0.2 mm. The posterior end is curved ventrally and has a single copulatory spicule 100–140 µm long. There is no gubernaculum. The bursa is reduced and there are various caudal papillae. The males die after copulation and often appear in the faeces.

Another species, **E. gregorii** Hugot, 1983, is usually present together with *E. vermicularis* and has been described from France, England, Japan, New Guinea and South Korea (Hugot and Tourte-Schaefer, 1985; Chittenden and Ashford, 1987). Males of this species differ by having a shorter, simple, spicule (60–80 µm long rather than 100–140 µm) and other slight morphological differences. The eggs and females cannot be differentiated.

LIFE CYCLE

The gravid female migrates out of the anus in the evening or at night and lays numerous sticky eggs on the perianal and perineal skin. The female normally dies after oviposition. Often she bursts, releasing all the eggs, which number about 11,000 (4000–17,000).

The eggs measure 50–60 (average 54) µm × 20–30 µm and have a thin semi-transparent shell composed of an outer albuminous layer, two chitinous layers and an inner lipoidal membrane. They are ovoid and flattened on one side (Fig. 123). Eggs are usually laid partially embryonated and contain infective rhabditiform larvae in 4–7 h at 35°C (they require oxygen for complete development and do not develop below about 22°C). However, if the female has burst, eggs may be only at the four-celled stage and then require about 48 h at 25°C to become infective. The outer albuminous layer of the egg is very sticky and in sensitized individuals can cause an intense itching, as does the adult female. This often leads to scratching and eggs then lodge under the fingernails. They are also carried in dust and, when ingested, the larvae (measuring 145 µm × 10 µm) hatch in the duodenum. From comparison with other members of the order, they are presumably at the third stage. The larvae lodge in the crypts of the

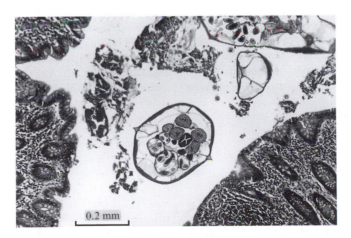

Fig. 73. Section of appendix with adult female *Enterobius vermicularis* in lumen.

ileum and moult twice. The young adults move down to the colon, attach to the mucosa and become mature in 15–43 days.

Retroinfection can occur if the larvae hatch on the perianal skin and migrate back up the anus. The adult females live for 5–13 weeks and males for 7 weeks, but infection in humans is usually maintained for very much longer by repeated reinfection. Retroinfection is more common in adults than in children and results in recurrent infections with a few worms every 40–50 days.

Biologically, this group of nematodes is interesting since it appears to be the only endoparasitic haplodiploid taxon, i.e. females are diploid while males are haploid and derived from unfertilized eggs (Adamson, 1989).

CLINICAL MANIFESTATIONS

The majority of cases are symptomless, although children often suffer from loss of appetite and irritability; it is usually regarded as primarily an infection of children.

The most common symptoms are due to the pruritus ani, which can be very severe and lead to disturbed sleep. In females the vulva can also be involved from vaginal migration of adult worms and in girls is the commonest cause of pruritus vulvae; there may also be acute urinary tract infection. Scratching may lead to secondary infection of the anal region.

Mild catarrhal inflammation, with nausea and diarrhoea, sometimes occurs and symptoms of appendicitis have been reported. Low eosinophilia of 4–12% may be found, but eosinophilia is not so pronounced as in many other intestinal nematodes, perhaps because there is no tissue phase.

If female worms reach the peritoneal cavity from intestinal perforations or following migration into the female reproductive tract, worms can die and become surrounded by granulomas (Gilman *et al.*, 1991).

PATHOGENESIS

Little internal pathology can be directly attributed to the presence of *Enterobius*, apart from a mild inflammation. Ulcerative and haemorrhagic lesions of the small and large intestine have been reported but may be coincidental.

The relationship of pinworm infection to acute appendicitis has not been clearly demonstrated, although *Enterobius* has been found in many patients with symptoms of appendicitis and where no other cause has been found. Sometimes eosinophilic granulomas are found (Al Rabia *et al.*, 1996), but recent large-scale examinations have not supported an association between *Enterobius,* or any other helminth, and appendicitis. In one study in Venezuela, 3500 removed appendices were examined and *Enterobius* found in 11%, *Trichuris* in 33% and *Ascaris* in 25%, but there were just as many in normal organs as in diseased ones (Dorfman *et al.*, 1995). Indeed, in another study in Denmark, looking at 2267 appendices, 4.1% had *E. vermicularis* but in 72% they were in normal organs and only 7.4% were in inflamed organs. Possibly *E. vermicularis* is the cause of appendicitis-like symptoms (pseudo-appendicitis) or, on the other hand, worms may leave an appendix that is inflamed (Addiss and Juranek, 1991). A few cases of perianal mass have been reported with recurrent cellulitis. Occasionally worms lodge in ectopic sites, such as the Fallopian tubes or the ovary and in peritoneal granulomatous nodules. In about 20% of infected young girls gravid female worms migrate into the vagina and uterus, occasionally evoking an endometritis (Sun *et al.*, 1991). Eggs are sometimes found in cervical Papanicolaou smears.

DIAGNOSIS

Adult worms are often observed on the surface of stools. Sometimes they can also be seen around the anus or in the vulva in the evening.

Ova are rarely found in the faeces and are better looked for in the perianal and perineal regions, using a swab technique. The National Institutes of Health cellophane swab has been in use since 1937, but nowadays cellophane is replaced by adhesive tape (Sellotape or Scotch tape). The tape is usually stuck by one end to a micro-scope slide and turned back over a tongue depressor or finger to make a swab (Graham swab). The sticky tape is rubbed over the anal region and stuck to the slide. A very convenient single-use flexible plas-tic slide is manufactured in Japan. In Russia an adhesive-covered glass ocular spatula is stated to be more sensitive and cheaper. Ideally the swab should be taken first thing in the morning and repeated for 7 days before a negative diagnosis can be made (and even then only at about the 90% level). If it is necessary to confirm whether the eggs are viable, the slide can be gently heated, when the enclosed larvae should become active. Where there is a lot of extraneous material, a drop of toluene may be placed on the slide first to increase transparency.

TREATMENT

Enterobius is one of the easiest of helminth infections to treat and a wide range of anthelminthics are effective. The benzimi-dazole compounds inhibit microtubule function and glycogen depletion and are the most effective. However, whichever drug is used, it is advisable to treat the entire family or group on several occasions; otherwise reinfection is almost inevitable. Where the cost is important, treatment is probably not worthwhile for symptomless cases unless used primarily for other helminths.

Albendazole. The standard treatment of a single dose of 400 mg, or a divided dose of 200 mg twice a day, usually gives 100% cure rates in children over 2 and adults (but should not be given to pregnant women).

Mebendazole. At a single dose of 100 mg with the same proviso, this is equally effec-tive.

Pyrantel pamoate. Given in a single dose of 10 mg kg^{-1} body weight or with a repeat dose 1 week later, this is also effective.

Ivermectin. At a single dosage of 50–200 µg kg^{-1} body weight or two doses of 100–200

µg kg^{-1}, has given about 85% activity in clinical trials.

Levamisole (2.5 mg kg^{-1} body weight in a single dose) and piperazine adipate (9 mg kg^{-1} daily for 7 days) have been used for many years and can still be employed.

EPIDEMIOLOGY

Enterobiasis is particularly a group infec-tion, being most common in large families and in institutions, such as boarding-schools, hospitals, mental homes and orphanages. Transmission may be termed contaminative, as the eggs are immediately infective, and normally takes place indoors; this is in contrast to the soil-transmitted geohelminths, in which the eggs or larvae continue development in the soil. Eggs may be found in large numbers inside houses, particularly in soiled bed-clothes, in night clothes and in dust in bed-rooms and lavatories (up to 50,000 m^{-2}). Once embryonated (at above 22°C), the eggs can survive for 6–8 weeks under cool, moist, conditions but are killed in a few days by a dry atmosphere. Direct contami-nation from anus to fingers to mouth is also a common mode of infection.

Recent estimates of infection rates in various countries using sticky tape are: preschool institutes in Azerbaijan 36%; Brisbane, Australia 43% (adults 23%); mental patients in Tasmania, Australia 19%; Bulgaria 6.5%; Chile 16–22%; chil-dren's homes in Santiago in Chile 87%; Denmark 12.5%; the Dominican Republic 12.5%; Shoubra, Egypt 45%; children in hospital in England 55%; Germany 34%; Greece 22%; adults in Bengal, India 12%; Tamil Nadu, India 14%; Basrah, Iraq 18%; children in Lithuania 21%; Macao 23%; Penang, Malaysia 58%; Quetta, Pakistan 4%; children in Peru 43%; Poland 30%; South Korea 20–77%; orphanages in South Korea 74–84%; Slovenia 40%; children in Moscow, Russia 30%; Tainen City, Taiwan 38%; Turkey 40–97%; primary schools in California, USA 12–22%; Venezuela 12.5%. Numerous other studies have been carried out using faecal examination only and these have given much lower infection rates.

As with other intestinal nematode infections, there appears to be a predisposition to infection, with a small percentage of patients having very heavy infections and being responsible for most of the eggs reaching the environment (Haswell-Elkins *et al.*, 1987a, b).

Enterobius eggs have also been found in 10,000-year-old coprolites from caves in Tennessee and Utah, USA, and Chile, so it is a well-established human parasite.

PREVENTION AND CONTROL

Hygienic measures are of primary importance and include frequent washing of hands and changing and washing of sheets and night garments every morning during an outbreak. The area around the anus should be washed every morning. Dust should not be allowed to collect and there should be good ventilation. The eggs are very light and easily become airborne.

ZOONOTIC ASPECTS

None. Almost exclusively a parasite of humans, although monkeys (chimpanzee, baboon, gibbon and marmoset) have been found infected in zoos. Other species are found in apes and monkeys and related genera occur in rabbits, rats, mice and horses.

Syphacia obvelata (Rudolphi, 1802) Seurat, 1916, is a common and cosmopolitan parasite of rats and mice, both in the wild and in the laboratory. Three cases have been reported from children in the Philippines.

Order Enoplida

Family Trichuridae

Trichuris trichiura
(Linnaeus, 1771) Stiles, 1901

SYNONYMS

Trichocephalos trichiura (Goeze, 1782) *Trichocephalus trichiurus* (Shrank, 1788); *T. dispar* (Rudolphi, 1802); *T. hominis* (Shrank, 1788); *T. intestinalis*; (Hooper, 1799) *Ascaris trichiura* (Linnaeus, 1771).

The generic name *Trichocephalus* is probably more correct as the original description by Roederer and Wagler in 1761 naming the organism *Trichuris* did not obey the rules of binary nomenclature and probably represented the species name. The fact that the name *Trichuris* ('hair tail') is not so apt as the later correction *Trichocephalus* ('hair head') is irrelevant to the argument, however. The name *Trichuris* is preferred in this edition partly because it was chosen by the Committee on Nomenclature of the American Society of Parasitologists in 1941 (although there has been no ruling from the International Commission on Zoological Nomenclature) but mainly because it is becoming more firmly established each year, except perhaps in eastern Europe.

DISEASE AND POPULAR NAME

Trichuriasis or trichuriosis, trichocephaliasis; whipworm infection. One of the geohelminths.

LOCAL NAMES

Cacing kerawit (Bahasy Malay), Njowni (Luo), Keeri pulu (Tamil), Wakanabbyo (Japanese).

GEOGRAPHICAL DISTRIBUTION

Cosmopolitan but more common in warm humid countries. There are about 800 million (Bundy and Cooper, 1989) to 1300 million (Chan *et al.*, 1994) cases in the world, with one individual in about 500 showing evidence of morbidity and 10,000 deaths annually (8–13%; Bundy, 1994).

LOCATION IN HOST

The adults usually occur in the caecum but may also be present in the appendix, rectum and upper colon with the thin anterior end embedded in the mucosa (Figs 74–76).

MORPHOLOGY

The male measures 30–45 mm, with a tightly coiled posterior end and a single spicule. The female is slightly longer (30–50 mm) and both sexes have a narrow anterior portion and a much wider posterior end (hence the popular name of whip-

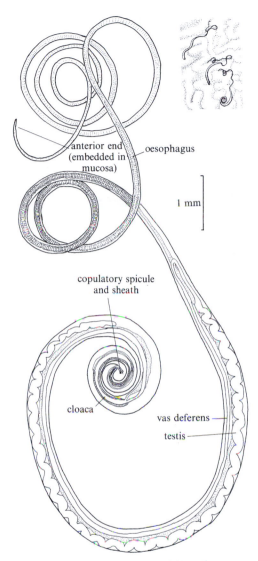

anterior end (embedded in mucosa)

oesophagus

1 mm

copulatory spicule and sheath

cloaca

vas deferens

testis

Fig. 74. Adult male of *Trichuris trichiura*. Insert shows two females and a male (with coiled tail) attached to the mucosa of the colon by their anterior ends.

worm, as they resemble the coaching whip once used in Europe or a stock-whip (Fig. 74). The mouth is simple, without lips, but with a stylet for penetration of the mucosa. In the living worm the stylet is constantly probing and slashing, like a fencer wielding a rapier. The mouth is followed by a simple non-muscular oesophagus, surrounded by a single row of cells with an intracellular lumen and extending about two-thirds from the anterior end. (The whole row is called a stichosome and each cell is known as a stichocyte.) The oesophagus opens into the midgut at the end of the anterior thin part of the worm. The anus is terminal. These features are typical of the class Adenophorea, which have no phasmids.

In the female the vulva opens at the junction of the oesophagus and intestine, the reproductive organs being confined to the wider posterior portion. The uterus contains about 60,000 eggs at one time.

LIFE CYCLE
The female lays about 2000–20,000 eggs 24 h^{-1}. The characteristically shaped egg is barrel-shaped with transparent terminal polar prominences with a high chitin content, and measures 57–58 µm × 26–28 µm, with an outer, brown bile-stained, shell and two inner shells (Fig. 123). The very resistant egg contains an unsegmented ovum when laid, which takes from 2 weeks to many months to develop in moist soil, depending on the ambient temperature (4–6 months at 15°C, 3–4 weeks at 26°C, 17 days at 30°C, 11 days at 35°C). Embryonated eggs are usually ingested on contaminated food, such as salad vegetables, or ingested in soil by infants. The contained second-stage larvae, measuring 260 µm × 15 µm, hatch in the distal portion of the small intestine or colon. They penetrate the crypts of Lieberkühn of the colon or caecum, where they live coiled up and after about a week move under the epithelium to the tip of the villus. The thin anterior end of each worm remains buried in a tunnel in the mucosa, while the rest emerges and hangs freely in the lumen. After the usual four moults, the females mature and lay eggs about 60–90 days after ingestion of the eggs.

The adult worms normally live for about 1–2 years where there is repeated reinfection, but can survive for much longer in some circumstances.

CLINICAL MANIFESTATIONS
In the great majority of infected individuals, only a few eggs can be found in a faecal

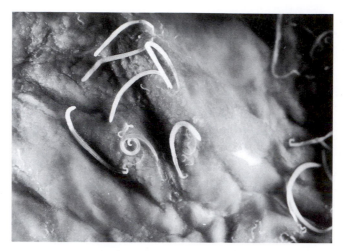

Fig. 75. Adults of *T. trichiura* in colon showing the slender anterior ends 'threaded' beneath the epithelium.

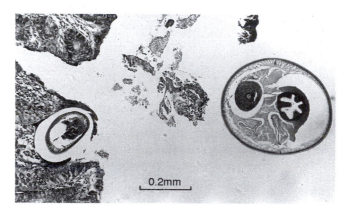

0.2mm

Fig. 76. Section of colon with adult *T. trichiura*. Note thinner anterior end embedded in mucosa.

sample and no overt symptoms can be attributed to the presence of the worms, except perhaps for diarrhoea; there is also usually an eosinophilia of up to 25% in the early stages. In heavy infections, *Trichuris* causes dysentery with blood in the stools, abdominal or epigastric pain, headache, anorexia and weight loss, with prolapse of the rectum in children (in about 30% of cases) (Plate 22). Iron-deficiency anaemia, pallor, malnutrition, stunting of growth, clubbing of fingers and poor school performance are associated with heavy chronic infections in children (Forrester *et al.*, 1990; Simeon *et al.*, 1994;

Cooper *et al.*, 1995; Ramdath *et al.*, 1995; Gardner *et al.*, 1996).

PATHOGENESIS

The anterior portions of the worms embedded in the mucosa cause petechial haemorrhages and there is evidence that the presence of *T. trichiura* predisposes to amoebic dysentery, presumably because the ulcers provide a suitable site for tissue invasion by *Entamoeba histolytica*, and it may also be involved in the spread of viral and bacterial pathogens (particularly *Shigella*). Cases have been reported in which the lumen of the appendix was filled with worms and consequent irritation and inflammation has led to appendicitis (but see p. 163) or granulomas. The mucosa of the large intestine becomes chronically inflamed, the extent depending on the number of worms present. In heavy infections there may be at least 1000 adult worms present (with about 30,000 eggs g^{-1} faeces), which can cause an insidious chronic colitis, similar to Crohn's disease, with inflammation extending to the rectum. A flexible fibre-optic colonoscope shows that the wall of the caecum and ascending colon is also hyperaemic and oedematous, with ulceration and bleeding. The bleeding might be partly due to blood ingestion by the parasites but is mainly caused by enterorrhagia. Blood loss has been estimated at about 0.005 ml per worm day^{-1}. The rectal prolapse results from straining (tenesmus) consequent on irritation and oedema of the lower colon simulating a full bowel (Plate 22).

Immune responses in humans have only recently been demonstrated; ES antigens of 16–17 kDa appear to be immunogenic in children (Needham and Lillywhite, 1994). Previously all knowledge on immunology of infection was based on *T. muris* in the mouse. In this host, parasites are rapidly expelled, with subsequent immunity to challenge infection, unlike the situation in human infection. However, predisposition to infection has been demonstrated for all the geohelminths, some individuals not becoming infected in spite of being exposed as much as those who do (Crompton, 1998). The immunology of all the intestinal nematodes is discussed on p. 122.

DIAGNOSIS
This is by finding the characteristic eggs in the faeces. In very light infections concentration techniques can be used. More than 1000 eggs in a 50 mg Kato–Katz faecal smear (20,000 eggs g^{-1} faeces) (p. 257) represents a heavy infection with overt symptoms. It has been estimated that 2000 eggs g^{-1} faeces indicates the presence of 5–15 adult worms but the relationship is not reliable. Each female worm produces about 200–370 eggs g^{-1} stool 24 h^{-1}.

In heavy infections sigmoidoscopy may show the white bodies of adult worms hanging from the inflamed mucosa – the so-called coconut-cake rectum.

TREATMENT
This is entirely by chemotherapy and, because of the sites of the adults, complete elimination used to be difficult. Recently, the newer benzimidazoles are proving to be very effective.

Albendazole is given at a single oral dose of 200 mg but for symptomatic cases should be given each day for 3 days. It is not recommended for pregnant women or infants under 1 year old (Savioli, 1999). Combined treatment with albendazole and ivermectin, as recommended for filariasis (p. 199), appears to have a synergistic effect also in trichuriasis.

Mebendazole at a single oral dose of 400–500 mg is similarly effective.

Oxantel pamoate with pyrantel (for other intestinal nematodes), at 10–15 mg kg^{-1} body weight, has the advantage that it does not cause ectopic migration of *Ascaris,* but it does require weight measurements – chemical formula: (E)-3-(2-(1,4,5,6-tetrahydro-1-methyl-2-pyrimidinyl)-ethenyl)-phenol.

Thiabendazole is unpleasant to take and not very effective and is no longer recommended.

EPIDEMIOLOGY
Trichuris infection is very common in many countries where there is heavy rainfall, dense shade and a constant temperature between 22 and 28°C.

Recent estimates of infection rates are: 25% in South and Central America, 31% in Africa (with 76% in Nigeria and 70% in Cameroon), 12% in the Middle East, 12% in southern India, 36% in Bangladesh, 58% in South-East Asia except China and 0.01% in Japan.

Fertile eggs are ingested with soil or on salad vegetables. This is similar to the mode of infection in *Ascaris* and the two worms are commonly present together. They are both particularly common where human faeces is used as a fertilizer ('night-soil'). The larvae inside the eggs develop only under moist conditions and are killed by direct sunlight or a low relative humidity. Under conditions of poor sanitation both infections are peridomestic and the areas around houses may be heavily contaminated with eggs (Plate 2) up to a depth of 20 cm; the habit of eating earth is an important reason why infants are often infected by the age of 1. In the past, infection was also common in temperate countries, even though the eggs took a long time to become infective in the soil. Infection is overdispersed with a small proportion of the infected population having a high worm burden and producing most of the eggs reaching the environment (Bundy and Medley, 1992).

Eggs of *Trichuris* were found in the rectum of the Alpine 'ice man', who lived about 5300 years ago. He also had a bag containing a fungal purgative and anthelminthic (Capasso, 1998).

PREVENTION AND CONTROL
Personal protection is by the thorough washing of salad vegetables.

Until recently, control was almost entirely by sanitary disposal of faeces, but mass chemotherapy has recently become much more practical, with the development of broad-action agents that can be used in a standard single oral dose against many intestinal helminths, and campaigns are taking place against all the soil-transmitted nematodes (see p. 135).

Sanitation measures are likely to be very slow to act. For instance, a campaign in northern Italy in the 1950–1960s took 25 years to reduce prevalence from 25 to 5% in schoolchildren. The basic reproductive rate of *Trichuris* is much higher than that of hookworms or *Ascaris,* which makes it more resistant to control. Children acquire approximately 90 new parasites per year and, in the absence of constraints, each female worm would produce four to six new egg-laying females (Bundy and Cooper, 1989).

ZOONOTIC ASPECTS
The same species occurs in monkeys and primates, such as lemurs, catarrhine monkeys and the orang-utan, but they are of no importance as reservoir hosts. The pig parasite, *T. suis* Schrank, 1788, is almost identical to the human parasite, although the eggs are stated to be slightly larger (64 μm × 30 μm). Experimental infections in humans are possible and it is likely that natural infections also occur where there is intensive pig farming. A few cases of human infection with the dog and fox whipworm, *T. vulpis* (Froelich, 1789), have been reported. Other species occur in sheep and cattle (*T. ovis*) and mice (*T. muris*) and over 70 species have been reported altogether; all from mammals.

References

Adamson, M.L. (1989) Evolutionary biology of the Oxyurida (Nematoda): biofacies of a haplodiploid taxon. *Advances in Parasitology* 28, 175–228.

Addiss, D.G. and Juranek, D.D. (1991) Lack of evidence for a causal association between parasitic infections and acute appendicitis. *Journal of Infectious Diseases* 164, 1036–1037.

Albonico, M., Crompton, D.W.T. and Savioli, L. (1998) Control strategies for human intestinal nematode infections. *Advances in Parasitology* 42, 278–343.

Al Rabia, F., Halim, M.A., Ellis, M.E. and Abdulkareem, A. (1996) *Enterobius vermicularis* and acute appendicitis. *Saudi Medical Journal* 17, 799–803.

Anderson, R.C., Chabaud, A.C. and Willmott, S. (eds) (1974–1983) *CIH Keys to the Nematode Parasites of Vertebrates,* Vols. 1–10. CAB International, Wallingford, UK.

Anderson, R.M. and Schad, G.A. (1985) Predisposition to hookworm infection in humans. *Science* 228, 1537–1540.

Anderson, T.J.C. and Jaenike, J. (1997) Host specificity, evolutionary relationships and macrogeographical differentiation among *Ascaris* populations from humans and pigs. *Parasitology* 115, 325–342.

Ashford, R.W., Barnish, G. and Viney, M.E. (1992) *Strongyloides fuelleborni kellyi*: infection and disease in Papua New Guinea. *Parasitology Today* 8, 314–318.

Blotkamp, J., Krepel, H.P., Kumar, V., Baeta, S., Van't Noordende, J.M. and Polderman, A.M. (1993) Observations on the morphology of adults and larval stages of *Oesophagostomum* sp. isolated from man in northern Togo and Ghana. *Journal of Helminthology* 67, 49–61.

Borkow, G. and Beutwich, Z. (2000) Eradication of helminthic infections may be essential for successful vaccination against HIV and tuberculosis. *Bulletin of the World Health Organization* 78, 1368–1369.

Boschetti, A. and Kasznica, J. (1995) Visceral larval migrans induced eosinophilic cardiac pseudotumour: a cause of sudden death in a child. *Journal of Forensic Sciences* 40, 1097–1099.

Bradley, M. (1990) Rate of expulsion of *Necator americanus* and the false hookworm *Ternidens deminutus* Railliet and Henry, 1909 (Nematoda) from humans following albendazole treatment. *Transactions of the Royal Society of Tropical Medicine and Hygiene* 84, 720.

Bundy, D.A.P. (1994) Immunoepidemiology of intestinal helminthic infection. 1. The global burden of intestinal nematode disease. *Transactions of the Royal Society of Tropical Medicine and Hygiene* 88, 259–261.

Bundy, D.A.P. and Cooper, E.S. (1989) *Trichuris* and trichuriasis in humans. *Advances in Parasitology* 28, 108–174.

Bundy, D.A.P. and Medley, G.F. (1992) Immunoepidemiology of human geohelminthiasis: ecological and immunological determinants of worm burden. *Parasitology* 104 (suppl.), S105–S119.

Bundy, D., Sher, A. and Michael, E. (2000) Helminth infections may increase susceptibility to TB and AIDS. *Parasitology Today* 16, 273–274.

Capasso, L. (1998) 5300 years ago the Ice Man used natural laxatives and antibiotics. *Lancet, British Edition* 352 (9143), 1864.

Chan, M.S., Medley, G.F., Jamison, D. and Bundy, D.A.P. (1994) The evaluation of potential global morbidity attributable to intestinal nematode infections. *Parasitology* 109, 373–387.

Chittenden, A.M. and Ashford, R.W. (1987) *Enterobius gregorii* Hugot, 1983: first report in the UK. *Annals of Tropical Medicine and Parasitology* 81, 195–198.

Chye, S.M., Yen, S.M. and Chen, E.R. (1997) Detection of circulating antigen by monoclonal antibodies for immunodiagnosis of angiostrongyliasis. *American Journal of Tropical Medicine and Hygiene* 56, 408–412.

Conway, D.J., Atkins, N.S., Lillywhite, J.E., Bailey, J.W., Robinson, R.D., Lindo, J.F., Bundy, D.A.P. and Bianco, A.E. (1993) Immunodiagnosis of *Strongyloides stercoralis* infection: a method for increasing the specificity of the indirect ELISA. *Transactions of the Royal Society of Tropical Medicine and Hygiene* 87, 173–176.

Conway, D.J., Lindo, J.F., Robinson, R.D. and Bundy, D.A.P. (1995) Towards effective control of *Strongyloides stercoralis*. *Parasitology Today* 11, 420–427.

Cook, G.C. (1994) *Enterobius vermicularis* infection. *Gut* 35, 1159–1162.

Cooper, E.S., Duff, E.M.W., Howell, S. and Bundy, D.A.P. (1995) 'Catch up' growth velocities after treatment for the *Trichuris* dysentery syndrome. *Transactions of the Royal Society of Tropical Medicine and Hygiene* 89, 653.

Croese, J., Loukas, A., Opdebeeck, J., Fairley, S. and Prociv, P. (1994) Human enteric infection with canine hookworms. *Annals of Internal Medicine* 120, 369–374 (also *Gasteroenterology* 106, 3–12).

Crompton, D.W.T. (1998) Gastrointestinal nematodes. In: Cox, F.E.G., Kreier, J.P. and Wakelin, D. (eds) *Topley and Wilson's Microbiology and Microbial Infections. Vol. 5. Parasitology*, 9th edn. Arnold, London, UK, pp. 561–584. .

Crompton, D.W.T. (2000) *Ascaris* and ascariasis. *Advances in Parasitology* 48, 286–376.

Crompton, D.W.T., Nesheim, M.C. and Pawlowski, Z.S. (1989) *Ascariasis and its Prevention and Control*. Taylor and Francis, London, UK.

Cross, J.H. (1987) Public health importance of *Angiostrongylus cantonensis* and its relatives. *Parasitology Today* 3, 367–369.

Cunningham, C.K., Kazacos, K.R., McMillan, J.A., Lucas, J.A., McAuley, J.B., Wozniak, E.J. and Weiner, L.B. (1994) Diagnosis and management of *Baylisascaris procyonis* infection in an infant, with nonfatal meningoencephalitis. *Clinical Infectious Diseases* 18, 868–872.

de Aguilar Nasumento, J.E., Silva, G.M., Tadano, T., Valadores Filho, M., Akiyama, A.M.P. and Castelo, A. (1993) Infection of the soft tissue of the neck due to *Lagochilascaris minor*. *Transactions of the Royal Society of Tropical Medicine and Hygiene* 87, 198.

Dorfman, S., Talbot, I.C., Torres, R., Cardozo, J. and Sanchez, M. (1995) Parasitic infestation in acute appendicitis. *Annals of Tropical Medicine and Parasitology* 89, 99–101.

Forrester, J.E., Scott, M.E., Bundy, D.A.P. and Golden, M.H.N. (1990) Predisposition of individuals and families in Mexico to heavy infection with *Ascaris lumbricoides* and *Trichuris trichiura*. *Transactions of the Royal Society of Tropical Medicine and Hygiene* 84, 272–276.

Garcia, M., Moneo, I., Audicana, M.T., del Pozo, M.D., Munoz, D., Fernandez, E., Diez, J., Etxenagusia, M.A., Ansotegni, I.J. and de Corres, L.F. (1997) The use of IgE immunoblotting as a diagnostic tool in *Anisakis simplex* allergy. *Journal of Allergy and Clinical Immunology* 99, 497–501.

Gardiner, C.H., Koh, D.S. and Cardella, T.A. (1981) *Micronema* in man: third fatal infection. *American Journal of Tropical Medicine and Hygiene* 30, 586–589.

Gardner, J.M., Grantham-McGregor, S., Baddeley, A. and Meeks-Gardner, J. (1996) *Trichuris trichiura* infection and cognitive function in Jamaican schoolchildren. *Annals of Tropical Medicine and Parasitology* 90, 55–63.

Geissler, P.W., Mwaniki, D., Thiong'o, F. and Friis, H. (1998) Geophagy as a risk factor for geo-helminth infections: a longitudinal study of Kenya schoolchildren. *Transactions of the Royal Society of Tropical Medicine and Hygiene* 92, 7–11.

Genta, R.M. (1992) Dysregulation of strongyloidiasis: a new hypothesis. *Clinical Microbiology Reviews* 5, 345–355.

Gibson, D.I. (1983) Ascaridoid nematodes – a current assessment. In: Stone, A.R. and Khalil, L.F. (eds) *Concepts in Nematode Systematics*. Academic Press, London, UK, pp. 321–338.

Gillespie, S.H. (1988) The epidemiology of *Toxocara canis*. *Parasitology Today* 4, 180–182.

Gillespie, S.H. (1993) The clinical spectrum of human toxocariasis. In: Lewis, J.W. (ed.) *Toxocara and Toxocariasis: Clinical, Epidemiological and Molecular Perspectives*. Institute of Biology, London, UK, pp. 55–61.

Gillespie, S.H., Dinning, W.J., Voller, A. and Crowcroft, N.S. (1993) The spectrum of ocular toxocariasis. *Eye* 7, 415–418.

Gilman, R.H., Marquis, G.S. and Miranda, E. (1991) Prevalence and symptoms of *Enterobius vermicularis* infections in a Peruvian shanty town. *Transactions of the Royal Society of Tropical Medicine and Hygiene* 85, 761–764.

Goldsmid, J.M. (1991) The African 'hookworm' problem: an overview. In: Macpherson, C.N.L. and Craig, P.S. (eds) *Parasitic Helminths and Zoonoses in Africa*. Unwin Hyman, London, UK, pp. 101–137.

Grove, D.I. (1996) Human strongyloidiasis. *Advances in Parasitology* 38, 251–309.

Hall, A. and Holland, C. (2000) Geographical variation in *Ascaris lumbricoides* fecundity and its implication for helminth control. *Parasitology Today* 16, 540–544.

Hall, A., Conway, D.J., Anwar, K.S. and Rahman, M.D. (1994) *Strongyloides stercoralis* in an urban slum community in Bangladesh: factors independently associated with infection. *Transactions of the Royal Society of Tropical Medicine and Hygiene* 88, 527–530.

Haswell-Elkins, M.R., Elkins, D.B. and Anderson, R.M. (1987a) Evidence for predisposition in humans to infection with *Ascaris*, hookworm, *Enterobius* and *Trichuris* in a South Indian fishing community. *Parasitology* 95, 323–338.

Haswell-Elkins, M.R., Elkins, D.B., Manjula, K., Michael, E. and Anderson, R.M. (1987b) The distribution and abundance of *Enterobius vermicularis* in a South Indian fishing community. *Parasitology* 95, 339–354.

Hotez, P.J. and Prichard, D.I. (1995) Hookworm infection. *Scientific American* 272, 42–48.

Hugot, J.P. and Tourte-Schaefer, C. (1985) Etude morphologique des deux oxyures parasites de l'homme: *Enterobius vermicularis* et *E. gregorii*. *Annales de Parasitologie Humaine et Comparée* 60, 57–64.

Ishikura, H., Kikuchi, K., Nagasawa, K., Ooiwa, T., Takamiya, H., Sato, N. and Sugane, K. (1992) Anisakidae and anisakidosis. In: *Progress in Clinical Parasitology*, Vol. 3. Springer Verlag, New York, USA, pp. 43–102.

Jelinek, T., Maiwald, H., Nothdurft, H.D. and Loscher, T. (1994) Cutaneous larva migrans in travellers: synopsis of histories, symptoms and treatment of 98 patients. *Clinical Infectious Diseases* 19, 1062–1066.

Kagei, N. and Isogaki, H. (1992) A case of abdominal syndrome caused by the presence of a large number of *Anisakis* larvae. *International Journal for Parasitology* 22, 251–253.

Kayes, S.G. (1997) Human toxocariasis and the visceral larval migrans syndrome: correlative immunopathology. In: Freedman, D.O. (ed.) *Chemical Immunology,* Vol. 66. S. Karger, Basle, pp. 99–124.

Kazacos, K.R. (1983) *Raccoon Roundworms (*Baylisascaris procyonis*): a Cause of Animal and Human Disease.* Bulletin No. 422, Agriculture Experimental Station, Purdue University, West Lafayette, USA.

Kliks, M.M. and Palumbo, N.E. (1992) Eosinophilic meningitis beyond the Pacific basin: the global dispersal of a peridomestic zoonosis caused by *Angiostrongylus cantonensis,* the nematode lung-worm of rats. *Social Science and Medicine* 34, 199–212.

Mangali, A., Chaicumpa, W., Nontasut, P., Chantavanij, P. and Viravan, C. (1991) Enzyme-linked immunosorbent assay for diagnosis of human strongyloidiasis. *Southeast Asian Journal of Tropical Medicine and Public Health* 22, 88–92.

Marti, H., Haji, H.J., Savioli, L., Chwaya, H.M., Mgeni, A.F., Ameir, J.S. and Hatz, C. (1996) A comparative trial of a single-dose ivermectin versus three days of albendazole for treatment of *Strongyloides stercoralis* and other soil-transmitted helminth infections in children. *American Journal of Tropical Medicine and Hygiene* 55, 477–481.

Mizgajska, H. (1993) The distribution and survival of eggs of *Ascaris suum* in six different natural soil profiles. *Acta Parasitologia* 38, 170–174.

Morera, P. (1994) Importance of abdominal angiostrongylosis in the Americas. In: Özcel, M.A. and Alkan, M.Z. (eds) *Parasitology for the 21st Century.* CAB International, Wallingford, UK, pp. 253–260.

Muller, R. (1983) *Ancylostoma, Necator* and ancylostomiasis. In: Feachem, R.G., Bradley, D.J., Garelick, H. and Mora, D.D. (eds) *Sanitation and Disease: Health Aspects of Excreta and Wastewater Management.* John Wiley & Sons, Chichester, UK, pp. 359–373.

Murrell, K.D., Eriksen, L., Nansen, P., Slotred, H.C. and Rasmussen, T. (1997) *Ascaris suum*: a revision of its early migratory path and implications for human ascariasis. *Journal of Parasitology* 83, 255–260.

Needham, C.S. and Lillywhite, J.E. (1994) Immunoepidemiology of intestinal helminthic infections. 2. Immunological correlates with patterns of *Trichuris* infection. *Transactions of the Royal Society of Tropical Medicine and Hygiene* 88, 262–264.

Pawlowski, Z.S., Schad, G.A. and Stott, G.J. (1991) *Hookworm Infection and Anaemia: Approaches to Prevention and Control.* World Health Organization, Geneva, Switzerland.

Peng Weidong, Zhou Xianmin and Crompton, D.W.T. (1998) Ascariasis in China. *Advances in Parasitology* 41, 109–148.

Petithory, J.C., Pangam, B., Buyet-Rousset, P. and Pangam, A. (1990) *Anisakis simplex,* a co-factor of gastric cancer? *Lancet* 336, 1002.

Phelps, K.R. and Neva, F.A. (1993) *Strongyloides* hyperinfection in patients coinfected with HTLV-I and *Strongyloides stercoralis. American Journal of Medicine* 94, 447–449.

Pit, D.S.S., de Graaf, W., Snoek, H., de Vlas, S.J., Baeta, S.M. and Polderman, A.M. (1999) Diagnosis of *Oesophagostomum bifurcum* and hookworm infection in humans: day-to-day and within-specimen variation of larval counts. *Parasitology* 118, 283–288.

Polderman, A.M. and Blotkamp, J. (1995) *Oesophagostomum* infections in humans. *Parasitology Today* 11, 541–456.

Polderman, A.M., Krepel, H.P., Baeta, S., Blotkamp, J. and Gigase, P. (1991) Oesophagostomiasis, a common infection of man in Northern Togo and Ghana. *American Journal of Tropical Medicine and Hygiene* 44, 336–344.

Polderman, A.M., Krepel, H.P., Verweij, J.J., Baeta, S. and Rotmans, J.P. (1993) Serological diagnosis of *Oesophagostomum* infections. *Transactions of the Royal Society of Tropical Medicine and Hygiene* 87, 433–435.

Polderman, A.M., Anemana, S.D. and Asigri, V. (1999) Human oesophagostomiasis; a regional public health problem in Africa. *Parasitology Today* 15, 129–130.

Prichard, D.I. (1993) Immunity to helminths: is too much IgE parasite- rather than host-protective? *Parasite Immunology* 15, 5–9.

Prociv, P. (1989) *Toxocara pteropodis* and visceral larva migrans. *Parasitology Today* 5, 106–109.

Prociv, P. and Croese, J. (1996) Human enteric infection with *Ancylostoma caninum*: hookworms reappraised in the light of a 'new' zoonosis. *Acta Tropica* 62, 23–44.

Prociv, P., Spratt, D.M. and Carlisle, M.S. (2000) Neuro-angiostrongyliosis: unresolved issues. *International Journal for Parasitology* 30, 1295–1303.

Ramdath, D.D., Simeon, D., Wong, M.S. and Grantham-McGregor, S.M. (1995) Iron status of school-children with varying intensities of *Trichuris trichiura* infection. *Parasitology* 110, 347–351.

Ross, R.A., Gibson, D.J. and Harris, E.A. (1989) Cutaneous oesophagostomiasis in man. *Journal of Helminthology* 63, 261–265.

Sakti, H., Nokes, C., Hertanto,W.S., Hendratno, S., Hall, A., Bundy, D.A.P. and Satoto (1999) Evidence of an association between hookworm infection and cognitive function in Indonesian school children. *Tropical Medicine and International Health* 4, 322–334.

Sato, Y., Toma, H., Kiyuna, S. and Shiloma, Y. (1991) Gelatin particle indirect agglutination test for mass examination for strongyloidiasis. *Transactions of the Royal Society for Tropical Medicine and Hygiene* 85, 515–518.

Savioli, L. (1999) Treatment of *Trichuris* infection with albendazole. *Lancet (British edition)* 353 (9148), 237.

Simeon, D., Callender, J., Wong, M., Grantham-McGregor, S.M. and Ramdath, D.D. (1994) School performance, nutritional status and trichuriasis in Jamaican school children. *Acta Pediatrica* 83, 1188–1193.

Sohn, W.M. and Seol, S.Y. (1994) A human case of gastric anisakiasis by *Pseudoterranova decipiens* larva. *Korean Journal of Parasitology* 32, 53–56.

Sugane, K., Sin, S. and Matsuura, T. (1992) Molecular cloning of the cDNA encoding a 42 kDa antigenic polypeptide of *Anisakis simplex* larvae. *Journal of Helminthology* 66, 25–32.

Sun, T., Schwartz, N.S., Sewell, C., Lieberman, P. and Gross, S. (1991) *Enterobius* egg granuloma of the vulva and peritoneum: review of the literature. *American Journal of Tropical Medicine and Hygiene* 45, 249–253.

Thien Hlang (1993) Ascariasis and childhood malnutrition. *Parasitology* 107, S125–S136.

Udonsi, J.K. and Atata, G. (1987) *Necator americanus*: temperature, pH, light, and larval development, longevity, and desiccation tolerance. *Experimental Parasitology* 63, 136–142.

Wakelin, D. (1994) Host populations: genetics and immunity. In: Scott, M.E. and Smith, G. (eds) *Parasitic and Infectious Diseases*. Academic Press, London, UK, pp. 83–100.

Wakelin, D. (1996) *Immunity to Parasites: How Parasitic Infections are Controlled*. Cambridge University Press, Cambridge, UK.

Wariyapola, D., Goonesinghe, N., Priyamanna, T.H.H., Fonseka, C., Ismail, M.M., Abeyewickreme, W. and Dissanaike, A.S. (1998) Second case of ocular parastrongyliasis from Sri Lanka. *Transactions of the Royal Society of Tropical Medicine and Hygiene* 92, 64–65.

Xingquan, Z., Chilton, N.B., Jacobs, D.E., Boes, J. and Gasser, R.B. (1999) Characterisation of *Ascaris* from human and pig hosts by nuclear ribosomal DNA sequences. *International Journal for Parasitology* 29, 469–478.

Zhou Xianmin, Peng Weidong, Crompton, D.W.T. and Xing Jianquin (1999) Treatment of biliary ascariasis in China. *Transactions of the Royal Society of Tropical Medicine and Hygiene* 93, 561–564.

Further Reading

Bundy, D.A.P., Chan, M.S., Medley, C.F., Jamison, D. and Savioli, L. (2001) Intestinal nematode infections. In: Murray, C.J.L. and Lopez, A.D. (eds) *The Global Epidemiology of Infectious Diseases*. Harvard University Press, Cambridge, Massachusetts, USA (in press).

Farthing, M.J.G., Keusch, G.T. and Wakelin, D. (eds) (1995) *Enteric Infections 2: Intestinal Helminths*. Chapman and Hall, London, UK.

Gilles, H.M. and Ball, P.A. (eds) (1991) *Hookworm Infections. Human Parasitic Diseases*, Vol. 4. Elsevier, Amsterdam, The Netherlands.

Grove, D.I. (ed.) (1989) *Strongyloidiasis: a Major Roundworm of Man*. Taylor and Francis, London, UK.

Holland, C. (1987) Neglected infections – trichuriasis and strongyloidiasis. In: Stephenson, L.S. (ed.) *Impact of Helminth Infections on Human Nutrition*. Taylor and Francis, London, UK, pp. 161–201.

Miller, T.A. (1979) Hookworm infection in man. *Advances in Parasitology* 17, 315–384.

Sakanari, J.A. and McKerrow, J.H. (1989) Anisakiasis. *Clinical Microbiology Reviews* 2, 278–284.

Schad, G.A. and Warren, K.S. (eds) (1990) *Hookworm Disease: Current Status and New Directions*. Taylor and Francis, London, UK.

Tissue Nematodes

All the nematodes considered in this section invade the tissues of the host, including those of the intestine, and have a life cycle involving an intermediate host. Members of the first group, including *Trichinella*, are only distantly related to all the rest and have vertebrate intermediate hosts, in contrast to the others where these are always arthropods and all of which belong to the order Spirurida.

Order Enoplida

Family Trichuridae

Aonchotheca philippinensis
(Chitwood, Velasquez and Salazar, 1968)
Moravec, 1982

SYNONYM
Capillaria   philippinensis   Chitwood,
Velasquez and Salazar 1968.

DISEASE AND COMMON NAME
Intestinal capillariasis or capillariosis; a cause of non-vibrio cholera.

GEOGRAPHICAL DISTRIBUTION
This parasite was first described 30 years ago from villages bordering the China Sea on the west coast of the island of Luzon in the Philippines. It has been reported since from the islands of Bohol, Mindanao and Leyte. Numerous cases have also been found in Thailand and others from Egypt, India, Indonesia, Iran, Japan and South Korea.

LOCATION IN HOST
The adults become embedded in the mucosa of the small intestine, especially the jejunum.

MORPHOLOGY
Aonchotheca is related to *Trichinella* and *Trichuris* and there are many species of capillarids that are parasites of a wide range of vertebrates. The adult worms are very small, females measuring 2.5–5.3 mm in length and males 1.3–3.9 mm. In the female, the vulval opening is just behind the oesophagus and the male has a single very long spicule in a sheath. Both sexes have a small spear at the anterior end.

LIFE CYCLE
The life cycle has been determined experimentally in monkeys and Mongolian jirds. Freshwater fishes indigenous to the Philippines were fed eggs from patients embryonated for 5–10 days in water. Larvae hatched in the intestines of the fish and reached the infective stage in about 3 weeks but could live for months; larvae developed into adults in 12–14 days when fed to monkeys or jirds.

Following copulation and fertilization, the females produce larvae. The first-generation larvae are retained and develop into second-generation males and females in another 2 weeks. The second-generation females produce eggs passed out in the faeces about 26 days after fertilization.

Autoinfection occurs in jirds and almost certainly in humans, as all stages of development, including viviparous and larviparous females, have been found at autopsy. In one experiment, two larvae from fish produced 5353 worms in a jird.

Several species of freshwater and brackish-water fish have been experimentally infected; *Hypeleotris bipartita*, *Ambassis miops* and *Eleotris melanosoma* are often eaten raw in the Philippines and *Cyprinus carpio* in Thailand.

The natural definitive hosts are probably fish-eating birds, which can be infected experimentally and one bittern has been found naturally infected.

CLINICAL MANIFESTATIONS
In the initial epidemic in 1967, when over 100 people died, all patients with eggs in the faeces had intermittent diarrhoea, with borborygmi and diffuse recurrent abdominal pain. The syndrome resembled tropical sprue, with five to ten voluminous stools per day. Weight loss, anorexia and vomiting were common. Patients who recovered from the initial attack usually suffered several relapses and, in a study conducted 3

years after the initial epidemic, patients who were still symptomatic were found to have depression of the D-xylose test and impairment of fat and protein digestion and absorption. A mortality rate of 35% in untreated males and 19% in untreated females was reported from one village in the initial epidemic.

Nowadays, only the early symptoms of borborygmi, diarrhoea and abdominal pain are present before treatment is sought.

PATHOGENESIS

The stools contain large amounts of fat, protein and minerals, particularly potassium, which results in a marked protein-losing enteropathy. Malabsorption also occurs. Muscle wasting, emaciation, weakness and cardiopathy were reported from 73% of early patients. Without treatment, death often ensues 2 weeks to 2 months after the onset of symptoms, due to cardiac failure or to intercurrent infection.

Necropsy studies on ten Philippinos showed the presence of adults and larvae embedded in the mucosa of the jejunum, together with numerous eggs (Fig. 77).

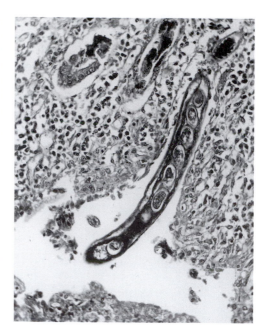

Fig. 77. Section of ileum with female *Aonchotheca* (cut tangentially) invading the villi and containing many unembryonated thick-shelled eggs in the vagina. A section of the same worm above shows a portion of the stichosome and oesophagus.

DIAGNOSIS

Clinical. The early symptoms are typical and easily recognized.

Parasitological. Eggs, larvae and adults may be found in the faeces. Eggs measure 36–45 μm and have a flattened bipolar plug at each end (Fig. 124). They could be mistaken for the eggs of *Trichuris* but differ in having a pitted shell, a more ovoid shape, a slightly smaller size and no protuberance of the plugs. Some eggs may contain larvae. The eggs of both parasites may be found together in the faeces.

Serological. ELISA, double diffusion and indirect haemagglutination assay (IHA) have been tried but are not satisfactory.

TREATMENT

Mebendazole at 400 mg day^{-1} in divided doses for 20–30 days is the current drug of choice. If treatment is curtailed there is likely to be a relapse, since larvae may not be affected and there is multiplication within the host.

Albendazole: In the few patients treated this drug appears to affect larvae as well as adults at a dose of 200 mg twice daily for 14–21 days and may be more effective.

Thiabendazole can be given at 25 mg kg^{-1} body weight day^{-1} for at least a month, but relapses are common.

EPIDEMIOLOGY

Raw fish are a popular item of diet in the Philippines and Thailand and were implicated in the cases in Japan and Iran.

Presumably infection could be prevented by thorough cooking of fish or even by removing the intestines.

Capillarid eggs passed over a period by a patient in Irian Jaya differed in size from those of all the species considered here (Bangs *et al.*, 1994).

Calodium hepaticum
(Bancroft, 1893) Moravec, 1982

SYNONYMS
Trichocephalus hepaticus Bancroft, 1893; *Hepaticola hepatica* (Bancroft, 1893) Hall, 1916; *Capillaria hepatica* (Bancroft, 1893) Travassos, 1915.

DISEASE AND POPULAR NAMES
Hepatic capillariasis or capillariosis; the capillary liver worm.

GEOGRAPHICAL DISTRIBUTION
About 25 human cases have been reported from many countries, including Brazil, England, Germany, India, Italy, South Korea, Mexico, Nigeria, Slovakia, South Africa, Turkey, continental USA and Hawaii. *C. hepaticum* is a natural parasite of the liver tissues of rats, mice, prairie dogs, muskrats, beavers, hares and monkeys.

CLINICAL MANIFESTATIONS AND PATHOGENESIS
Female worms measure about 70 mm long by 0.12 mm wide, males 22 mm by 0.05 mm. The anterior portion of the worm contains the stichosome, oesophagus and bacillary bands, the posteror part the intestine and reproductive organs. Eggs measure 48–66 µm × 28–38 µm (larger than those of *Trichuris*) and are thick-shelled, with surface pits and bipolar caps that do not protrude. The adults live in the liver parenchyma. The females lay eggs in the tissues and these accumulate and form large whitish spots under the liver surface. The eggs do not pass out in the faeces but reach the soil after the death of the host or after the host is eaten by another and the eggs are passed in the faeces.

Clinical symptoms resemble those of visceral larva migrans, with an initial hepatitis. The liver is tender and enlarged, with persistent fever, anorexia, weight loss and a very high (over 90%) eosinophilia. There is focal destruction of parenchyma and fibrosis in chronic infections.

Diagnosis is by needle liver biopsy or usually at post-mortem. The presence of eggs in the faeces is evidence of a spurious infection from eating an infected animal liver. A recent case was treated successfully with albendazole at 10–20 mg kg^{-1} body weight day^{-1} for 20 days and then thiabendazole at 25 mg kg^{-1} day^{-1} for 27 days, although hepatomegaly was still present 2 years later (Choe *et al.*, 1993). Most infections have been in children and a recent case in a 14-month-old girl was treated. Eggs are presumably ingested in vegetables or on soil after passing through the gut of a predator.

Eucoleus aerophilus
(Creplin, 1839) Dujardin, 1845

SYNONYM AND DISEASE
Capillaria aerophila Creplin, 1839. Pulmonary capillariasis or capillariosis.

CLINICAL MANIFESTATIONS AND PATHOGENESIS
This is a worldwide parasite of wild carnivores and 11 human cases have been reported from France, Iran, Morocco and Russia. Adults live buried under the mucosa of the respiratory tract, the female measuring 20 mm × 0.1 mm and the male 18 mm × 0.07 mm. Eggs reach the intestine from the lungs and are passed out in the faeces. Infection is common in dogs in the USA but this might be a separate species (*E. boehmi*).

Clinical symptoms include a painful dry cough, fever, dyspnoea and acute tracheobronchitis. There is some eosinophilia. In one biopsy there were numerous small granulomatous lesions in the wall of a small bronchus. Ivermectin at 200 µg kg^{-1} has had encouraging results and repeated doses of thiabendazole have been tried.

Three cases of ***Anatrichosoma cutaneum*** (Swift, Boots and Miles, 1922) Chitwood and Smith, 1956, a parasite of the rhesus monkey, have been reported from humans in Japan, Malaysia (Marwi *et al.*, 1990) and Vietnam. Adults and eggs are found in lesions in the skin. Eggs removed from the facial skin were similar to those of *Trichuris* but larger (59 µm × 28 µm).

Family Trichinellidae

Trichinella spiralis
(Owen, 1835) Railliet, 1895

SYNONYM
Trichina spiralis Owen, 1835.

DISEASE AND POPULAR NAME
Trichiniasis or trichinellosis, trichinosis; trichina worm infection.

GEOGRAPHICAL DISTRIBUTION
Infection with *Trichinella* species is worldwide in carnivorous or scavenging animals but is particularly important in humans in Alaska and Canada in Inuit, Chile, eastern Europe, Kenya and Russia. Other endemic areas include Central and South America (including the Caribbean), central and western Europe, China, Indonesia, Japan, New Zealand, the Pacific area (particularly Hawaii) and the Aleutians.

LOCATION IN HOST
The short-lived adults are partially embedded in the mucosa of the ileum. The larvae are present in cysts in all the striated muscles.

MORPHOLOGY
The adults are minute, threadlike worms, the females measuring 2.8 (2.4–3.4) mm × 0.06 mm and the males 1.5 (1.3–1.6) mm × 0.03 mm. Both sexes are wider posteriorly than anteriorly. The oesophagus differs from that of all other animal-parasitic nematodes (apart from *Trichuris* and capillarids), as its posterior part is non-muscular but is surrounded by a column of cuboidal cells, known as a stichosome or cell body (Zellenkörper), with an intracellular canal. The oesophagus connects with a thin-walled intestine, which ends in a terminal anus. The male has two copulatory appendages at the posterior end but no spicules. The reproductive system of the female consists of a single ovary, oviduct, seminal receptacle, uterus, vagina and vulva. *Trichinella* is ovoviviparous, so that in the mature female the uterus is filled with larvae (Figs 78–80).

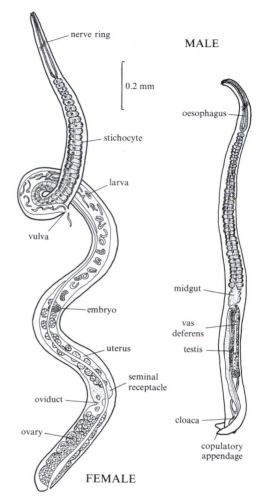

Fig. 78. Adult female and male of *Trichinella spiralis*.

LIFE CYCLE
The muscle cysts containing larvae are ingested in raw or semi-cooked meat. The cyst wall is digested out in the stomach and the larvae emerge in the duodenum. The released first-stage larvae invade the mucosa of the duodenum and jejunum and undergo four moults. The immature worms emerge into the lumen of the intestine 22–24 h after ingestion of cysts and, in mice, fertilized females have been observed at 30 h. In most experimental hosts, approximately twice as many females as males are present and both sexes re-enter

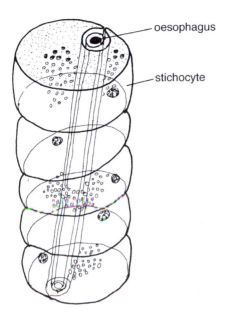

oesophagus

stichocyte

Fig. 79. Portion of the stichosome of *T. spiralis*.

the mucosa. The female begins to produce first-stage larvae (measuring 80–129 μm × 5–6 μm) approximately 5 days after ingestion of cysts. Each female produces 200–2000 larvae during its lifetime. The larvae are deposited in the mucosa and reach the active skeletal muscles, travelling by the lymphatics and blood-vessels. After reaching the muscles and penetrating the sarcolemma with the help of a stylet, the larvae grow, measuring about 1 mm in length 17–20 days after infection. The sexes can be differentiated at this time. The larvae coil and by 17–21 days after infection are capable of transmission to a new host, as they can resist the action of digestive juices. The normal lifespan of the female worms in the intestine of humans is not known but from autopsy studies appears to be less than 2 months.

From the point of view of the parasite, humans are dead-end hosts. Transmission normally takes place from one flesh-eating animal (including carrion eaters) to another, often of the same species, as with rats and mice.

CLINICAL MANIFESTATIONS

The first signs and symptoms can be caused by the development of the adults and production of larvae in the intestine; in heavy infections they can be protean and infection is often misdiagnosed. With about 1000 larvae g^{-1} muscle tissue, there may be a sudden onset of illness, with nausea, vomiting, epigastric pain and severe watery diarrhoea, followed by pyrexia (38–40°C), myalgias, facial or generalized

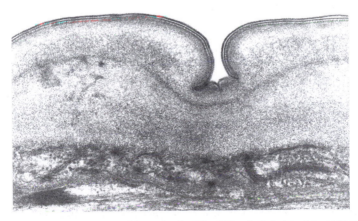

Fig. 80. An electron micrograph of the cuticle and epicuticle of *T. spiralis* (original magnification × 82,000).

oedema (Plate 23) and urticarial manifestations. There are also likely to be cardiovascular, renal and central nervous system symptoms. Eosinophilia is often the first clinical sign and becomes apparent about 10 days after infection, reaching a maximum (usually 25–50%, but may be as high as 90% with 4000 eosinophils mm^{-3}) during the 3rd or 4th week, and slowly diminishing over a period of months. There is also some degree of leucocytosis. When only a few cysts are ingested, these may be the only signs and symptoms, and the majority of cases of trichiniasis are diagnosed only at routine autopsy.

Larvae in the muscles can cause many effects (Fig. 81). Transient cardiac manifestations (feeble pulse, cardiac dilatation and apical systolic murmur and palpitations), various nervous system manifestations (meningitis or meningoencephalitis, hemiplegia, coma and neuritis with muscular paralysis) and pulmonary manifestations (effort dyspnoea, cough, hoarseness, bronchopneunomia, chest pain and pulmonary oedema) are all possible (Capo and Despommier, 1996). Ocular signs and symptoms occur in over one-third of clinical cases and characteristically include orbital oedema and waxy yellow chemosis of the bulbar conjunctiva, with photophobia and blurred vision. Scleral or retinal haemorrhages with pain on pressure or movement of the eyes and diplopia may also occur.

Flame-shaped splinter haemorrhages under the fingernails are sometimes seen and are almost diagnostic.

About 90% of infections are light, with fewer than ten larvae g^{-1} of muscle. One of the heaviest infections known was a fatal one in a young boy in East Africa, who had over 5000 cysts g^{-1} of tongue muscle and 6530 cysts g^{-1} in another boy (see *T. nelsoni* below). With massive infections like this, there is a greater volume of cyst substance than of muscle fibre. However, death may result with as few as 100 cysts g^{-1}, the severity of the reaction probably being more important than the number of larvae present. In very heavy infections, death is more likely between the 4th and 8th weeks, from exhaustion, pneumonia or cardiac failure.

Some infections in Inuit in northern Canada and Alaska from eating raw walrus or seal show atypical symptoms of prolonged diarrhoea, with no fever or oedema, short myalgia, but a high eosinophilia (this is caused by *T. nativa* – see below); this possibly occurs in patients who have been previously infected (infections are likely to

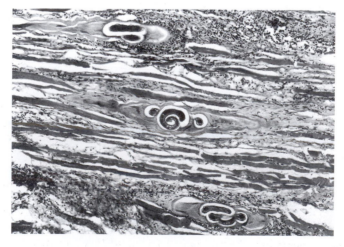

Fig. 81. Section of skeletal muscle with cysts of *Trichinella* and interstitial inflammatory cells between the muscle cells. From a fatal case with severe myositis (original magnification × 65).

be high since they are almost entirely meat eaters).

There is usually eventual complete recovery in most patients, but muscular pain (in 60% of sufferers), fatigue (in 52%) and cardiovascular pains may persist for 1–6 years. The presence of two cysts per gram of muscle is likely to result in mild clinical symptoms.

A few cases are recorded where death has occurred about 10 days after infection owing to the action of the stages in the intestine.

PATHOGENESIS

In the early stages the mucosa of the digestive tract may be hyperaemic, with inflammation consisting of eosinophils, neutrophils and lymphocytes and petechial haemorrhages at the site of attachment. Antigen–antibody complexes form in the tissues and are probably involved in the occasional severe gut reactions found in heavy infections (antibodies are produced particularly to the stichocyte contents).

Most of the important pathology is due to the larval stages in the muscles. These cause myositis, which makes the muscle tougher than normal, and there may also be contractures. The extraocular muscles, masseter, muscles of the tongue and larynx, diaphragm, muscles of the neck, intercostal muscles, deltoid muscles and sites of attachment to tendons and joints are most often involved.

Larvae that invade other organs may be responsible for more specific pathology, as shown below.

Heart. Larvae often invade the myocardium but cardiac muscle cannot form nurse cells and cysts are never found. At autopsy of fatal cases, the myocardium is usually soft and flabby and there may be fatty degeneration.

Nervous system. Migratory larvae are often present in the cerebrospinal fluid and meninges and the brain substance becomes oedematous and hyperaemic. There may also be many punctate haemorrhages. Microscopic nodules, with a clear area of necrosis around each parasite are found in the subcortical white matter.

Lungs. There may be oedema, disseminated haemorrhages and eosinophilic abscesses surrounding larvae, indicative of an allergic response.

In general many more migrating larvae are destroyed in humans than in experimental animals and this is accompanied by more pronounced inflammatory changes.

Histopathology of muscle stages. Within 2 days of larval invasion, the muscle fibres lose their cross-striations and become more basophilic. The fibres are changed biochemically and become oedematous and swell. About 17 days postinfection, the remains of the muscle fibres become more dense and apparently help to form 'Nevinny's basophilic halo' surrounding each larva. This halo area is actually fluid and contains proliferating, enlarged and altered nuclei. The redifferentiation changes in the muscle fibres near each larva, with an increase in nuclear numbers and in mitochondria and with enlargement of the Golgi apparatus, are followed by an inflammatory response, with invasion by lymphocytes, polymorphs and histiocytes. The larvae become progressively encapsulated and the oedema subsides by the 5th week.

The outer homogeneous capsule that surrounds each larva is derived from the sarcolemma. It is usually translucent and is probably composed of collagen. The size of the cysts formed varies with the host and with the muscle involved. In humans, the cysts measure on average 0.4 mm × 0.26 mm. There is usually only one larva per cyst, but two may be present and infrequently even more. The *Trichinella* larvae in the cyst may live for years but the cyst walls usually calcify a few months or years after infection (Fig. 82).

The cysts in meat are very resistant and the larvae can probably remain viable until decomposition occurs (at least 10 days). They have large glycogen reserves and an anaerobic type of respiration.

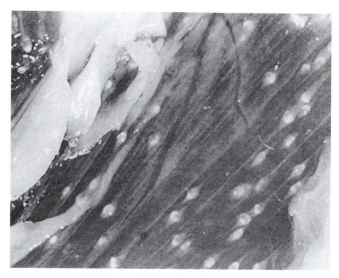

Fig. 82. Calcified cysts seen in the voluntary muscles of a silver fox.

Trichinella down-regulates the host immune response by antigen-dependent mechanisms (molecular mimicry, antigen shedding and renewal, anatomical seclusion of the larvae in the cysts and stage specificity) and by immunomodulation (Bruschi, 1999).

DIAGNOSIS

Clinical. Blood eosinophilia is usually the earliest sign and almost invariably has appeared by the 10th day of infection; the level can be extremely high (90%). It usually continues to rise for 2–5 weeks, remains stable for a further few weeks and slowly falls by the 9th week. The combination of eosinophilia, orbital oedema, muscle pain, fever and gastrointestinal disturbances following ingestion of pork is very suggestive. None the less, trichiniasis is often misdiagnosed as typhoid fever or influenza.

Parasitological. Occasionally adults and larvae can be seen in the stools and larvae in the blood during the 2nd to 4th weeks after infection. More certain is the recovery of larvae by muscle biopsy. A sample of 1 g of biceps or gastrocnemius is sufficient for compression of one half (Fig. 83) and sec-

tioning and staining of the other. The best time for obtaining a positive biopsy specimen is after the 4th week – rather late for chemotherapy aimed at killing the adult worms to be of much use. Digestion of pooled muscle samples is of use in epidemiological surveys of prevalence in animals or in autopsy material. It is carried out for 30 min in 1% pepsin in saline containing 1% HCl at 37°C and the freed larvae are examined under the lower power of the microscope.

Immunological. Because of the difficulties of parasitological diagnosis, particularly in the early stages, immunological methods are more important for individual diagnosis than in most other helminth infections.

Antibodies can be detected by an ELISA as early as 12 days after infection (Ljungstrom, 1983) and there is a commercial kit available, or by Western blotting of a characterized fraction of sonicated larvae in an immunoglobulin G (IgG) ELISA with a molecular mass of 109 kDa, reacted with specific antibodies (Chan and Ko, 1990). Recently the use of recombinant antigens (with an excretory/secretory (ES) antigen of 53 kDa) and of DNA probes has given encouraging results in trials.

larva

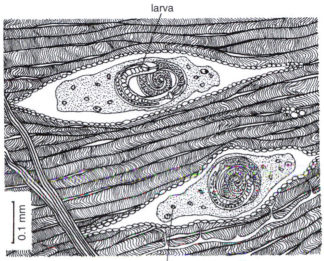

remnant of degenerated muscle fibre

Fig. 83. Cysts of *Trichinella* as seen in muscle squash.

TREATMENT

Albendazole (at 14 mg kg^{-1} or 400–800 mg daily for 3–8 days), albendazole sulphoxide or mebendazole (200 mg daily for 5 days) are effective in removing adult worms from the small intestine but unfortunately diagnosis is not usually made before the majority of larvae have already been produced and moved to the muscles (3–5 weeks after infection). Thiabendazole (at 25–45 mg kg^{-1} for 5–6 days) is equally effective but has more side-effects. Pyrantel pamoate at 5 mg day^{-1} for 5 days has also been used successfully.

Massive doses of corticosteroids (e.g. 40–60 mg daily of prednisolone, 200 units of adrenocorticotrophic hormone (ACTH) or 25 mg of cortisone, four times daily for 4–5 weeks) have been given to relieve the effects of the allergic response to the muscle phase but are most important for relieving neurological manifestations. Anthelminthics should always be given first, as corticosteroids could prolong the presence of adult worms in the intestine.

EPIDEMIOLOGY

Some estimates of prevalences are: Belarus 0.06%, Chile 0.26% (1989–1995), Bolivia 3.0% (locally by ELISA: this is a new endemic area), Lithuania 0.02% and Poland 0.03%. Infection is spreading in Belarus, Bulgaria, China (Yunnan Province), Lithuania, Romania, Russia, Ukraine (ten cases year^{-1} between 1984 and 1996), former Yugoslavian countries (there was an outbreak in Bosnia in 1996) and northern Canada. There have been recent epidemics in France (there were 538 cases in 1993 from a horse imported from Canada) and Italy from eating raw horsemeat; the horses had probably been fed on animal products. A recent outbreak in Lebanon was caused by eating 'kubeniye', a local uncooked pork dish, at New Year and a source in China is from eating undercooked pork dumplings. Infection is common in pigs in some countries: 11% in Bolivia, up to 2% in Chile, up to 57% in China, 4% in Costa Rica, up to 22% in Croatia, 4% in Egypt, up to 30% in Mexico, 7% in Nigeria and up to 4% in Poland (Murrell and Bruschi, 1994).

While various strains of *Trichinella* have been recognized for many years based on infectivity to domestic or wild animals (Fig. 84), recent studies based on biological, biochemical and genetic data of 300 geographical isolates indicate that there are five separate species (Pozio *et al.*, 1992; Kapel *et al.*, 1998), although more conservative authorities (e.g. Bessonov, 1998) believe that there are only the two generally agreed (*T. spiralis* and *T. pseudospiralis* Garvaki, 1972), while the others are subspecies of *T. spiralis*.

Trichinella britovi has a sylvatic cycle in wild carnivores in Europe (Estonia, France, Italy, Netherlands, Poland and Spain), often in national parks with no exposure to humans. This species (or subspecies) is similar to *T. nativa* but is less resistant to freezing for 3 weeks, differs in distribution and genetic make-up and has less severe intestinal symptoms.

T. nativa is found in holarctic sylvatic animals (polar bear, Arctic fox, mink, wolf, seal and walrus), but not in mice, rats or pigs. It has a high resistance to freezing. It has still not been proved how marine mammals become infected; seals may possibly eat infected amphipod crustaceans that ingest larval cysts in fragments of meat when feeding on dead walruses or polar bears.

T. nelsoni is found only in Africa in wild suids and has no resistance to freezing. It is also found in many large wild carnivores in East Africa (hyena, jackal, leopard and lion), while human infection is from eating uncooked bushpig or warthog.

T. pseudospiralis is cosmopolitan in wild birds and mammals and has no resistance to freezing. This form differs from all others, as the larvae do not form cysts in the muscles. It is not common in humans but can cause muscle pain and fatigue with polymyositis and a raised creatine kinase level (Andrews *et al.*, 1994).

T. spiralis is cosmopolitan, mainly in domestic pigs and sometimes rodents, and is responsible for the great majority of human cases, the symptoms and pathogenesis of which are described above.

There have been recent outbreaks from eating wild boar in Croatia (5.7% boars infected), Ethiopia, France, Italy, Poland (0.5%), Spain (0.2%), northern Canada and the USA. In the USA, bear and cougar 'jerky' are another source of infection in hunters.

PREVENTION AND CONTROL

Larvae in pork are killed by heating above 55°C or (for *T. spiralis*) by deep-freezing at −15°C for 20 days. The number of cases in the USA has dropped recently (with only 38 cases each year for 1991–1996, with three deaths), chiefly because most pork is deep-frozen and pig swill is sterilized. However, it is estimated that inspection costs $1000 million annually in the USA and $570 million in the European Union (Murrell and Pozio, 2000).

Pork can be examined for infection by means of the trichinoscope at the abattoir; this is a projection microscope that projects an image of cysts in compressed samples of muscle (best from the tongue). A pooled digestion technique with muscle samples from groups of pigs has replaced the trichinoscope in those countries which still undertake routine examinations, since it is more suitable for low prevalences. An ELISA test is good for diagnosing infection in live animals. It is not possible to recognize infected pigs from clinical symptoms, as there is often an absence of morbidity, even with large numbers of cysts.

Most developed countries now have laws to prevent feeding pigs with uncooked swill (primarily to control vesicular erythema in pigs) and this has lowered the incidence of infection. Rats in piggeries should be destroyed and meat from wild carnivores should never be fed to pigs.

All pork and pork products should be thoroughly cooked, as should the meat from wild suids or carnivores.

ZOONOTIC ASPECTS

This is an entirely zoonotic infection, except possibly among the Turkana of East Africa, who put dead bodies out to be eaten by wild carnivores.

Rats and other rodents are frequently infected with *T. spiralis* subspecies, but are not usually important in transmission; dogs and cats may become infected from ingesting them but do not maintain transmission. However, wild carnivores are important in transmitting *T. nativa* and *T. nelsoni*. *T. murrelli* has recently been described from wildlife in the USA (Pozio

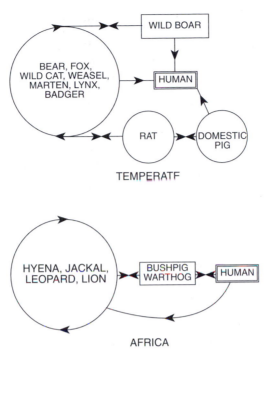

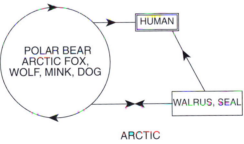

Fig. 84. Life cycles of *Trichinella* species from various regions. Top: *T. spiralis*; centre: *T. nelsoni*; bottom: *T. nativa*.

and La Rosa, 2000), although not so far from humans.

In some areas, more than one species (or subspecies) is present: for instance in Europe, *T. spiralis* and *T. britovi* occur in France and Spain, *T. britovi* alone in Italy and Switzerland, *T. spiralis* alone in Belgium and Germany, *T. spiralis*, *T. britovi* and *T. nativa* in Sweden, *T. nativa* in Norway and *T. spiralis* and *T. nativa* in Finland (Pozio, 1998).

Experimentally a wide range of mammals can be infected, but cysts do not form in Chinese hamsters.

Another non-cyst-forming species, *T. papuae*, has been recently described from pigs in Papua New Guinea, but not so far from humans (Pozio *et al.*, 1999).

Family Dioctophymidae

Dioctophyma renale
(Goeze, 1782) Stiles, 1901

SYNONYMS, DISEASE AND POPULAR NAME
Dioctophyme renale; Eustrongylus gigas (Rudolphi, 1802) Diesing, 1951. Dioctophymosis. Giant kidney worm infection.

CLINICAL MANIFESTATIONS AND PATHOGENESIS
Dioctophyma is a natural parasite of the pelvis of the kidney or the body cavity of carnivores, including the dog, fox, mink, ottter, racoon and rat. About 20 human cases have been reported from Europe, North and South America, Iran, China and Thailand.

These are very large nematodes, reddish in colour when alive. The female measures 20–100 cm × 5–12 mm and the male 14–20 cm × 4–6 mm. The male has a single spicule set in the middle of a posterior bursal cup. The unembryonated eggs (measuring 64–68 µm × 40–44 µm) have a thick, deeply pitted shell (Fig. 124) and are passed out in urine. Embryonated eggs must reach water for further development, where they are ingested by aquatic oligochaetes. These are then ingested by final hosts; fish or amphibians may also act as paratenic hosts and this is probably the source of human infections.

Adult worms in the kidney cause renal colic and later dysfunction, the worms eating the kidney tissue. Larvae have also been found in subcutaneous nodules.

A related parasite, ***Eustrongylides ignotus*** (or ***E. tubifex***), a parasite of fish-eating birds and with larvae in oligochaetes and fish has been reported from humans a few times along the Atlantic coast of the USA. Symptoms of acute pain in the right lower quadrant with vomiting, diarrhoea and fever indicating acute abdomen or appendicitis, required surgery. Red-coloured fourth-stage larvae measuring 4–6 cm have been removed from a perforated caecum and from the peritoneum. One patient in New York had eaten raw oysters and goose barnacles (Wittner *et al.*, 1989) and others raw fish. In one patient in New Jersey, raw minnows were eaten when being used as fish bait – 48% of the minnows in the area contained larvae (Eberhard *et al.*, 1989).

Superfamily Mermithoidea

The mermithids are free-living, aphasmid nematodes with larvae that are parasitic in insects. There have been occasional reports of recovery of larvae from humans (*Agamomermis hominis* once in faeces, *A. restiformis* once in the urethra, *Mermis nigrescens* once in the mouth, *Mermis* sp. once in urine), but these are probably spurious infections (Hasegawa *et al.*, 1996), with one presumably genuine report of a male mermithid beneath the tunica in a case of hydrocele of the scrotum in a Nigerian (Hunt *et al.*, 1984); one can only speculate how this occurred.

Order Spirurida

Superfamily Gnathostomoidea

Gnathostoma spinigerum
Owen, 1836

DISEASE AND POPULAR NAMES
Gnathostomiasis or gnathostomosis; a cause of visceral larva migrans and of creeping eruption (the latter usually due to another species, *G. hispidum*).

GEOGRAPHICAL DISTRIBUTION
Most common in Japan (Kyushu, Shikoku and south Honshu) and Thailand (Daengsvang, 1980); occasional cases occur in Bangladesh, Burma, China, Ecuador, India, Indonesia, Malaysia, Mexico, New Guinea and Vietnam.

LOCATION IN HOST
Adults live in small nodules in the stomach wall of carnivores but are rarely found in humans. Third-stage larvae in humans migrate through the tissues, usually subcutaneously, and may be present in any part of the body.

MORPHOLOGY

Adults measure 1.1–3.3 cm and have a characteristic head bulb with eight rows of hooks (Fig. 85). The mouth has two large lips. The anterior part of the body is covered with cuticular spines. Third-stage larvae migrating in humans measure about 4 mm and also have a head bulb with fewer rows of hooks (Fig. 86).

LIFE CYCLE

The eggs in the faeces of carnivores are yellowish-brown and contain an ovum. In the one- or two-celled stage. They measure 69 (62–79) μm × 39 (36–42) μm and have a finely granulated surface and a characteristic polar thickening (Fig. 124). The eggs develop in water and the first-stage larvae hatch in 7 days at 27°C. The larvae are ingested by species of cyclopoid copepods (e.g. *Cyclops varicans*, *C. vicinus*, *C. strenuus*, *Eucylops agilis*, *E. serrulatus*, *Mesocyclops leuckarti*, *Thermocyclops* sp.), which live in ponds, moult in the body cavity in 7–10 days (Plate 34), and develop further when the freshwater microcrustaceans

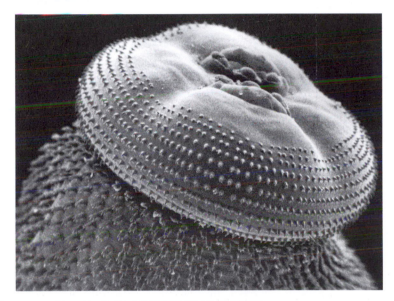

Fig. 85. Stereoscan of head bulb of adult *Gnathostoma hispidum*.

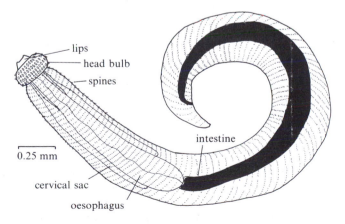

Fig. 86. Third-stage larva of *G. spinigerum* removed from human subcutaneous tissues.

are ingested by a second intermediate host. These are usually freshwater fish, frogs (such as *Rana limnocharis*) or snakes. The second-stage larvae pierce the gastric wall and moult in about 1 month, and the third-stage larvae are eventually surrounded by a cyst in the muscles, measuring around 1 mm in diameter. The natural definitive hosts are the dog, cat and large carnivores, such as the tiger and leopard, which are infected by eating fish or by eating a paratenic host (possibly a rodent) that has eaten fish. Suitable paratenic hosts are other fish, amphibians, snakes, rats, mice or chickens, new cysts being formed in these. Twenty-five species of animals from all vertebrate classes can act as paratenic hosts and multiple transfers are also possible.

Prenatal transmission of larvae from mother to offspring can occur in mice and may account for human cases of gnathostomiasis reported from babies.

The adult worms take about 100 days to become mature in the stomach of carnivores.

CLINICAL MANIFESTATIONS AND PATHOGENESIS

Many patients suffer from epigastric pain, fever, nausea and diarrhoea 24–48 h after ingestion of the larvae, presumably caused by the larvae penetrating through the intestinal wall. There is often a very high eosinophilia of up to 90%, with leucocytosis.

Some of the pathology is apparently caused by toxic substances secreted by *Gnathostoma* larvae; these include a haemolytic substance, acetylcholine, hyaluronidase-like substances and a proteolytic enzyme.

The larvae migrate through the liver and cause disturbances of liver function. They then usually reach the subcutis, moving at a rate of about 1 cm h^{-1}, where they cause a painless, migrating oedema. The oedema is generally erythematous and remains for about 2 weeks in one place (Plate 25). A few cases of ocular and pulmonary gnathostomiasis have also been reported and most importantly, an eosinophilic myelencephalitis, in which the cerebrospinal fluid is grossly bloody or xanthochromic. Some fatal cases have presented with paraplegia.

Mature adult worms in intestinal nodules have also been reported in a few cases.

DIAGNOSIS

Clinical. A painless, migrating, intermittent, subcutaneous oedema is characteristic, particularly when there is an eosinophilia of over 50%.

Immunological. A purified antigen from advanced third-stage larvae (L_3s) of 24 kDa can be used in an indirect ELISA, which is stated to be 100% sensitive and specific (Nopparatana *et al.*, 1991). A Western immunoblot technique with an antigen of 16 kDa has also given good results.

TREATMENT

Surgical excision of worms is often possible when they are in subcutaneous sites.

Albendazole at 400 mg twice daily for 10–21 days has been used successfully in a few cases (Kraivichian *et al.*, 1992) and is stated to stimulate larvae to move to the surface so that they can be easily excised (Suntharasamai *et al.*, 1992). Mebendazole at 300 mg daily for 5 days was also effective in one case.

EPIDEMIOLOGY AND PREVENTION

Infection in humans usually follows eating raw fish dishes, such as 'sashimi' in Japan, 'somfak' in Thailand or 'ceviche' (if made with freshwater fish) in Latin America. Important species of food fish in Japan are crucian carp, *Ophiocephalus* spp. or goby (*Acanthogobius hasta*); chicken can also be a source of infection to humans. The encysted larvae in fish are killed by cooking for 5 min in water at 70°C or by pickling in vinegar for 6 h. Skin penetration is possible experimentally in cats and might occur during preparation of fish dishes.

Prevention is by thorough cooking of fish and chicken.

There are at least seven other species of *Gnathostoma* that could infect humans. **G. doloresi** Tubangui, 1925, and **G. hispidum** Fedchenko, 1872, are parasites of pigs in Asia and there have been a few cases of human infection in China and Japan following ingestion of raw freshwater fish or snakes, usually causing creeping eruption, sometimes accompanied by stomach convulsions (Akahane *et al.*, 1998). In one case *G. doloresi* caused colonic ileus, due to eosinophilic nodular lesions. **G. nipponicum** Yamaguti, 1941, has been recently described from humans in Japan, where it has caused itching and creeping eruption after eating freshwater fish. (Ando, 1989; Ando *et al.*, 1991). There has been a 'rash' of cases of creeping eruption in Japan recently after eating raw marine fish or squid, with one patient having larvae in the eye ('type x' spirurid larvae).

Larvae of the different species can be differentiated, although this is likely to be impossible in tissue sections (Ando *et al.*, 1991).

Other Spirurids

Thelazia callipaeda Railliet and Henry, 1910, is a parasite of the conjunctival sac and lachrymal ducts of dogs in the Far East. It has been recorded about 60 times from humans in China, Indonesia, Japan, Korea, Thailand and Russia (Siberia). The adults of both sexes are filariform and have a serrated cuticle. The female measures 7–19 mm, the male 4–13 mm. The movement of the adults under the eyelids in the conjunctival sac causes intense irritation and the scratching of the cornea can lead to scar formation and opacity. Worms can be removed after local anaesthesia.

The intermediate hosts are dipteran flies, including *Musca domestica* (Shi *et al.*, 1988).

Thelazia californiensis Price, 1930, an eye parasite of ruminants, particularly deer, has been reported five times from humans in the USA, causing keratoconjunctivitis, and is also transmitted by flies.

Gongylonema pulchrum Molin, 1857 (the gullet worm), is a natural parasite of the oesophagus of herbivores (sheep, cattle, goats, camels, equines, pigs and deer). It has been reported about 40 times from humans in Austria, Bulgaria, China, Hungary, Italy, Morocco, New Zealand, Russia, Serbia, Sri Lanka and the USA. Adult females measure about 145 mm × 0.5 mm, males 63 mm × 0.3 mm and the anterior end of both sexes is covered with cuticular thickenings. The worms live in serpentiginous tunnels in the squamous epithelium of the oesophagus and oral cavity, where they can cause painful abscesses of the buccal mucosa (Jelinek and Loscher, 1994), sometime accompanied by pharyngitis, vomiting and irritability. Eggs produced in these tunnels reach the mouth cavity and are passed out fully embryonated in the faeces. The eggs from natural hosts containing first-stage larvae are ingested by dung-beetles or, experimentally at least, cockroaches, which act as intermediate hosts. Adults take about 80 days to develop when third-stage larvae are ingested inside these insects. Diagnosis is by identifying the characteristic tunnels and by extracting adult worms after giving anti-inflammatory drugs (Jelinek and Loscher, 1994): eggs have been seen in sputum but not in faeces.

Abbreviata (= ***Physaloptera***) ***caucasica*** (von Linstow, 1902), is a natural parasite of monkeys in the tropics. The adult females measure 20–100 mm × 2.5 mm, males 14–34 mm × 1.0 mm, and both live with their heads embedded in the mucosa of the stomach or intestinal wall. Cockroaches and grasshoppers can act as experimental intermediate hosts. It has been reported from humans in Brazil, Colombia, Congo Republic (Zaire), India, Indonesia, Israel, Namibia, Panama, Zambia and Zimbabwe. In a recent case in an Indonesian woman, adult worms were recovered from the biliary duct, where they had caused biliary pain, jaundice and fever. Another species, ***Physaloptera transfuga*** Marits and Grinberg, 1970, a parasite of cats and dogs, has been recovered once from the lip of a woman in Moldova.

Cheilospirura sp. Diesing, 1861 (or ***Acuaria*** sp.), a parasite of the gizzard of birds with insect intermediate hosts, has been recovered once from a nodule on the conjunctiva of a Philippine farmer.

Spirocerca lupi (Rudolphi, 1809) is a common parasite of dogs and other carnivores in warm countries, forming tumours in the stomach wall, with dung-beetles as intermediate hosts and birds or mammals as paratenic hosts. It has been found once embedded in the wall of the ileum of a newborn baby in Italy; it is assumed that infection was prenatal.

Rictularia spp. Froelich, 1802, are parasites of rodents or bats, and a gravid female worm has been recovered once from a section of an appendix of a man in New York.

Superfamily Filarioidea: the Filariae

Members of the superfamily Filarioidea of the order Spirurida are tissue-dwelling nematodes, responsible for some of the most important helminth diseases of humans. Bancroftian filariasis (caused by infection with *Wuchereria bancrofti*) and onchocerciasis (due to *Onchocerca volvulus*) in particular are the cause of much morbidity and the former shares with schistosomiasis the dubious distinction among helminth infections of increasing in incidence each year. All human filariae are transmitted by the bite of a bloodsucking insect (Fig. 87). The adults are ovoviviparous and the early first-stage larvae, known as microfilariae, are found in the blood or skin. Microfilariae measure from 150 to 350 µm in length and some retain the much expanded eggshell as a thin sheath; their specific identification can be of great importance in diagnosis (Figs 88 and 89).

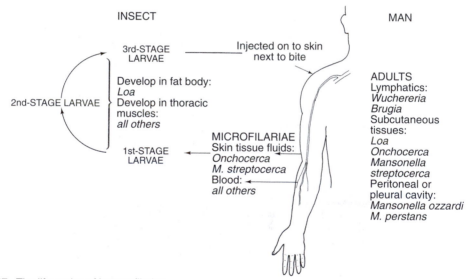

Fig. 87. The life cycles of human filariae.

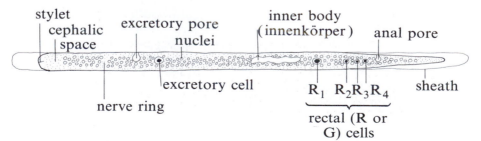

Fig. 88. A generalized microfilaria showing the features of use in identification (some features can be seen only with special staining techniques and the stylet and sheath are not always present).

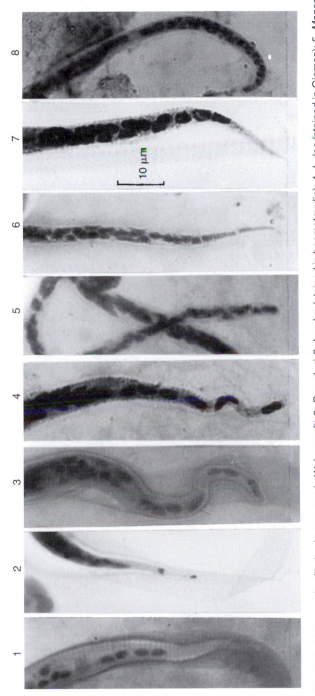

Fig. 89. The tails of human microfilariae in smears: 1. *W. bancrofti*; 2. *B. malayi*; 3. *Loa loa* (stained in haematoxylin); 4. *L. loa* (stained in Giemsa); 5. *Mansonella perstans*; 6. *M. ozzardi*; 7. *Onchocerca volvulus*; 8. *M. streptocerca*.

Wuchereria bancrofti
(Cobbold, 1877) Seurat, 1921

SYNONYMS

Filaria sanguinis hominis; *Filaria bancrofti* Cobbold, 1877; *Wuchereria pacifica*.

DISEASE

Lymphatic filariasis or filariosis (LF); Bancroftian filariasis or filariosis; cause of elephantiasis.

LOCAL NAMES

Jakute (Burmese), Etow = hydrocele and Barawa gyeprim = elephantiasis (Fanti), Wagaga or Wagana (filarial fever) (Fijian), Tundermi (Gwaina = hydrocele) (Hausa), Kusafurui (filarial fever) or Kusa in Kyushu and Ryuku Island (Henki, Senki or Oogintama = hydrocele) (Japanese), Apipa = elephantiasis (Luo), Mumu (filarial fever) (Samoan), Watharoga = hydrocele (Singalese), Sheelo = hydrocele and Lugo marodi = elephantiasis (Somali), Matende (Mshipa = hydrocele) (Swahili), Fee fee and Mariri (Tahitian), Yanaikal (Tamil), Gypeym (Etwo = hydrocele) (Twi).

GEOGRAPHICAL DISTRIBUTION

It has been estimated recently that 119 million people are infected with LF, of whom 107 million are due to *W. bancrofti*.

Infection is present in most equatorial countries of tropical Africa between 20°N and 20°S and in Madagascar, Asia (Bangladesh, China, India, Indonesia, Japan, Korea, Myanmar, Pakistan, Philippines, Sri Lanka, Thailand), the Pacific (New Guinea, Melanesia, Polynesia, including Fiji, Samoa, Tahiti), the West Indies and northern South America.

LOCATION IN HOST

The adults live in the lymphatics, either of the lower limbs and groin region or of the upper limbs, and breasts in women. Sheathed microfilariae are found in the bloodstream.

MORPHOLOGY

Like all filariae of humans the adults of *Wuchereria* are long, threadlike worms (hence the name 'filaria' from Latin). The head end is slightly swollen and has two rows of ten sessile papillae. The cuticle is smooth, with very fine transverse striations, and the posterior end of the female is finely tuberculated. The female measures 80–100 mm × 0.25 mm, the male 40 mm × 0.1 mm. The ovoviviparous female has two posterior ovaries; from these two oviducts lead into the paired uteri, which coil back and forth through the greater part of the body before they fuse and open by a short vagina at the vulva, 0.8 mm from the anterior end. The proximal portions of the uteri are filled with eggs and embryos, while near the vulva the microfilariae are crowded and remain in the sheath formed by the elongation of the egg membrane. Cross-sections of females of all human filariae show this double-uterine structure. The male has the posterior end curved ventrally and on the ventral surface of the tail are 12–15 pairs of sessile papillae. There are two unequal spicules, measuring 0.6 and 0.2 mm, and a gubernaculum (the number and arrangement of the papillae and the structure and lengths of the spicules of the male worms are of great taxonomic importance among the filariae).

The microfilariae are found in the bloodstream and can live for 3–6 months; they measure 210–320 µm by 7.5–10 µm (the mean lengths of microfilariae from various geographical regions vary from 250 to 290 µm). The anterior end is rounded and the posterior end pointed. Each microfilaria is surrounded by a long sheath, which stains pale pink in Giemsa stain. In wet preparations the microfilaria moves vigorously in a serpentine manner; in stained preparations it often assumes graceful curves. The posterior end is free of nuclei and thus differs from the microfilarial larvae of *Brugia malayi* (Fig. 90) and *Loa loa*.

The microfilariae have various structures (nerve ring, excretory pore and cell, inner body or innenkörper, rectal cells and anus) whose size and position can be of help in recognition. However, it must be remembered that these features are only of use in well-fixed and stained preparations and some individual variation may occur.

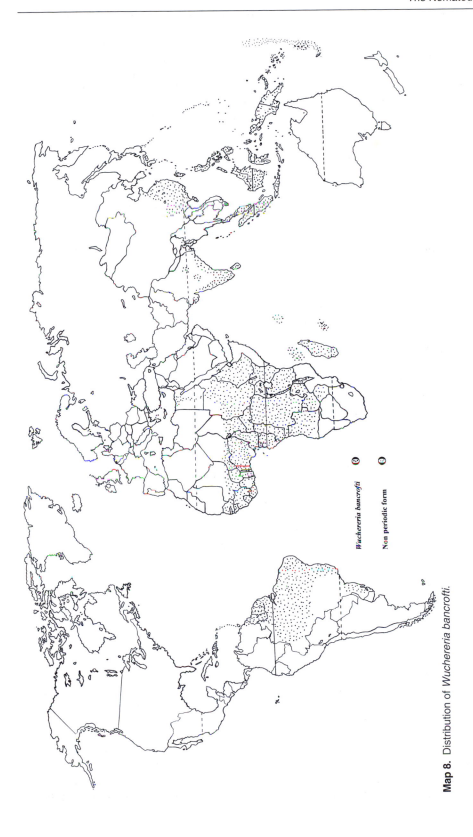

Map 8. Distribution of *Wuchereria bancrofti*.

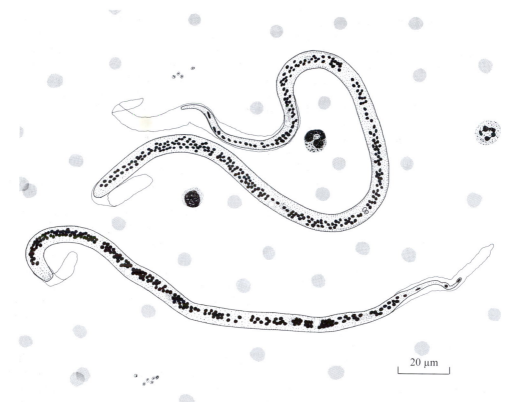

20 μm

Fig. 90. Microfilariae of (top) *Wuchereria bancrofti* and (bottom) *Brugia malayi*.

Microfilariae described from eastern Madagascar (Malagasy Republic) had some characters resembling *W. bancrofti* and others resembling those of *Brugia malayi* and were designated as belonging to *W. bancrofti* var. *vauceli*.

LIFE CYCLE

The sheathed microfilariae circulate in the bloodstream and, in most parts of the world, show a marked periodicity; they are found in the peripheral circulation from 22.00 to 02.00 h, while during the day they hide in the capillaries of the lungs. In areas of the Pacific east of longitude 160°, such as Fiji, Samoa and Tahiti, where the vectors are day-biting mosquitoes, the periodicity is partially reversed and the strain is said to be diurnally subperiodic. Investigations on the mechanism of microfilarial periodicity have shown that during the day, in the periodic form, the microfilariae are held up in the small blood-vessels of the lungs principally because of the difference in oxygen tension between the arterial and venous capillaries in the lungs. Perhaps the peripheral circulation represents an unfavourable environment and the microfilariae remain there for the minimum time necessary to maintain transmission.

When the microfilariae are ingested with a blood meal by a suitable species of mosquito, they lose their sheath within 15–30 min in the stomach of the insect. A proportion manage to penetrate the stomach wall before the formation of a peritrophic membrane and migrate to the thoracic muscles in 1–24 h. Two days later they have metamorphosed into sausage-shaped larvae, measuring 150 μm × 10 μm, and by the end of a week (usually at 5 days) the larvae have moulted, the alimentary canal is developed and the second-stage larvae then measure 250 μm × 25 μm. During the 2nd week

(9–10 days) the larvae moult again, grow much longer (1.2–1.8 mm) and migrate to the head, where they enter the labium and emerge through the tips of the labella while the mosquito is feeding. The infective third-stage larvae can be differentiated from other filarial larvae, if the mosquito is dissected in a drop of saline, by size and by the three subterminal papillae (Fig. 91) (there may be larvae of various animal filariae in mosquitoes, such as *Dirofilaria* and *Setaria*). The parasite cannot be transmitted from one person to another until the larvae have undergone this essential development to the infective stage in the mosquito.

Optimal conditions for filarial development in mosquitoes are about 26°C (range 16.5–31°C) and 90% relative humidity. Many mosquitoes are killed by heavy infections and in others larvae often fail to mature, so that the infection rate in mosquitoes is usually low (below 0.5%), though under some conditions it can be much higher.

Development in the mosquito takes 11 or more days and the infective larvae escape through the labella when the insect bites a new individual and enter the skin through the puncture wound (this is likely to be more successful in areas of high humidity, where the skin will be moist, although the mosquito does deposit a drop of fluid on the skin while feeding). After entering the skin of a human, the larvae migrate to the lymph vessels and glands, where they moult twice

more and mature and the females produce microfilariae within 1 year (206–285 days in experimental infections in leaf monkeys). The adult female worms probably produce microfilariae for about 5 years (Vanamail *et al.*, 1996), although greater longevity has been reported in the past (10–17 years).

CLINICAL MANIFESTATIONS

It has been estimated that currently about 44 million people suffer from overt manifestations of lymphatic filariasis. The other 76 million cases appear to be symptomless, a condition that may last for years, and the only overt evidence of infection is the presence of microfilariae in the blood. However, recent studies using lymphoscintigraphy indicate that even these apparently symptomless cases are probably suffering from subclinical lymphatic and renal damage (Freedman *et al.*, 1994; Noroes *et al.*, 1996).

Acute disease. From the 3rd month after entry of the larvae, there may be recurrent attacks of acute lymphangitis (inflammation of the lymph ducts), with inflamed, tender lymph nodes, headache, nausea and sometimes urticaria ('filarial fever'), each attack lasting from 3 to 15 days. At this time microfilariae vanish from the blood (amicrofilaraemia) and there may be many attacks in a year. There is often eosinophilia accompanied by chyluria (the

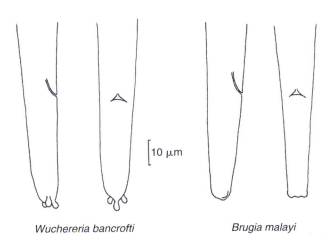

Wuchereria bancrofti   Brugia malayi

Fig. 91. Tails of third-stage larvae of *W. bancrofti* and *B. malayi* from mouth-parts of mosquito.

presence of whitish lymph containing fatty acids from the intestinal lymph vessels in the urine). In many areas acute symptoms start at the age of about 6, with a peak at age 25. In many areas infection probably occurs in very young children. In a study in Haiti, 6% of 2-year-olds and 30% of 4-year-olds had filarial antigens but only one child was microfilaraemic; some of these children already had dilated lymphatics, shown by ultrasound (Lammle *et al.*, 1998). The most serious clinical manifestations are due to disturbances of the lymphatic system (Fig 92), which may result in lymphadenitis (inflammation of the lymph nodes), lymphoedema, lymphoceles, lymphuria, chyluria and, in males, genital lesions, including hydrocele and lymph scrotum, in which lymph drips from the spermatic cord. In Ghana, hydrocele but not adenolymphangitis was associated with a high infection prevalence and intensity (Gyapong, 1998).

Chronic disease. True elephantiasis, in which the oedema is hard and non-pitting, takes about 10–15 years to develop. Secondary bacterial and fungal infection often follows, with the develop of verrucous growths (Fig. 93).

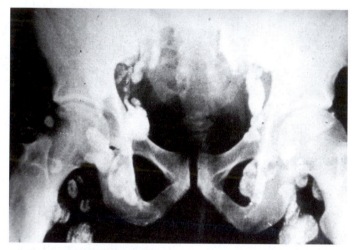

Fig. 92. Radiograph showing blocked lymph ducts.

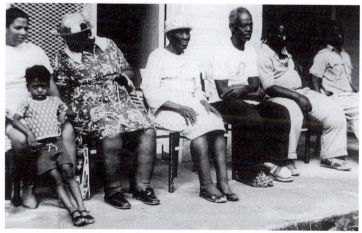

Fig. 93. Cases of elephantiasis in Guyana caused by *W. bancrofti*. It is not so evident in males because of the trousers worn. In the man third from the right there are verrucous lesions of the foot ('mossy foot').

The changes in the lymphatics are often stated to be due to blockage caused by the dead worms but recent experimental studies indicate that it is caused mainly by an allergic response to the still-living worms.

The nature of the lesions varies in different parts of the world, reflecting particularly the different sites of obstruction. In India, chyluria is rarely reported, but it was common in Japan. In Africa, elephantiasis is less common than in the Pacific and is usually confined to the legs. Hydrocele (Figs. 94 and 95), with probable reduction in fertility, is particularly common in males in East Africa (up to 50% of infected individuals) and India (with about 27 million cases) and has very serious social/sexual implications (Dreyer *et al.*, 1997). In West Africa, there are often high microfilarial rates (40–50% of the population) but few clinical manifestations. In those Pacific islands where the subperiodic strain of the parasite occurs, slowly developing gross elephantiasis of the arms, legs, breasts, scrotum or vulva was common until transmission was reduced in the last few years.

Tropical pulmonary eosinophilia is caused by an abnormal host reaction to the

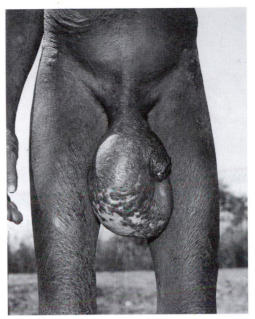

Fig. 94. A case of filarial hydrocele.

presence of a lymphatic filarial infection and is sometimes known as occult filariasis. The symptoms include bouts of severe, paroxysmal, dry, wheezy coughing, resembling an asthma attack, with dyspnoea,

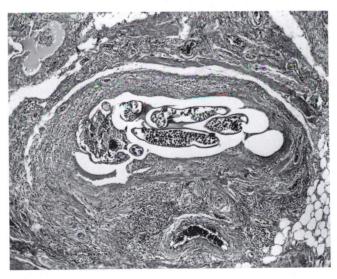

Fig. 95. Section of dilated lymphatic of the testis with adult female of *W. bancrofti*. The vessel wall is thickened and there is a granulomatous reaction to the worm (magnification × 55).

chest pain and fever, resulting from dense eosinophilic infiltrations in the lungs lasting for weeks or months. It occurs particularly in India or Singapore (in persons of Indian extraction). Patients are amicrofilaraemic but have strong filarial serology, with a high eosinophilia (about 35%).

A similar reaction is known as Meyers–Kouwenaar's syndrome, found in the Pacific and East Indies. There is a benign lymphadenitis with enlargement of the lymph nodes, liver and spleen and with pulmonary symptoms but no microfilaraemia. Histologically the lymph nodes are hyperplastic with dead microfilariae surrounded by eosinophils and then hyaline material to form nodular, granulomatous, abscesses ('M–K bodies'). The condition can easily be mistaken for Hodgkin's disease and the symptoms of both filarial conditions are diagnostically rapidly alleviated by treatment with diethylcarbamazine (DEC).

PATHOGENESIS
The first phase of clinical disease is characterized by dilatation of the afferent lymphatic vessels reacting to the presence of masses of adult worms. Initially the sinuses of the smaller lymph vessels increase in size (lymphangiectasia), but following the repeated attacks of adenolymphangitis the enlarged lymph nodes become progressively firm and fibrotic. The nodes become hyperplastic and microscopical sections show inflammation of the endothelial lining, with many lymphocytes, plasma cells and particularly eosinophils, and there may be foci of necrosis, with sections of adults in the lumen. Lymphatics often become invaded by bacteria, but some clinical (Dissanayake *et al.*, 1995) and experimental (Denham and Fletcher, 1987; Lawrence, 1996) studies indicate that this is not the primary cause of pathogenesis, which is caused by an allergic reaction to the adult worms, allied to cofactors such as a high worm burden, lymphangiectasia, location of adult worm nests (e.g. in spermatic cord) and chronology of adult worm deaths. However, recurrent secondary bacterial infections superimposed on the damage to the lymphatics probably play an important part in the development of lymphoedema and elephantiasis (Dreyer *et al.*, 2000). In chronic infections, lymphoid aggregates and germinal centres develop and eventually cause complete occlusion of the lumen, so that the lymph vessels are no longer functional. Worms die and become surrounded by fibrotic tissue, which eventually calcifies. It is not known what triggers the initial inflammatory response. Chyluria is caused by rupture of lymph varices into any part of the urinary tract, with fatty lymph appearing in the urine. In cases of renal chyluria there may be passage between the renal pelvis and a dilated lymphatic to the cisterna chyli. Such cases show up on intravenous or retrograde pyelograms but are not serious and do not require surgery. The rupture of varicose lymph vessels near the skin of the scrotum results in lymph oozing on to the surface (lymph scrotum).

Adults of *Wuchereria* and *Brugia* contain a bacterium, *Wohlbachia*, in the lateral cords and it has recently been postulated that these bacteria are responsible for inflammatory responses, inducing cytokines (Fig. 96). The chronic release of *Wohlbachia* might lead to desensitization of the innate immune response and the bacterial catalase may protect the filariae from the action of hydrogen peroxide-mediated damage (Taylor, 2000). The presence of the bacterium appears to be essential for the long-term survival of the filaria.

Immune responses. Many of the symptoms associated with filarial infection (e.g. eosinophilia, urticaria, lymphangitis and lymphoedema) are immunological in origin and confirm that infection induces strong immune responses. Epidemiological studies show that, in endemic areas, there are individuals who appear to be parasitologically negative, despite evidence of exposure to infection (the so-called endemic normals). A key question is whether immune responses have the potential to be host-protective as well as pathogenic. Analysis of immune responses has been

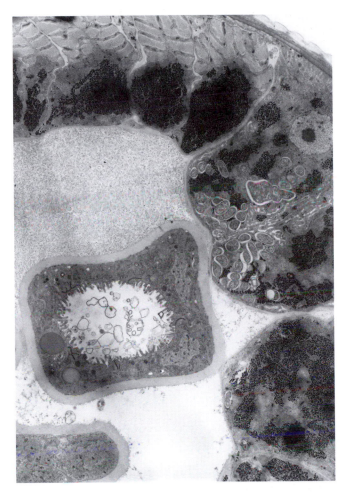

Fig. 96. Section of *W. bancrofti* with the bacterium *Wohlbachia* in the lateral cords (the numerous bodies on right side of electron micrograph).

carried out in many infected populations and there has been a large amount of laboratory research with experimental models. However, it has to be said that no clear picture has emerged.

Immunological relationships between filarial nematodes and their hosts are complex and the cause of much contention. Particular difficulties are caused by the fact that in filarial-infected populations some individuals apear to be immune, others suffer immune-infected pathology, while yet others (microfilaraemic individuals) show a depression of responses to filarial antigens that is reversed after chemotherapy. T cells appear to be impor-

tant in all of these phenomena and there have been many attempts to explain each in terms of differential T-helper 1 (Th1) and Th2 responses. However, there is no straightforward relationship between subset activity and host response. It is true that patients with high microfilarial loads tend to show reduced Th1 responses and high Th2 (e.g. reflected in high IgG4 levels, possibly acting as blocking antibody), but not all type 2 cytokines are produced normally. T cells from microfilaraemic individuals show much reduced proliferation to worm antigens, but can still release interleukin 4 (IL-4), though IL-5 responses are reduced. The cytokine IL-10 may be involved in down-regulating proliferative responses, although antigen overload from the large numbers of circulating microfilariae may also be involved. Filarial worms are also thought to release immunomodulatory molecules that depress specific T-cell functions, such as proliferation, gamma interferon (IFN-γ) secretion and, surprisingly, IL-5 production. Children born to mothers who are microfilaraemic may show a profound T-cell unresponsiveness, both Th1 and Th2 responses being down-regulated, which presumably results from placental transfer of antigen or immunomodulatory factors.

Immune-mediated protection against infection may act independently against the three major life-cycle stages (infective L$_3$s, adults and microfilariae). Individuals who remain uninfected in endemic areas tend to show Th1-biased responses, and mice lacking the capacity to make IL-4 (a major Th2 cytokine) retain the ability to kill incoming infective larvae of *B. malayi*. However, neither Th1 nor Th2 responses appear to eliminate adult *B. malayi* from the body cavity. It is clear that the different stages also induce quite different patterns of host responses. Thus, in mice, adult worms and L$_3$s elicit Th2 responses with high IL-4 and IgG4 production, as well as IgG1 and IgE antibodies (although IgE responses are depressed), whereas exposure to microfilariae alone can induce Th1 responses, with high initial IFN-γ production and IgG2 antibody. How worms are killed is still controversial, despite clear evidence from *in vitro* studies that antibody and antibody-dependent cellular cytotoxic (ADCC) mechanisms can damage or eliminate parasites. Eosinophils participate in ADCC mechanisms against infective L$_3$s, and IgM and IgG2a antibody can clear microfilariae. It is likely that nitric oxide mechanisms are important in attacks against larvae (Maizels *et al.*, in Nutman, 2000). People probably become resistant following repeated reinfection and, as in schistosomiasis, may develop a state of concomitant immunity, with existing adult worms remaining alive but invading larvae being destroyed.

DIAGNOSIS

Parasitological. Routine diagnosis is by finding microfilariae, usually in stained thick blood films (see p. 262 for various techniques). Blood should be taken from the ear or finger at 22.00–02.00 h for the nocturnally periodic forms and at 10.00–14.00 h for the subperiodic Pacific form. Microfilariae can sometimes be obtained during the day by taking blood smears about 1 h after giving two tablets (100 mg) of diethylcarbamazine (DEC) (provocation test). Concentration techniques can be employed (counting chamber or Nuclepore filter (p. 264)).

Clinical. Lymphangitis, lymphadenitis or manifestations of lymph stasis in a patient in an endemic area, often with eosinophilia, are very suggestive. Recent studies, particularly in Brazil, using ultrasound have enabled direct visualization of adult worms in the lymphatics (Amaral *et al.*, 1994; Noroes *et al.*, 1996). It has been found that the worms are in ceaseless movement, undergoing what has been termed a 'filarial dance'.

Immunological. These tests are most successful in cases without microfilariae in the blood. A new simple immunochromatographic test (ICT) card kit is commercially available, using 100 μm of whole-blood finger-prick samples (or serum or plasma), which can be taken at any time by untrained staff and put on a nitrocellulose layer on a sample pad (Weil *et al.*, 1997). The pink sample pad contains a dried polyclonal antibody (AD12.1) specific to *W. bancrofti* attached to colloidal gold and migrates up the pad to reach a specific monoclonal antibody immobilized in a line on the pad; this traps free antibody–antigen complexes to form an intense pink line, which can be compared with a control line. The test takes 5–15 min and detects early infections in children, which is very important for assessing the success of any control campaign, as well as for individual diagnosis, and is negative for all filarial infection apart from Bancroftian filariasis (this kit is commercially available from www.amrad.com.au or amradict@amrad.com.au). A commercially available dot ELISA with monoclonal antibodies (usually Og4C3), using whole dried blood samples, can even give an indication of the number of parasites present but is not easy to use in the field (from JCU Tropical Biotechnology, Townsville, Queensland). Circulating parasite DNA detection by a PCR is both sensitive and specific, particularly when microfilariae are present, but is highly labour-intensive and expensive.

TREATMENT

Chemotherapy. Recent ultrasonic studies have enabled the action of chemotherapeutic agents to be directly observed and worm nests can be surgically removed and worms examined to ascertain drug-induced changes in somatic tissues or in the ability to produce new larvae (embryogenesis) (Dreyer *et al.*, 1995). Previously the effects on adult worms required studies over many years.

DEC has been used for the last 50 years, usually at an oral dose of 72 g over 3 weeks, and was thought to kill microfilariae but not adults. Recent studies indicate that it does kill about 50% of adult worms as well. Recently, much smaller doses (6 mg kg^{-1}) have been found to be effective. However, it cannot be used in patients from Africa (see p. 201). *In vitro* DEC has no effect on microfilariae and its action may be mediated by platelets; excreted filarial antigens are also necessary to trigger the reaction.

Ivermectin at an oral dose of 400 µg kg^{-1} every fortnight for 6 months (total dose of 4.8 mg kg^{-1}) completely inhibits production of microfilariae but has no effect on adults when examined by ultrasonography, even at the end of long-term treatment. For mass chemotherapy, 200 µg kg^{-1} once yearly has been advocated. It probably acts by binding to glutamate-gated chloride channels.

Albendazole in a single oral dose of 400 mg can be given with DEC or ivermectin and appears to have some action against adults (possibly synergistic).

Long-term treatment with antibiotics, such as rifampicin or oxytetracycline, is showing promise in research and clinical trials (Townson *et al.*, 2000).

Surgical. Traditionally hydrocele has been treated by adding sclerosing agents and lymphoedema by bandaging and elevation of limbs. Radical surgery has also been used to remove adventitious tissue in elephantiasis. Recently, regular washing and hygienic care of inflamed lymph vessels and hydroceles has been shown to resolve manifestations and prevents further development. Following 5 years of chemotherapy and simple medical treatment in New Guinea, 87% of patients were cured of hydrocele and in 69% lymphoedema had resolved.

EPIDEMIOLOGY

Of the 107 million cases of Bancroftian filariasis in the world, 49% are in South-East Asia (particularly India, with an estimated 48 million infections), 31.3.% in Africa, 16% in the western Pacific, 3.4% in the Americas and 0.3% (or now probably nil) in the eastern Mediterranean; altogether it occurs in over 80 countries, where 750 million people are at risk. The geographical distribution of the disease is determined largely by climate, being found in areas with a hot, humid climate; the local distribution can be forecast by geographical information systems (GIS) imaging (Brooker and Michael, 2000) and by the distribution of the vectors, but other factors may be involved, such as local variations in the density, susceptibility, longevity and human-biting habits of the vector and in the density, sleeping habits and natural and acquired resistance of the human population.

Many species of mosquitoes have been shown to act as vectors in various parts of the world (WHO, 1992; Kettle, 1995; Service, 2001), including at least 31 species of *Anopheles* (*An. aquasalis, bellator, darlingi* in the Americas; *An. funestus, gambiae, arabiensis, bwambae, melas, merus, nili* in Africa; *An. aconitus, anthropophagus, kewiyangensis, nigerrimus, sinensis* complex, *letifer, whartoni, flavirostrus, minimus, candidiensis, balabacensis, leu-cosphyrus, maculatus, philippinensis, sub-pictus, tesselatus, vagus* in Asia; *An. bancrofti, farauti, koliensis, punctulatus,* in Papua New Guinea), five species of *Culex* (*C. quinquefasciatus* in the Americas, Africa and Asia; *C. pipiens molestus* in the Middle East; *C. bitaeniorhynchus, sitiens* complex*, pipiens pallens* in Asia; *C. pipiens pallens* in the western Pacific; *C. annulirostris, bitaeniorynchus* in Papua) 15 species of *Aedes* (*Ae. scapularis* in the Americas; *Ae. niveus* group*, harinasutai, togoi, poicilius* in Asia; *Ae. togoi* in the western Pacific; *Ae. fijiensis, oceanicus, samoanus, vigilax, futunae, polynesiensis, pseudoscutellaris, tabu, tongae, upolensis* in the South Pacific) and two species of *Mansonia* (*M. titillans* in the Americas; *M. uniformis* in Asia and Papua).

Vector *Anopheles* species breed in ponds, slow-flowing streams, rice paddies and fresh- or salty-water swamps, and LF transmitted by them is principally a rural disease. Members of the *An. gambiae* group (*An. gambiae, arabiensis, melas, merus*) are very susceptible vectors and show facilitation, whereby the penetration of one larva through the stomach wall facil-itates the entry of others; this can result in high mortality of mosquitoes when microfi-larial rates are high (Dye, 1992). In rural areas of East Africa, infection rates of 1–1.5% are found in *An. gambiae, An. ara-biensis* and *An. funestus,* but 0–0.3% in *C. quinquefasciatus* (although this is the only vector in urban areas). In West Africa, transmission is entirely due to *Anopheles*; although *C. quinquefasciatus* is common in urban areas, it cannot be infected.

Culex quinquefasciatus is the most important vector in urban areas of Asia and East Africa, as it can breed in very small bodies of water contaminated with organic matter (especially leaking septic tanks, pit latrines and drains). The adult females readily enter houses, tend to rest indoors and are night biters; they can sometimes fly for up to 1 km. They are almost entirely anthropophilic and in Singapore infection rates of 20% occur. *Culex* species show the phenomenon of limitation, whereby pene-tration of one larva inhibits the passage of others, so that only a few larvae are usually found in each mosquito (it also has a pha-ryngeal armature, which destroys many microfilariae). However, there may be many mosquitoes biting each night (over 100 per night is common) and in Calcutta it has been estimated that one person may be bit-ten by 6000–7000 infected *C. quinquefas-ciatus* per year. This species is extending its range alarmingly in both Asia and Africa.

On Polynesian islands (east of longitude 160°), such as Fiji, Samoa and Tahiti, a diurnally periodic form of LF occurs and the vectors are species of *Aedes,* which can breed in small bodies of water, such as opened coconut shells, leaf bracts, crab holes and manufactured containers, such as pots, tin cans and car tyres. In Thailand there is a nocturnally periodic form of LF transmitted by *Ae. niveus.*

To determine transmission rates in mos-quitoes they can be dissected individually (Davies, 1995) or, where rates are very low, a pool method using 1000–2000 (possibly dried) mosquitoes can be employed and the presence of larvae shown by DNA determination after PCR amplification.

PREVENTION AND CONTROL

Lymphatic filariasis was identified recently as one of six potentially eradicable diseases by an International Task Force (1993), and the World Health Organization (WHO) is coordinating campaigns to eliminate it as a public health problem in the next few years (Ottesen *et al.*, 1997; WHO, 1999; see also WHO web site: www.filariasis.org). The reason for optimism is partly because of new regimes of chemotherapy and from the success of campaigns already carried out in various countries. It is possible that there is a window of opportunity such as in retrospect can be seen to have con-tributed to the success of the smallpox campaign: just after its eradication mass vaccination would not have been possible because of the spread of AIDS.

Control is aimed at both alleviating the suffering caused by the disease (morbidity control) and stopping the spread of infec-tion (transmission control).

Morbidity control. Mass treatment campaigns with DEC have been tried with varying degrees of success over the last 40 years. China, where compliance is good, is now in the final stages of a long-term campaign: in 1950 there were estimated to be 30 million cases, while there were only about 1.65 million in 1995. In China and other countries, such as Samoa, Solomon Islands and Tahiti and particularly in the Ryuku Islands (Japan), South Korea and Taiwan, DEC has been added to cooking salt (at a dose of about 3 mg kg^{-1}) and has greatly reduced disease. In the past it was thought that DEC only acted against microfilariae (at a total dose of 72 g usually given over 12 days), but recently studies have indicated that a single annual dose is effective and also has some action against adults. If microfilarial rates fall below a critical breakpoint, then infection should die out (this level probably differs in different areas and with different populations).

The real breakthrough in mass treatment was the recent finding that combined treatment schedules are much more effective than the use of a single drug (Ottesen *et al.*, 1999; Plaisier *et al.*, 2000). In the new WHO initiative two main regimes are recommended:

1. All areas except sub-Saharan Africa:
(a) DEC (6 mg kg^{-1} body weight) combined with albendazole (400 mg) once yearly for 4–6 years is the preferred regime;
(b) or DEC (6 mg kg^{-1}) once a year for 4–6 years alone (this has fewer side-effects than the traditional 12-day treatment;
(c) or DEC in salt (0.2–0.4% w/w) for 6–12 months.
2. Sub-Saharan Africa:
DEC cannot be given because there may also be infections with loiasis or onchocerciasis and this drug can then be dangerous (see p. 210) or very unpleasant (see p. 218).
(a) Single yearly dose of ivermectin (200 μm kg^{-1}) plus albendazole (400 mg) for 4–6 years (optimal);
(b) or ivermectin alone at same dose.

Campaigns using these schedules have started in American Samoa and western Samoa and Niue (25 countries by August 2001). It is intended that 50 million individuals will have been treated at least once by the end of 2001 and that the disease will be eliminated as a problem in any country by 2020. There is a concerted campaign starting in all Pacific islands that hopes to eliminate infection there by 2010. This area consists of 22 island states with a total population of 7 million but extends over one-third of the world's surface. The manufacturers of both albendazole (GSK) and ivermectin (Merck) have donated enough of these agents to carry out the programme. It is very important in ivermectin treatment that coverage and pattern of attendance at mass clinics should be satisfactory (Plaisier *et al.*, 2000).

To treat adenolymphangitis and hydrocele, thorough and frequent washing and possibly antibiotic and antifungal treatment can help to prevent bacterial infection and this appears to prevent subsequent elephantiasis also.

Transmission control. There is no animal reservoir host and so all efforts can be directed to breaking the human transmission cycle.

1. Insecticide-impregnated (usually permethrin) bed nets and curtains, as used for malaria control, which can be effective for months even if the net has a few holes. Spraying walls is not as popular as it once was, as many mosquitoes, particularly *Culex* species, are exophilic and do not rest inside houses. Screening of doors and windows and provision of ceilings reduced the biting rate from 200 to 5 per night in a trial in Tanzania.
2. The use of long-lasting polystyrene beads in enclosed breeding sites, such as latrines, cesspools and ponds to prevent the air breathing of mosquito larvae and pupae. The ventilated improved pit (VIP) latrine with a screened air pipe, which traps emerging *C. quinquefasciatus* adults as they move towards the light, can help in controlling mosquito numbers. New

biocides, such as *Bacillus sphaericus*, a self-reproducing, toxin-producing bacterium specific against *C. quinquefasciatus*, will also kill larvae.

3. Environmental engineering can be designed to prevent open drains and sewage systems and to remove unwanted water and solid waste safely to prevent mosquito breeding. Cesspools should also be covered. Measures against *Culex* are often welcomed by the local population as it is an important nuisance biter (Plate 26). Where the same *Anopheles* vectors are involved, malaria control measures can help to control LF also and, indeed, in the Solomon Islands the latter has almost vanished in this way, although malaria is still common. The situation is similar in Vanuatu, which at present has a prevalence of 2.8%. In Polynesia, clearing up small containers containing water or adding safe organophosphorus insecticides to drinking-water pots can help to control *Aedes* vectors.

The use of larvivorous fish has long been advocated and might have a limited effect against *Anopheles* vectors.

Integrated control measures are likely to be necessary for successful control schemes, involving community participation and possibly primary health-care initiatives.

4. Chemotherapy also plays a large part in reducing transmission and in New Guinea the annual transmission potential (ATP) of the vector *Anopheles punctulatus* was reduced enormously after the first year's treatment.

ZOONOTIC ASPECTS
None, although microfilariae of Wuchereria type have been reported once from a potto (*Peridicticus potto*). In experimental infections, complete development has been obtained in leaf monkeys (*Presbytis cristata*) and macaques (*Macaca cyclopis*) and slight development in male jirds. Another species, *W. kalimantani,* is a natural parasite of the leaf monkey in Kalimantan (Borneo) and is used in drug trials but has not been recorded from humans. Microfilariae from humans in

Brazil differ in nuclear number and were given the name *W. lewisi* Schacher, 1969, but no differences have been found in adults recovered from the same area.

Brugia malayi
(Brug, 1927) Buckley, 1960

SYNONYM
Wuchereria malayi Brug, 1927.

DISEASE
Lymphatic filariasis or filariosis (LF), Malayan filariasis or filariosis, cause of elephantiasis.

LOCAL NAMES
As for *W. bancrofti*. Baku (Japanese in Hachijo Koshima Island).

GEOGRAPHICAL DISTRIBUTION
Infection is confined to Asia and occurs in Cambodia, southern China, southern India, Indonesia, Korea, Laos, Malaysia, Philippines (Palawan Islands), Vietnam and until recently in Japan.

LOCATION IN HOST
The adults inhabit the lymphatic glands and lymph vessels, usually of the lower limbs and groin. Sheathed microfilariae occur in the peripheral bloodstream.

MORPHOLOGY
The adults are very similar to those of *W. bancrofti* but there are small differences in the papillae and spicules at the tail end of the male worm.

The sheathed microfilariae in the blood can be clearly differentiated from those of *W. bancrofti*. They measure 170–260 µm × 5–6 µm and in stained smears appear stiff and kinky, unlike the smooth curves of *W. bancrofti* microfilariae (Fig. 90). The sheath is much longer than the body and stains bright pink in Romanowsky stains, such as Giemsa, at a pH of 6.8 (the sheaths of microfilariae are sometimes lost in the process of making a smear, so more than one should be examined). The round

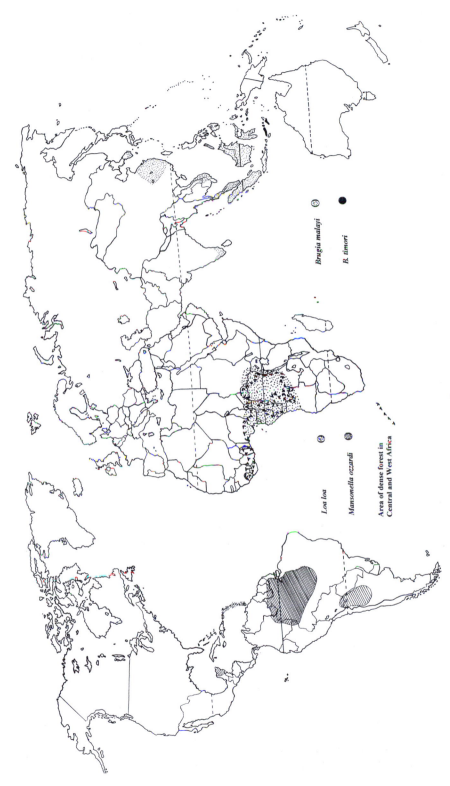

Map 9. Distribution of *Brugia malayi*, *B. timori*, *Loa loa* and *Mansonella ozzardi*.

anterior end is free of nuclei for 12–16 μm and has a double stylet process. The tail is pointed and has two distinctive nuclei at the posterior extremity. Of the complete 100 Mb genome of *B. malayi*, 33% has now been deposited in a database (Williams and Johnston, 1999).

LIFE CYCLE

The microfilariae are usually nocturnally periodic: a subperiodic form occurs in peninsular Malaya, the Palawan Islands, Sabah and Thailand.

On being ingested by a mosquito vector from the blood capillaries of an infected person, the microfilariae lose their sheaths in the stomach and penetrate the wall of the gut. The larvae develop similarly to those of *W. bancrofti* and moult twice in the thoracic muscles before migrating to the labium in 6–12 days. Infective third-stage larvae, measuring 1.3–1.7 mm in length, migrate out through the tips of the labella when the mosquito bites another individual and enter the skin through the puncture wound (Figs 91 and 97). The larvae reach the lymph glands, moult twice more and reach maturity in about 3 months.

CLINICAL MANIFESTATIONS AND PATHOGENESIS

Brugia malayi causes similar disturbances of the lymphatic system to those already described under *W. bancrofti*. Elephantiasis is usually confined to the lower leg below the knee and is a common complication in Malaysia (Plate 27), while hydrocele is uncommon in males. There is also a higher proportion of apparently symptomless carriers than with bancroftian filariasis (probably because of a lower intensity of infection).

In animals experimentally infected with *Brugia* species, developing worms can cause dilatation of the lymph vessels and enlargement of the nodes within weeks of infection (Denham and Fletcher, 1987); ultrasound studies could help to determine whether this occurs in humans.

DIAGNOSIS

As for *W. bancrofti,* although new commercial immunological tests for the former do

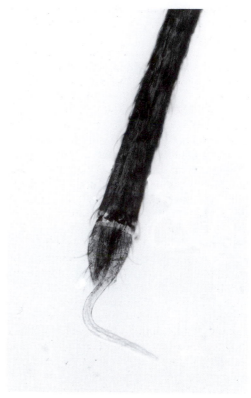

Fig. 97. Infective larva of *Brugia* emerging from labella palp of mosquito.

not cross-react. Specific tests for *B. malayi* are also being investigated, one of which uses recombinant ES antigens (Kumari *et al.*, 1994).

In blood films microfilariae of the nocturnally periodic form often lose their sheaths, which can be seen separately.

TREATMENT

As for bancroftian filariasis, except that with DEC only one-third of the normal dose should be given on the first 2 days, due to likely febrile reactions. These are probably more severe in malayan filariasis because the drug is more effective against their microfilariae and the count is usually higher.

EPIDEMIOLOGY

In all endemic areas of malayan filariasis except for Sulawesi (Borneo), bancroftian filariasis also occurs. However, the infection patterns of the two infections differ, as explained below.

The nocturnally periodic form of malayan filariasis is transmitted by night-biting species of mosquito; by *Mansonia uniformis* in most areas, by *Anopheles barbirostris* and *Anopheles campestris* in southern China, India and Japan, and by *Aedes togoi*, which breeds in swampy areas, in Cheju Island (Korea) and coastal areas of China. Species of *Mansonia* (*M. anullifera, indiana, uniformis*), which transmit the nocturnally periodic form of infection, lay their eggs in small batches on the undersurface of the leaves of water-plants, such as the water hyacinth in Assam, mangrove in western Malaysia or water lettuce (*Pistia stratiotes*) in southern India and Sri Lanka. The larvae and pupae attach to the underwater stems of these plants by the specially adapted respiratory siphon through which they obtain air from the plant. This form of *B. malayi* is also transmitted by species of *Anopheles* (*An. aconitus, anthropophagus, barbirostris, campestris, donaldi, kewiyangensis, nigerrimus, letifer, sinensis* complex, *whartoni*) and by *Aedes togoi*. These species, unlike the *Culex* vectors of *W. bancrofti*, cannot breed in small temporary bodies of water and so malayan filariasis is a more rural disease than bancroftian. The periodic form is highly adapted to humans and reservoir hosts are not important.

The subperiodic form, with microfilariae occurring in the peripheral circulation during the day, is transmitted by species of *Mansonia* (*M. annulata, annulifera, bonnae, dives, indiana, uniformis*), which bite by day as well as by night and are predominantly zoophilic. This form is probably a natural parasite of monkeys and civet cats and human infections occur when rice-fields adjoin areas of, often cleared, forest.

PREVENTION AND CONTROL

Clearing of the water-weeds necessary for the development of *Mansonia* larvae can be difficult as they re-establish so quickly. However, in Sri Lanka, they have been removed from the ponds used for treating copra and, with the help of weed-killers and insecticides against adults (used principally for malaria control), infection has been virtually eliminated. Unfortunately, bancroftian filariasis is still spreading in Sri Lanka.

The worldwide measures being started against LF should be particularly effective against the nocturnally periodic form of malayan filariasis: a mass treatment campaign in north-west Malaysia reduced microfilarial rates from 26% to below 1%.

ZOONOTIC ASPECTS

Subperiodic *B. malayi* is one of the most catholic of filarial worms and natural infections have been reported from four species of monkeys (particularly the leaf monkey, *Presbytis obscurus*), civet cats, domestic cats and pangolins. Experimentally it will also develop to maturity in various rodents.

Brugia pahangi (Buckley and Edeson, 1956) is a natural parasite of cats and wild carnivores in western Malaysia and has developed to maturity in humans in experimental infections. The different forms of *B. malayi* may reflect the presence of a species complex with the sibling species *B. pahangi*. The microfilariae of subperiodic *B. malayi* occurring in wild animals can be differentiated from those of *B. pahangi* by the fact that only the former will develop in *Mansonia bonneae*.

Brugia timori Partano, Purnomo, Dennis, Atmosoedjono, Oemijati and Cross, 1977, causes timoran filariasis or filariosis in humans on the islands of Timor, Flores and Alor (see Map 9, p. 203). Microfilariae are nocturnally periodic and in blood smears can be differentiated from those of *B. malayi* as the sheath does not stain in Giemsa stain.

Clinical manifestations are similar to those of *B. malayi* but the presence of adult worms in the lymphatics often causes abscesses to develop in the groin region (Plate 28). It is transmitted by mosquitoes of the *Anopheles barbirostris* group (probably *An. campestris*).

Brugia beaveri Ash and Little, 1964, is a natural parasite of wild carnivores (bobcat, mink and racoon) in Louisiana, USA, and an adult male worm has been recovered once from an enlarged human lymph node (Schlesinger *et al.*, 1977).

Brugia guyanensis Orihel, 1964: adults have been reported once from a human cervical lymph node in Peru (Baird and Neafie, 1988). It is a natural parasite of the coatimundi (*Nasua nasua*).

Loa loa
(Cobbold, 1864) Castellani and Chalmers, 1913

SYNONYMS
Filaria oculi humani, Microfilaria diurna.

DISEASE AND POPULAR NAMES
Loiasis or loaosis; *Loa* filariasis or filariosis. Eye-worm infection. Cause of Calabar swellings.

LOCAL NAMES
Agan anya (Ibo), Aroro or Aján oju (Yoruba).

GEOGRAPHICAL DISTRIBUTION
Confined to forest areas of West and Central Africa, particularly where equatorial rain forest has been cleared and on the fringes of guinea savannah. In northern Angola, southern Cameroon, Central African Republic, Congo, Democratic Republic of Congo (Zaire), Gabon, Ghana, Guinea-Bissau, Ivory Coast, Nigeria (Niger delta region), Sierra Leone, southern Sudan and western Uganda, with a few infections reported from Ethiopia (see Map 9, p. 204).

LOCATION IN HOST
Adults are found in the subcutaneous connective tissues and the sheathed microfilariae circulate in the peripheral blood during the day.

MORPHOLOGY
The adults are thin transparent worms, the females measuring 70 mm × 0.5 mm, the males 30–35 mm × 0.3–0.4 mm. The head is truncated and has a ring of six papillae just behind the mouth. The cuticle has numerous, randomly arranged, smooth, round bosses; they are absent from the head end of the female and from both ends of the male (these bosses must be differentiated from the regular annulations found in *Onchocerca* (Fig. 98), as portions of either species could be found in biopsy material). The lateral cords are much more conspicuous than in other human filariae.

In the female the vulva opens 2.5 mm from the anterior end. The posterior end is rounded and has a pair of terminal papillae. The females are ovoviviparous, the twin uteri containing all stages of developing eggs and larvae enclosed in egg membranes (the sheath). The male has a tail curved ventrally, with two lateral, posteriorly placed, cuticular expansions and five pairs of asymmetrically placed, pedunculated papillae around the cloaca and three pairs of small, sessile papillae. There are two unequal spicules, measuring 150 and 100 µm.

The microfilariae are sheathed and measure 250 (230–300) µm × 6–8 µm. They have a kinked appearance in stained preparations (in contrast to the smooth curves of *W. bancrofti* microfilariae). The tail is short and relatively thick, with large nuclei continuing to the tip. The sheath does not stain with Giemsa or Wright's stain (although it does with haematoxylin) so that the microfilariae are sometimes mistakenly identified as being unsheathed (Figs 99 and 109).

LIFE CYCLE
Microfilariae found in the peripheral blood show a diurnal periodicity, being most plentiful from 08.00 to 17.00 h, when up to 40 ml^{-1} may be present.

The vectors are large (7 mm long), day-biting, tabanid flies, principally *Chrysops dimidiata* and *C. silacea* (also *C. centurionis, distinctipennis, langi, longicornis, zahrai* and possibly *streptobalius*). *Chrysops*, known as the mango, mangrove or softly-softly fly, usually bites (painfully) below the knee and is a pool feeder. The

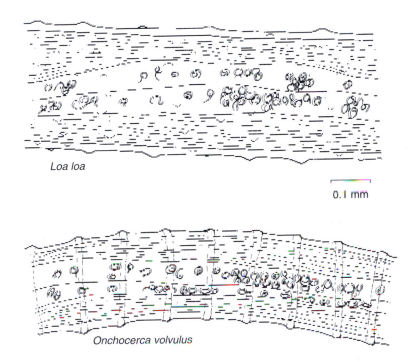

Loa loa

0. I mm

Onchocerca volvulus

Fig. 98. Portions of *Loa* and *Onchocerca* as may be recovered in tissue biopsies.

microfilariae are picked up in a blood meal, lose their sheaths inside the stomach of the fly and penetrate the gut wall after about 6 h. They develop in the cells of the fat body and moult twice. The third-stage larvae, measuring 2 mm × 25 µm, migrate first to the thorax and then to the head and are infective after 10–12 days. The larvae move down the labium when the fly bites a new host and enter at the site of the wound. Because the vector takes such a large blood meal, up to 100 larvae can be found in one fly. They migrate through the human subcutaneous connective tissues and muscle fasciae, moulting twice and developing into adults in 6–12 months. The adults live for 4–17 years.

CLINICAL MANIFESTATIONS

A weal appears at the site of the bite if the individual has been previously infected.

The adult worms migrate through the connective tissues in any part of the body, the resulting hypersensitivity reaction sometimes causing painless Calabar swellings, which disappear in a few hours or days to reappear elsewhere. These non-pitting oedematous swellings, which can be easily differentiated from onchocercal nodules by their fugitive nature, appear 6–12 months after infection, most commonly in the hand or ankle, and reappear at intervals for another year or so. The Calabar swellings are sometimes accompanied by intense itching, with arthralgia, pruritus and fever, and, if near a joint, may cause difficulty in flexion. In chronic infections the worms go deeper and may migrate through all the viscera of the body; they do not then cause swellings and microfilariae may no longer be found in the blood, but there have usually been often undiagnosed symptoms of fatigue, recurrent fever and perhaps arthritic pains for a long time. In general, indigenous inhabitants have higher micro-filaraemias but fewer swellings and symptoms than visitors or expatriates. Adult worms sometimes cross the conjunctiva at a rate of about 1 cm min^{-1} and can then be extracted (Fig. 100); they usually pass

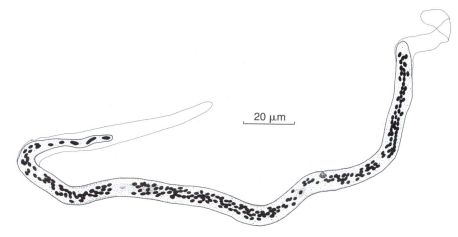

Fig. 99. Microfilaria of *Loa loa* (stained in haematoxylin – compare Fig. 109).

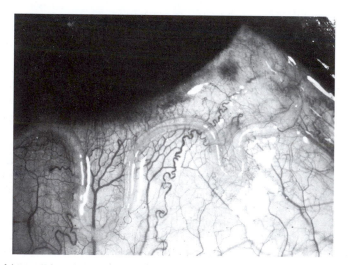

Fig. 100. Adult of *Loa* moving under the conjunctiva.

across the eye in minutes but can remain for days, causing considerable discomfort. In most cases loiasis is a relatively benign disease with a good prognosis.

A hypereosinophilia of 60–90% (20,000 –50,000 eosinophils mm^{-3}) is frequently found and may contribute to the endocardial fibrosis sometimes reported; pulmonary infiltrations have also been reported rarely. IgE levels are typically raised, although it is not clear what role this plays in the host response.

PATHOGENESIS

Biopsy sections of swellings sometimes show adults in the centre of an oedematous reaction. In chronic cases the skin may become lichenified. Dying worms in the subcutaneous tissues can cause a chronic abscess, followed by a granulomatous reaction and fibrosis (Fig. 101); worms have been excised from many parts of the body.

It is likely that in chronic sufferers who are amicrofilaraemic, microfilariae are being destroyed by immune responses in these

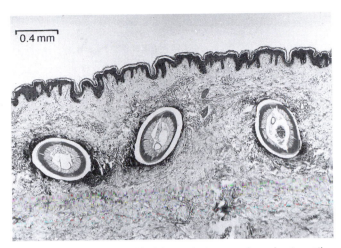

0.4 mm

Fig. 101. Section of subcutaneous tissues with dying male *Loa* causing a host reaction.

hypersensitized individuals, and the endo-myocardial fibrosis and nephrotic syndrome sometimes reported from such cases resemble the situation in the collagen diseases.

Various visceral lesions have been attributed to loiasis, but the most serious complication is meningoencephalitis, which can be fatal and is not uncommon in areas of high endemicity. It may be accompanied by retinal haemorrhages and is associated with DEC in patients with very high microfilaraemia. Microfilariae may be found in the cerebrospinal fluid of such cases and encephalitis is presumably caused by an allergic reaction to dead or dying microfilariae obstructing the capillaries of the brain (Pinder, 1988).

The relatively mild pathology usually associated with this infection includes a number of allergic manifestations. These may include pruritus, oedema and arthritis, all indicative of immune-mediated reactions to the parasite. Studies in mandrills have shown both Th1 and Th2 responses during infection, although there is some stage specificity (L_3s preferentially stimulated Th2, while microfilariae provoked both Th2 and Th1 cytokines). The adverse reactions to DEC seen in loiasis patients are, as in onchocerciasis patients, associated with immunological hyper-responsiveness to microfilarial antigens (Wahl and Georges, 1995).

DIAGNOSIS

The most common method of diagnosis is by finding microfilariae in thick blood smears taken during the day. In chronic infections and those in visitors, microfilariae may be very scanty and concentration techniques can be used (see p. 263). The microfilariae also live for many years and can continue to circulate even after adults are dead.

The presence of the fugitive ('wasp sting') swellings with high eosinophilia in a patient who lives in or who has visited an endemic region is characteristic of an early infection. Biopsy sections of swellings sometimes show portions of adults in the centre of an oedematous reaction. Adult worms seen moving across the conjunctiva can be removed and identified.

Detection of antibodies is possible but is not very specific. Recently, methods for detection of circulating antigens have been more successful. An ELISA using parasite-specific IgG4 can recognize specific *Loa* antigens of low molecular mass (12–30 kDa) and works in patients with or without microfilaraemia. The test can also differentiate from other filarial infections, particularly *Mansonella perstans* (Akue *et al.*, 1994). Antigen detection by coelectrosynerisis (Co-ES) has also shown promise. A PCR amplification method to detect *Loa* DNA using a Southern blot technique is stated to be very sensitive and specific (Toure *et al.*, 1997).

TREATMENT

Chemotherapy. DEC kills both adults and microfilariae when given at 2–6 mg kg^{-1} (usually 300 mg for an adult) for 14–21 days. However, side-reactions, such as transient oedema, generalized eruptions, arthralgia, nausea, diarrhoea and fever, often occur and, where there is a high microfilaraemia (over 1000 mm^{-3}), more serious effects are possible, such as meningo-encephalitis, coma and renal damage. It is wise to commence treatment at a very low dosage in all patients with more than 20 microfilariae ml^{-1}, perhaps under corticosteroid cover.

Ivermectin (200 μg kg^{-1} body weight every 3 months for 2 years) decreased microfilarial levels by 90% and reduced prevalence from 30% to 10% in a trial in Cameroon, but these slowly returned to previous levels after about 2 years. Side-effects of pruritus, headache, arthralgia and maybe fever are common (Chippaux *et al.*, 1992). Rare reports (1 per 10,000 persons treated in one trial) of encephalopathy, coma and renal damage have been noted. The use of a single dose of ivermectin (200 μg kg^{-1}) to reduce microfilaraemias before DEC treatment has also been advocated.

Albendazole (200 mg twice daily for 21 days) causes microfilarial numbers to fall slowly and may have an adulticidal (macrofilaricidal) action, since immunological tests become negative after a few months and eosinophilia falls.

Surgery. When a worm is seen moving across the eye, a curved, bayonet-edge, surgical needle can be passed under the worm and it can then be removed with a mounted needle. The conjunctiva and worm are first anaesthetized with a few drops of 10% novocaine.

EPIDEMIOLOGY

The disease is restricted to equatorial forest regions and prevalence is falling in some areas as forest is cleared. Recent estimates

of infection are 30% in Calabar and 10% in Gongola State in Nigeria, 30% in Cameroon, 19% in Bantu and 11% in pygmies in Congo, 10–70% in the Republic of Congo, 12% in Equatorial Guinea, 30% in Gabon; everywhere infection rates are higher in adults than in children.

Chrysops breeds in densely shaded streams covered with leaves, in which the sandy bottom is overlaid with mud and decaying vegetation, on which the slowly developing larvae feed. In West Africa, adult *Chrysops* are particularly common in the rainy season (June–September). The adult female flies live in the high canopy of the forest and possibly feed on monkeys. They are attracted to movement below or to wood smoke rising, and humans get bitten most often in cleared areas, such as rubber, cocoa, teak or oil-palm plantations on the forest fringes, where the flies can see a break in the canopy. *C. dimidiata* and *C. silacea* are the principal vectors in West Africa and *C. distinctipennis* in Central Africa. Flies bite during the day and (except sometimes for *C. silacea*) do not usually enter native houses as they are too dark inside. *Chrysops* ingests 10–20 μl of blood per meal; it probably feeds about once a fortnight, since it requires one full blood meal in each gestation period of about 12 days.

PREVENTION AND CONTROL

For individual protection, repellents and protective clothing can be used. It has also been reported that DEC kills infective larvae and 5 mg kg^{-1} daily for 3 days every month has been suggested as a prophylactic.

In the past dieldrin sucessfully controlled larvae and pupae in forest streams in Cameroon, but treatment (nowadays probably with temephos) is not practical over large areas. A mass campaign with DEC in Nigeria was not successful, but prevalence was reduced from 30% to 10% in an area of Cameroon after mass treatment with ivermectin.

ZOONOTIC ASPECTS

A sympatric but ecologically separate cycle of *Loa loa* is also found in many species of forest-dwelling primates, such as the drill (*Papio* = *Mandrillus leucophaeus*), the mona monkey (*Cercopithecus mona*) and the putty-nosed guenon (*C. nictitans*). However, the microfilariae in these hosts are larger and show a nocturnal periodicity, while the species of *Chrysops* acting as vectors (*C. centurionis* and *C. langi*) are also night biters. The parasite is sometimes given subspecific status as *L. loa papionis,* with the human parasite called *L. l. loa.* The monkey and human strains have been hybridized experimentally, but it is unlikely that humans become infected with the monkey strain, because the flies bite almost entirely in the upper canopy; there is also some evidence that humans cannot be infected with the monkey strain (or subspecies). It is possible, though, that monkeys living near the ground sometimes become infected with the human form and could then act as reservoir hosts.

A similar parasite, *Loaina* sp., of rabbits, transmitted by mosquitoes, has been recovered once from the anterior chamber of the eye in a man in Colombia (Orihel and Eberhard, 1998).

Onchocerca volvulus
(Leuckart, 1893) Railliet and Henry, 1910

SYNONYMS
Filaria volvulus Leuckart, 1893; *Onchocerca caecutiens* Brumpt, 1919.

DISEASE AND POPULAR NAMES
Onchocerciasis or onchocercosis; river blindness, craw-craw (West Africa), blinding filaria.

LOCAL NAMES
Amar eljur (N. Sudan), Aràn oju (Yoruba), Firkaw and Ekraw (Twi), Kirci (Hausa), Sowda (Yemen), Ungoujwa ya usinyi (Sambaa).

GEOGRAPHICAL DISTRIBUTION
Africa (including Angola, Benin, Cameroon, Central African Republic, Chad, Congo, Côte d'Ivoire, Equatorial Guinea, Ethiopia, Gabon, Ghana, Guinea, Liberia, Malawi, Mali, Nigeria, Republic of Congo, Senegal, Sierra Leone, Sudan, Tanzania, Togo and Uganda, with limited foci in Burkina Faso, Guinea-Bissau, Niger and Yemen) and Central and South America (Brazil, Guatemala, southern Mexico, Venezuela and possibly still Colombia and Ecuador). It is estimated that there are about 17.5 million cases in Africa and 140,000 in the Americas, of whom 0.8 million have visual impairment and 0.27 million are blind.

LOCATION IN HOST
The adult worms live in the subcutaneous tissues and in long-standing infections they form tangled masses inside fibrous nodules (onchocercomas). Microfilarial larvae are found in the skin (probably mostly in lymphatic channels in the dermis) but not usually in the blood.

MORPHOLOGY
Both ends of the filiform adults are tapered but the tail terminates bluntly. The anterior end has two circles of four papillae and a large lateral pair. The cuticle has conspicuous annular thickenings (rugae), which are important in identification as usually only portions of worms can be obtained from nodules (Fig. 98).

The adult female measures 300–500 mm × 0.25–0.4 mm and the male 20–40 mm × 0.15–0.20 mm. The vulva of the female opens about 0.85 mm from the anterior end and the uterus is bicornate. The male has a variable number of anal papillae and two unequal spicules.

The microfilariae measure 280–330 μm × 6–9 μm. They are unsheathed and have a tapered tail, and the head and tail are free of nuclei (Fig. 102). The head is characteristically expanded and the cuticle is striated. The microfilariae wander in the skin but are not usually found in the bloodstream, except after DEC treatment; they can survive for 6–24 months. Sometimes microfilariae are also present in the urine and sputum.

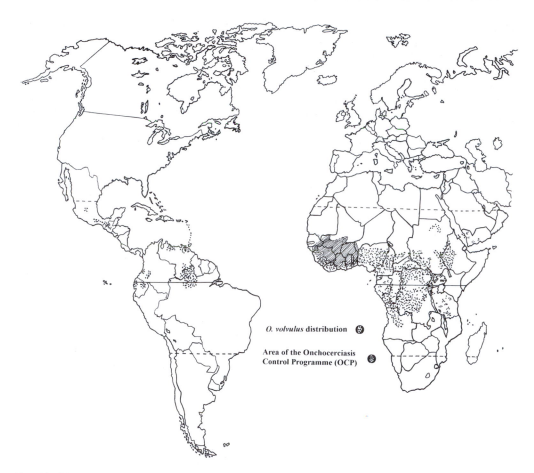

Map 10. Distribution of *Onchocerca volvulus*.

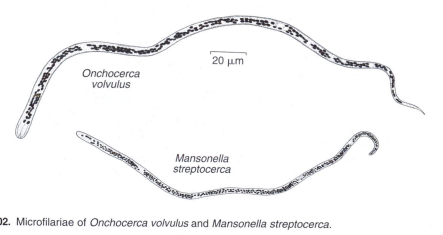

Fig. 102. Microfilariae of *Onchocerca volvulus* and *Mansonella streptocerca*.

LIFE CYCLE

Microfilariae in the skin are ingested by biting flies of the genus *Simulium* (known as black-flies or buffalo gnats. Figs 103 and 104). The microfilariae are probably attracted to the site of the bite by saliva injected into the puncture wound. The flies have a short scarifying proboscis and are pool feeders on tissue fluids released by their bite. Some of the microfilariae ingested by the fly leave the midgut before the formation of the peritrophic membrane and penetrate the thoracic muscle cells, particularly the flight muscles; others are trapped in the midgut and die. After two moults in the muscles of the fly, the first moult giving rise to a sausage stage, the few infective larvae move to the head and proboscis, complete development taking 6–12 days, depending on the ambient temperature (no development occurs below 18°C). For studies of transmission rates, the infective third-stage larvae must be differentiated from other animal filarial larvae found in *Simulium* (including the cattle species *O. ochengi*, which occurs in West Africa and has morphologically identical larvae); they measure 560 (440–700) μm × 19 μm and have a single small knob at the tail. These larvae probably enter through the puncture wound when an infected fly bites another individual. They migrate to the subcutaneous tissues, moult twice and reach sexual maturity in about 10–15 months. Microfilariae can first be found in the skin by 18 months after infection and take 4–6 weeks to reach the skin after leaving the vulva of the adult worm (about 1000 actively leave the vulva of each female per day). The adults live on average for 9–11 years and very rarely survive for more than 13 years, while microfilariae can live in the skin for up to 2 years.

CLINICAL MANIFESTATIONS AND PATHOGENESIS

Most of the severe manifestations are due to the presence of the microfilariae; the adults are of secondary importance (contrast

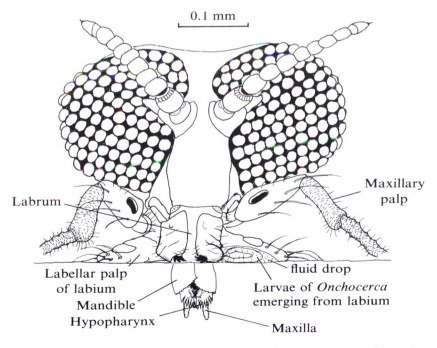

Fig. 103. Diagram of head of *Simulium* feeding on human skin with infective larvae of *O. volvulus* emerging from the labium (it is probable that they usually emerge from the posterior surface of the labium or from the hypopharynx).

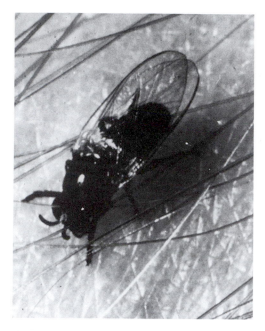

Fig. 104. The black-fly *Simulium damnosum* s.l. feeding on human.

infections with the lymphatic filariae). In long-standing infections the adults are often found in characteristic non-tender nodules, known as onchocercomata, which can be felt and often seen, especially over bony prominences (Fig. 105). There may be a single nodule or many present. In Africa nodules are usually found around the

pelvic region, knees and lateral chest and spine, while in the Americas (except for Venezuela) the nodules are more commonly seen in the upper part of the body, including the head.

Death of adult worms deep in the tissues can lead to the formation of an abscess and nodules on the scalp may erode the bone.

As in many helminth infections, there is a blood eosinophilia, in this case of 10–75% (usually with 700–1500 eosinophils mm^{-3} blood).

The majority of lightly infected indigenous individuals living in an endemic area show few or no signs, although at some time many will have pruritus, with skin lesions leading to the characteristic presbydermia. In the early stages, or in lightly infected persons, the presence of the adult worms cannot be detected, but the microfilariae usually cause pruritus with a persistent and intensely itchy rash of the skin in their vicinity (filarial itch), often confined to one anatomical quarter of the body. The rash consists of many raised papules, 1–3 mm in diameter, and often becomes secondarily infected following scratching ('craw-craw' or 'gale filarienne'). There is usually lymphadenopathy in the groin or axilla of the affected side, sometimes accompanied by aches and pains. The

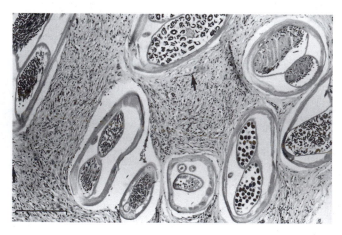

Fig. 105. Section of subcutaneous nodule with adult female and microfilariae (one arrowed) in the fibrous connective tissues.

onchodermatitis can lead in months or years to a secondary stage of thickening due to intradermal oedema (often giving a 'peau d'orange' effect) and to pachydermia (lichenification or crocodile skin). The loss of elastic fibres in the skin can lead to 'hanging groin', pendulous sacs containing inguinal or femoral glands (Fig. 106) or hernias, which are particularly found in males in East Africa, and probably to the leonine facies encountered in Guatemala. Elephantiasis of the scrotum can also occur in males but, in contrast to that caused by Bancroftian filariasis, there is not usually an associated hydrocele.

The last stage is characterized by atrophy of the skin, with loss of elasticity, giving a striking prematurely aged appearance and a paper-thin skin. Mottled depigmentation ('leopard skin'), particularly of the

shins, is common and can resemble leprosy (Fig. 106). Skin changes often mimic those seen in vitamin A deficiency. Progressive skin lesions can be roughly divided into stages: acute and then chronic papular onchodermatitis (Fig. 107); lichenified onchodermatitis; atrophy and depigmentation (Murdoch *et al.*, 1993).

In Central America, patients, particularly children, may have reddish-mauve lesions on the face, known as *erisipela de la costa*. The condition of 'sowda' is found in Yemen and in East and West Africa, in which there are very few microfilariae in the skin, but the skin of a localized area, usually one or both legs, is itchy, papular and pustular, hyperpigmented and thickened, with accompanying groin lymphadenopathy, distinguishable clinically from 'hanging groin'. This hyperreactive onchodermatitis, with frequent acute exacerbations, is also encountered in visitors or new residents to an endemic region.

The most important consequence of

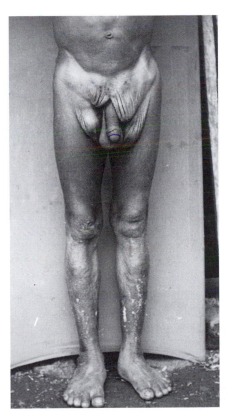

Fig. 106. A case of 'hanging groin' with loss of elasticity in the skin. There is also vitiligo of the shins ('leopard skin').

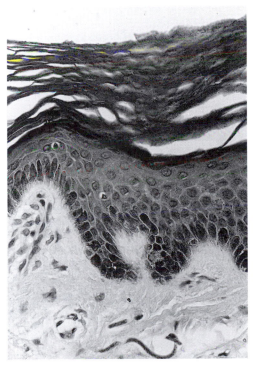

Fig. 107. Section of skin with marked dyskeratitis and presence of microfilariae of *O. volvulus*.

infection is blindness, which has led to the popular name for the disease of river blindness. Blindness occurs more commonly in savannah areas of Africa and America than in forest zones, where it is seldom over 1%. In some savannah areas of Africa and Guatemala, over 10% of the population may be completely blind and another 20% have impaired vision on account of onchocerciasis. In endemic savannah areas the sight of a small boy leading a band of blind men to their work in the fields is not uncommon. A few years ago there were reckoned to be about 70,000 adults with 'economic blindness' in the upper Volta basin.

The eye lesions can be separated into two types.

1. Anterior lesions are caused by microfilariae reaching the cornea from the skin of the face through the conjunctiva. By the use of the slit lamp, live microfilariae may sometimes be seen in the cornea, usually just below Bowman's membrane, without causing any reaction. When microfilariae die they first cause a punctate keratitis with numerous opacities, with a diameter less than 0.5 mm, around each dead microfilaria (Fig. 108). The fluffy opacities are often symptomless, but there may be photo-phobia and watering, with chronic conjunctivitis. This can be followed by a sclerosing keratitis, usually starting in the lower half of the cornea, with an 'apron' coming in from the sides and below (Plate 29). Microfilariae may also be seen in the anterior chamber of the eye and their death may produce iridocyclitis and uveitis, with loss of the pigment ruff and a distorted pupil. Secondary glaucoma and cataract may follow.

2. The aetiology of the posterior-segment lesions is not so clear but they are associated with heavy *O. volvulus* infection in both savannah and forest areas. The 'Ridley–Hissette' fundus is a well-defined patch, usually bilateral, in which all retinal elements have vanished except for the retinal vessels and in which the choroidal vessels may show marked sclerosis (Plate 30). Optical atrophy is of the postneuritic type, with dense sheathing of the retinal vessels. Active optic neuritis appears to be commoner than once thought (WHO, 1995) and lasts for several weeks to over 1 year, with scarring and pigment disturbance at the disc margin. It has a reported prevalence of 1–4% in hyperendemic communities in Cameroon and 6–9% in the guinea savannah of northern Nigeria. Complete blind-

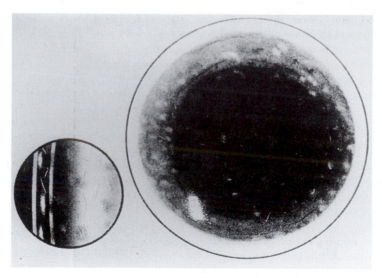

Fig. 108. Snowflake opacities in onchocercal keratitis (slit-lamp view and section).

ness may result or tubular vision may remain. Onchocerciasis can cause severe reduction in peripheral visual fields, so that functional blindness might be much higher than the standard 'below 3/60 visual acuity in the better eye' definition shows. A new field test, the Wu–Jones computerized visual function test, should make it easier to obtain accurate and reproducible measurements of paracentral visual fields, as well as acuity.

IMMUNOLOGY OF ONCHOCERCIASIS

There are some overall similarities between the immunobiology of onchocerciasis and lymphatic filariasis, but some important differences associated with the differences in parasite location.

As with lymphatic filariasis, infected individuals show a spectrum of pathological responses and these may reflect genetic as well as environmental influences. Individuals with high microfilarial loads may show a degree of both specific and non-specific immune unresponsiveness and low-grade skin inflammatory changes. A small percentage of patients show hyperreactive responses, with severe localized skin changes typical of sowda. When tested against worm antigens, patients with hyperreactive onchocerciasis showed evidence of a Th2 bias in their antibody responses – for example, making greater IgE and IgG1 and lower IgG4 and IgM responses than those with generalized onchocerciasis. These differences in classes of antibody associated with differences in pathology may also be relevant to protection – IgE and IgG1 participating in ADCC-mediated killing, while IgG4 and IgM antibodies may block effector activity. Th1-biased responses have been implicated in the development of immunity, although both infected patients and endemic normals appear to make mixed Th1/Th2 responses. Production of both Th1 and Th2 cytokines in putatively immune individuals may allow the involvement of both macrophages and eosinophils in ADCC-mediated killing of infective L_3 stages.

Chemotherapeutic treatment of onchocerciasis with drugs, such as DEC and iver-mectin, carries the risk of adverse reactions. In part, these follow increased production of proinflammatory mediators, such as IL-6, tumour necrosis factor-α (TNF-α) and C-reactive protein, but there are also changes in T cells and eosinophils.

Major histocompatibility complex (MHC)-linked influences on patterns of infection and pathology have been established and the interesting idea proposed that possession of one human leucocyte antigen (HLA) locus (DQB1*0501), associated with protection against severe malaria, may carry the cost of reduced resistance to onchocerciasis – an example of a trade-off between two endemic diseases in West Africa (Meyer and Kremsner, 1996).

DIAGNOSIS

Clinical. The acute pruritic onchocercal rash has to be distinguished from those caused by scabies, insect bites, prickly heat, contact dermatitis, hypersensitivity reactions, post-traumatic or inflammatory depigmentation, tuberculoid leprosy, dermatomycoses, trepanonemoses and the similar parasite *Mansonella streptocerca* (see p. 223). The presence of the typical nodules measuring 0.5–10 cm in diameter, from which portions of adult worms may be obtained on excision, allows a positive diagnosis to be made if no microfilariae can be found in skin snips. Ultrasound can also be used to confirm whether a nodule is onchocercal. The presence of nodules in more than 20% of young males over the age of 20 in a savannah area is estimated to give a sensitivity of 94% and specificity of 50% (Whitworth and Gemade, 1999) in epidemiological surveys, while skin depigmentation might give a better rapid, but rough, method in forest regions. In chronic infections, skin and eye changes are usually pathognomic.

The Mazzotti or DEC provocation test is still sometimes used, in which 50 mg of DEC is given orally and, hopefully short-lived, itching, rash and lymphadenitis occur 1–24 h later. A much better recent modification uses a DEC-impregnated patch and results in a small localized rash.

Parasitological. Microfilariae may some-times be seen in the cornea and anterior chamber of the eye and, in heavy infec-tions, in urine and blood.

The most widely used diagnostic proce-dure in onchocerciasis is the skin snip. After cleaning with spirit, a needle is used to raise a small cone of skin, which is then cut off under the needle point with a sharp razor-blade or fine pair of scissors (the Walser or Holth corneoscleral punch is used to give a standard-sized sample of skin and enables quantitative microfilarial counts to be made). It is important to take the snip from an area of maximum microfilarial density – from above the iliac crest in Africa, from the trapezius in Guatemala and from the lower calf in Yemen. The bloodless skin snip, measuring about 3 mm in diameter and 0.1–1 mm deep (preferably taken in the afternoon), is placed in a drop of physiological saline or water and, after gentle teasing, is allowed to stand for 30 min before being examined under the microscope. Microfilariae show active thrashing movements and in West Africa must be separated from those of *M. strepto-cerca*, also found in the skin. Microfilariae of the latter have a shivering mode of activ-ity and in stained smears have a thinner shape, small caudal space and non-over-lapping of the anterior nuclei (Fig. 102). Recently, skin scarification is being widely used as an alternative to skin snips.

Immunological. Superficial skin scrapings, which can be dried on microscope slides, can also be used in a PCR-based assay to show the presence of onchocercal DNA (Toe *et al.*, 1998), but is still expensive. This test can also be used to specifically identify infections in black-flies and to dif-ferentiate between savannah and forest strains of parasite (WHO, 1995).

Most immunological tests are more use-ful for epidemiological studies than for individual diagnosis. ELISAs using a cock-tail of recombinant antigens (e.g. MBP/10, 11 and 29) have been tested in many areas with different levels of endemicity (WHO, 1995; Bradley and Unnasch, 1996; Bradley *et al.*, 1998), and tests have been devised

for recognizing antigens in tears for ocular onchocerciasis, in dermal fluid for skin microfilariae and in urine for microfilariae (Ngu *et al.*, 1998).

TREATMENT

Surgery. Nodulectomy under local anaes-thetic (2% lignocaine) has been widely used in Central America and has been claimed to markedly reduce the number of microfilariae in the skin and more impor-tantly around the eyes (Plate 31). Results have not been so striking in Africa, where nodules are often impalpable or the larger ones are merely fibrous reactions around dead and dying worms.

Chemotherapy. Ivermectin (Mectizan – a macrocyclic lactone) is the only drug in widespread use and has completely replaced DEC, which is no longer advo-cated. It is given as a single oral dose of 150 µg kg^{-1} of body weight once or twice a year. It should not be given in cases of severe illness. Side-effects are very rarely severe but can include itching and rashes, fever and glandular pain (severe allergic reactions used to be common after treat-ment with DEC, which kills microfilariae more rapidly). Ivermectin appears to have little effect against adult female worms when given at the standard dose but does prevent the release of microfilariae from the uterus for over 6 months. Moxidectin, a promising long-persisting relation of iver-mectin, is now undergoing clinical trials, as is long-term treatment with antibiotics, probably directed against *Wohlbachia* (see p. 197. (Townson *et al.*, 2000).

Intravenous suramin (Antrypol or Bayer 205) is the only drug which has a clear macrofilaricidal effect, but it is toxic and should only be given rarely and under close medical supervision in hospital (WHO, 1995).

EPIDEMIOLOGY

Persons involved in agriculture and other outdoor activities, such as fishing, are at the highest risk, and in some parts of West Africa in the past onchocerciasis has rendered whole areas bordering rivers uninhabitable.

In Africa, the most important vectors are black-flies belonging to the *Simulium damnosum* complex, small (4 mm long) nematocerous flies, which breed on vegetation and on rocks in a great variety of river systems, including the largest rivers, such as the Niger, Volta and Nile, as well as small streams, provided that they are well oxygenated. Members of the *S. damnosum* subcomplex acting as vectors (*S. damnosum sensu stricto* (s.s.), *S. sirbanum*, *S. rasyani* and possibly *S. dieguerense*) are found in savannah areas, while those of the *S. sanctipauli* (*S. sanctipauli* s.s., *S. soubrense*, *S. leonense* and *S. konkourense*) and *S. squamosum* (*S. squamosum* s.s., *S. yahense*, *S. mengense* and *S. kilibanum*) subcomplexes are mostly found in forest areas. Most of these sibling species are morphologically identical and can only be differentiated by the banding patterns of the larval chromosomes; many other cytospecies not known to act as vectors have also been described. Members of the *S. neavei* complex (*S. neavei* s.s., *S. woodi* and *S. ethiopense*) are local vectors in eastern Congo Republic (Zaire), Tanzania and Ethiopia; all members breed in small highland streams and have an obligatory association with freshwater crabs or other crustaceans. *S. albivirgulatum* is a local vector in central Congo Republic.

In the Americas, members of the *S. ochraceum* complex are high-biting flies that are the principal and efficient vectors in highland foci in Mexico and Guatemala. They breed in small rivers, streams and small trickles of water flowing through highly wooded volcanic slopes of coffee-growing areas between 1000 and 2000 m above sea level. *S. callidum* and *S. metallicum sensu lato* (s.l.) are secondary vectors; the latter is low-biting and mainly zoophilic and is also found in Venezuela. Various other species (*S. exiguum* s.l., *S. guianense*, *S. incrustatum*, *S. oyapockense* s.l., *S. quadrivittatum* and probably *S. limbatum*) act as vectors in South America (WHO, 1995).

Variations in the localization of nodules in Africa and Central America are probably caused by differences in the biting habits of the species of black-flies.

Although all species of *Simulium* are confined to running water for breeding, adult flies have been found many kilometres from water and are probably carried by winds. In savannah areas of West Africa, flies have a shorter flight range than those in forest areas, so that infections tend to be heavier but more localized.

The epidemiology of onchocerciasis differs over its range because different disease patterns are associated with different strains of parasite, with differences in the abundance, anthropophilic nature and vector capacity of vectors and with differences in the responses of the human host to the parasite. Because of strain differences between parasites in Africa, microfilariae of savannah forms will not infect forest flies and vice versa; also, anterior eye lesions are more common in savannah than in forest areas in infections of comparable severity.

PREVENTION AND CONTROL

Control campaigns in the past have concentrated on the vectors. The disease was eradicated from Kenya and from large areas of Uganda in the 1950s by using the insecticide (dichlorodiphenyltrichloroethane: DDT). In Kenya the *Simulium* species responsible (*S. neavei*) has a short flight range and lived on land crabs which inhabited water-filled holes, and these were easy to treat. In Uganda infection was confined to the Nile, which could be treated.

The largest control campaign is that of the Onchocerciasis Control Programme (OCP) (funded principally by the World Bank, Food and Agriculture Organization (FAO), United Nations Development Programme (UNDP) and WHO), which commenced in 1974, dedicated to controlling the disease in savannah regions of seven West African countries of the Volta River basin, comprising a land area of 0.7 million km^2 (Benin, Burkina Faso, Côte d'Ivoire, Ghana, Mali, Niger and Togo). In some infected villages in the control area, more than 10% of the infected population was blind and as many as 30% had irreversible eye lesions. At first, control was entirely by the addition of the larvicide temephos (Abate) to rivers and streams, mostly from helicopters and fixed-wing aircraft (Plate 32). In 1980 insecticide resistance was encountered and the bacterial agent *Bacillus thuringiensis* H14 replaced it for a while until black-fly populations became susceptible again. By 1986 vector control had interrupted transmission almost completely in 90% of the area, with blindness reduced by 40%, while the incidence of infection in children was reduced by 99%. However, in the remaining 10% western area, reinvasion by flies borne on the monsoon winds occurred, so the control area was extended to a further four countries (Guinea, Guinea-Bissau, Senegal and Sierra Leone). Since 1987 the microfilaricide ivermectin (Mectizan) has been donated by the manufacturers and this has augmented the use of insecticides. To date, over 20 million people have received at least one dose and some up to nine doses. The drug is given at 150 μm kg^{-1} once or twice a year, as it does not kill adult worms. With the use of both regular Mectizan and larviciding, treatment needs to be continued for about 12 years to reduce infection by 99% (this represents the average lifespan of adult worms).

The campaign currently costs about $27 million per annum but is due to end in 2002, when responsibility will be handed over to the African Programme for Onchocerciasis (APOC). The maintenance phase of control will be almost entirely by repeated community-based administration of Mectizan (Remme, 1995) and a community-directed treatment programme is already under way in 19 African countries, which will become part of primary health care. It has been realized recently that the severe skin lesions, which also occur in the forest zones, can be very debilitating and treatment will be much more widespread than just the OCP area.

The benefits of the OCP to date can be enumerated as below (Samba, 1994).

1. 10 million children prevented from becoming infected.

2. 125,000–200,000 adults prevented from becoming infected, with 1.5 million having lost their infection.

3. 25 million ha that can now be used for agriculture – enough to support 17 million people.

4. Infection no longer being a problem in Burkina Faso, Niger, northern Benin, Côte d'Ivoire, Ghana, Togo or south-eastern Mali.

5. An estimated 20% return on the investment in the programme.

In Central America insecticidal control has not been successful because of the difficulties in treating all the small mountain streams in which *Simulium* larvae breed. However, mass treatment campaigns with Mectizan are proving very effective in both Central and South America.

ZOONOTIC ASPECTS

Probably none, although a natural infection has been found in a gorilla, and chimpanzees can be experimentally infected (an infection reported from a spider monkey appears to have been mistaken). Other species of *Onchocerca* are found in a wide range of herbivores (*O. gutturosa* in the nuchal cartilage, *O. lienalis* in the gastro-splenic region and *O. gibsoni* in the subcutaneous tissues of cattle and *O. cervicalis* and *O. reticulata* in the ligaments of horses occur in many parts of the world and *O. armillata* parasitizes the aorta of cattle in Africa and Asia). The horse species are transmitted by species of *Culicoides*, but the cattle species are transmitted by *Simulium* species and so could be confused with *O. volvulus* in the vector. This is most important for a subcutaneous cattle species in West Africa, *O. ochengi*, as the infective larvae are almost identical to those of the human species and are found in the same species of black-fly (differentiation requires DNA probes and can be carried out on large pooled samples of flies).

A few amicrofilaraemic infections, presumably zoonotic from cattle or horse species, have been reported from Canada, Japan, Russia, Switzerland and the USA.

Mansonella perstans
(Manson, 1891) Orihel and Eberhard, 1982

SYNONYMS
Filaria sanguinis hominis minor, F. s. h. perstans and *F. perstans* Manson, 1891; *Acanthocheilonema perstans* Railliet, Henry and Langeron, 1912; *Dipetalonema perstans* Yorke and Maplestone, 1926; *Tetrapetalonema perstans* Chabaud and Bain, 1976. This species and *M. streptocerca* (below) have had many rather confusing name changes. For many years they were included in the very large and heterogeneous genus *Dipetalonema* and were split off as *Tetrapetalonema* just before adults of *Mansonella ozzardi* were recovered from experimental animals, when they were all found to belong the same genus (Muller, 1987). *M. perstans* and *M. streptocerca* are included in the subgenus *Esslingeria* while *M. ozzardi* is in the subgenus *Mansonella*, i.e. the full names are *M. (Esslingeria) perstans, M. (Esslingeria) streptocerca* and *M. (Mansonella) ozzardi*.

DISEASE
Perstans filariasis or filariosis, mansonelliasis or mansonellosis perstans.

GEOGRAPHICAL DISTRIBUTION
West and Central Africa, including Benin, Cameroon, Congo, Republic of Congo, Equatorial Guinea, Ethiopia, Gabon, Ghana, Guinea, Guinea-Bissau, Mali, Mozambique, Nigeria, Sierra Leone, Togo, western

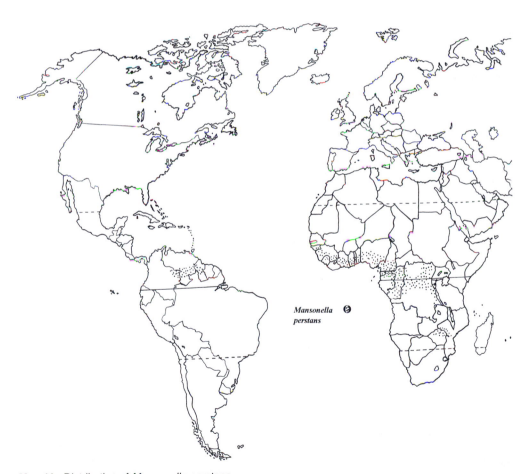

Mansonella perstans

Map 11. Distribution of *Mansonella perstans*.

Uganda, Zimbabwe and limited areas of South America (Colombia, Guyana and Venezuela).

LOCATION IN HOST

Adults inhabit the body cavities, mesenteric, retroperitoneal and perirenal tisues; unsheathed microfilariae can be found in the peripheral bloodstream at any time.

MORPHOLOGY

The adult females measure 70–80 mm × 0.12 mm, males 35–45 mm × 0.06 mm; both sexes have a smooth cuticle and a ventrally curved tail, which has a trilobed appearance (Baird *et al.*, 1987). The tail of the male has four pairs of preanal and one pair of postanal papillae and there are two, very unequal, rodlike spicules. The microfilariae in the blood are unsheathed and measure 200 (190–240) µm × 4.5 µm (they look appreciably smaller and thinner than the sheathed microfilariae of *Wuchereria*, *Brugia* or *Loa*); they assume graceful curves when fixed and stained. The tail ends bluntly and contains nuclei to the tip (Figs 89 and 109).

LIFE CYCLE

There is no marked periodicity but microfilariae are slightly more numerous in the peripheral circulation at night. The microfilariae are ingested in a blood meal by small (2 mm) female ceratopogonid midges of the genus *Culicoides*, which are pool feeders. The larvae enter the thoracic muscles, moult twice and reach the infective third stage by 9 days, when they migrate to the head. They exit from the labium of the midge while it is feeding. The parasites take a few months to become mature, moulting twice more, in the human body.

CLINICAL MANIFESTATIONS AND PATHOGENESIS

There are often none, but infection has been associated with allergic symptoms, such as itching, pruritus, joint pains, enlarged lymph glands and vague abdominal symptoms, accompanied by high eosinophilia.

DIAGNOSIS

By identification of the microfilariae in stained blood smears. More than ten microfilariae per millilitre may be present, often together with those of *L. loa* and *W. bancrofti*. Differences in the morphology of microfilariae in various African countries have resulted in the name *M. semiclarum* being given to a longer microfilaria (198 µm × 5.2 µm in thick films, 221 µm × 5.0 µm in thin) found in the blood of a man in Congo Republic (Dujardin *et al.*, 1982).

TREATMENT

DEC has no effect. Albendazole and mebendazole given for 10 days have given equivocal results. Ivermectin appears to

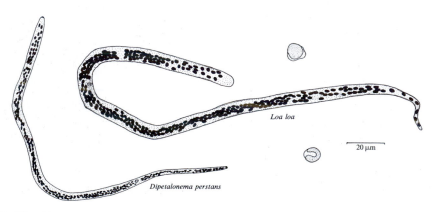

Loa loa

20 µm

Dipetalonema perstans

Fig. 109. Microfilariae of *Loa loa* and *Mansonella perstans* in same blood smear (stained in Giemsa so that sheath of *Loa* has not stained).

reduce microfilaraemia for a period but probably has no long-term effect.

EPIDEMIOLOGY

Recent reports of infection rates are southern Cameroon 15–27%, southern Congo 16% in Bantu and 81% in pygmies, Congo Republic (Zaire) 42%, Equatorial Guinea 52%, Gabon 25–80%, Abia and Imo States 29%, Bauchi State 1.4%, Gongola State 11%, Jos Plateau 13% (all in Nigeria).

In Africa the vector species are *Culicoides grahami* and *C. milnei*. These have a short flight range of about 100 m. Eggs are laid in mud or wet soil in batches or in water in banana stumps.

There is usually only one larva per infected midge, but midges are numerous and a high percentage may be infected. This results in a high infection rate in the human population, but almost all infections are light.

ZOONOTIC ASPECTS

Possibly identical microfilariae are found in chimpanzees and gorillas in Central Africa and similar ones in New World monkeys. Recently, new species have been reported from African primates.

Meningonema peruzzii has been described from the leptomeninges of *Cercopithecus* spp. in Zimbabwe. The microfilariae are almost identical to those of *M. perstans* but have an indistinct sheath that does not stain with Giemsa. Recently, a fourth-stage female larva of *Meningonema* was recovered from the cerebrospinal fluid of a patient in Cameroon (Boussinesq *et al.*, 1995). It is possible that the nervous manifestations reported from humans in Rhodesia (now Zimbabwe), with the presence of microfilariae in the spinal fluid, which led Patrick Manson to postulate that *M. perstans* was the cause of sleeping sickness, was due to this species.

Microfilariae found in the blood of a patient in Thailand may be of **Mansonella digitatum** (Sucharit, 1988).

Mansonella streptocerca
(Macfie and Corson, 1922) Orihel and Eberhard, 1982

SYNONYMS

Agamofilaria streptocerca Macfie and Corson, 1922; *Acanthocheilonema streptocerca* Faust, 1949; *Dipetalonema streptocerca* Peel and Chardome, 1946; *Tetrapetalonema streptocerca* Chabaud and Bain, 1976.

DISEASE

Streptocercal filariasis or filariosis; streptocerciasis or streptocercosis.

GEOGRAPHICAL DISTRIBUTION

Confined to the rainforest areas of Benin, Cameroon, Central African Republic, Congo, Congo Republic, Côte d'Ivoire, Equatorial Guinea, Gabon, Ghana, Nigeria, Togo and western Uganda.

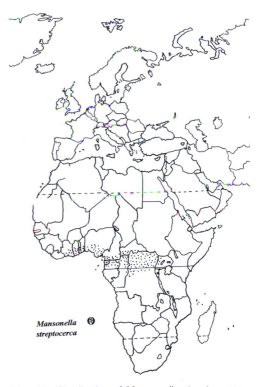

Mansonella streptocerca

Map 12. Distribution of *Mansonella streptocerca*.

LOCATION IN HOST

The adults are tightly coiled in the subcutaneous tissues of the dermis, microfilariae occur in the skin (Fig. 110).

MORPHOLOGY

Adult worms are very thin and females measure 27 mm × 0.08 mm. Males have been recovered only once from patients in the Congo Republic in the dermal collagen (Meyers *et al.*, 1977) and measured 17 mm × 0.05 mm. Microfilariae are unsheathed and measure 180–240 μm × 3–4 μm. The tail is tapered and curved to form a hook; it ends bluntly and has a quadrate nucleus to within 1 μm of its bifid end. The cuticle is striated.

LIFE CYCLE

Complete development has been observed experimentally in the midge *Culicoides grahami*. Ingested microfilariae moved rapidly to the thoracic muscles and moulted twice, and infective third-stage larvae, measuring 574 μm, were seen in the mouth-parts on the 8th day. Natural infection rates of up to 1% have been found in these insects.

CLINICAL MANIFESTATIONS AND PATHOGENESIS

Used to be regarded as non-pathogenic, but it is responsible for mild pruritus, with unpigmented spots (in about 60% of cases), papules and oedema, and thickening of the skin has been reported. Infection is often mistaken for onchocerciasis and sometimes leprosy.

DIAGNOSIS

By finding the microfilariae in skin snips taken in the shoulder region. Living specimens in saline can be differentiated from microfilariae of *Onchocerca* by their shivering mode of activity in contrast to the active twisting of the latter. In stained smears they are thinner with a hooked and bluntly rounded tail, small caudal space and non-overlapping anterior nuclei (Figs. 89 and 102).

TREATMENT

DEC (2–6 mg kg^{-1} body weight day^{-1} for 21 days) kills microfilariae and probably adults but can cause unpleasant itching. Ivermectin (150 μg kg^{-1}) effectively removes microfilariae for long periods.

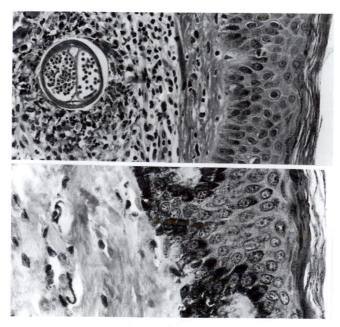

Fig. 110. Section of subcutaneous tissues with adult *M. streptocerca* above and microfilariae below (compare with Figs 105 and 107 showing microfilariae of *O. volvulus*).

EPIDEMIOLOGY

Infection rates were 36% in children in western Uganda, 0.4% in Nigeria (Bauchi State). *M. streptocerca* is transmitted by *Culicoides grahami* and possibly by *C. milnei*, so the epidemiology is similar to that of *M. perstans*.

ZOONOTIC ASPECTS

Adults have been found in chimpanzees and gorillas in Congo Republic, but it is unlikely that they act as reservoir hosts.

Sheathless microfilariae of ***Mansonella rodhaini***, measuring 300 µm × 2.2 µm, have been recovered from skin snips taken from both sexes in Gabon. It was impossible to determine pathogenicity since most also had *M. streptocerca* and *M. perstans* (Richard-Lenoble *et al.*, 1988). It is a natural parasite of chimpanzees in Congo Republic.

Mansonella ozzardi
(Manson, 1897) Faust, 1929

SYNONYMS

Filaria demarquayi Manson, 1897; *F. ozzardi* Manson, 1897; *F. tucumana* Biglieri and Araoz, 1917.

DISEASE

Mansonelliasis or mansonellosis ozzardi, Ozzard's filariasis or filariosis.

GEOGRAPHICAL DISTRIBUTION

Central America, including Mexico (Yucatán) and Panama; South America, including northern Argentina, Bolivia, Brazil, Colombia, Dominican Republic, French Guiana, Guyana, Surinam and Venezuela; Caribbean, including Desirade Island, Dominica, Guadeloupe, Haiti, Martinique, St Lucia, St Vincent and Trinidad (see Map 9, p. 203).

LOCATION IN HOST

Adults inhabit the abdominal mesenteries and subperitoneal tissues, microfilariae circulate in the blood.

MORPHOLOGY

Adult females from monkeys measure 49 mm × 0.15 mm, with a smooth cuticle and two lappets at the caudal extemity, while males measure 26 mm × 0.07 mm.

The unsheathed microfilariae in the blood are similar in size to those of *M. perstans*, measuring 175–240 µm × 4.5 µm. They differ in that the posterior end of the body is free of nuclei for 3–4 µm, giving the appearance of a sharp tail (Fig. 111).

LIFE CYCLE

The microfilariae in the blood show no periodicity.

The intermediate host in St Vincent is the minute (1 mm) female midge *Culicoides furens*, in Trinidad *C. phlebotomus* and experimentally in Argentina *C. paraensis*. However, in Brazil the vector is a member of the black-fly *Simulium amazonicum* complex. In this area microfilariae are also found in the skin as well as the blood.

The microfilariae penetrate the stomach wall of the insect and develop in the thoracic muscles, moulting twice. Infective, third-stage larvae migrate to the head and proboscis by 8 days. Nothing is known of the

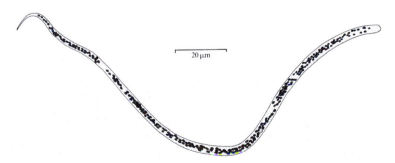

Fig. 111. Microfilaria of *M. ozzardi*.

20 µm

development in humans, but it has recently been followed experimentally in patas monkeys, in which patency took 163 days.

CLINICAL MANIFESTATIONS AND PATHOGENESIS
The majority of cases appear to be symptomless, but allergic reactions have been reported, particularly from Brazil. These include pruritus, joint pains, headache, hypopigmented blotchy papules and enlarged and painful inguinal lymph nodes, accompanied by a blood eosinophilia.

DIAGNOSIS
By finding the characteristic microfilariae in stained blood smears.

TREATMENT
DEC (2–6 mg kg^{-1} body weight for 21 days) kills microfilariae for a period. Ivermectin reduces microfilarial numbers greatly, but they often return after a few years. Side-effects are common but minor.

EPIDEMIOLOGY AND ZOONOTIC ASPECTS
Infection is most common in Amerindians living in rainforest areas. In Brazil it is found particularly in outdoor workers of both sexes but is rare in children under 8.

Infection rates of over 50% in the Roraima area of Brazil, 81–94% over the border in Venezuela and 22% in Trinidad have recently been reported. Older figures are 45% in Panama, 96% in Amerindians in forests of southern Colombia, 85% in Yucatán (Mexico) and 4–15% in Surinam.

Little is known of the epidemiology of this parasite in the Amazon basin. Although no reservoir host is known, monkeys can be experimentally infected.

Accidental filarial infections

DIROFILARIA
Those members of the genus *Dirofilaria* that have been found as parasites of humans are all natural parasites of dogs or, more rarely, primates in tropical and subtropical areas of the world. They can be divided into two groups, depending on their structure and on their location in the body:

1. Subgenus *Dirofilaria*: *Dirofilaria (Dirofilaria) immitis, D. (D.) magalhaesi, D. (D.) louisianensis* and *D. (D.) spectans.* These parasites have been recovered from the lungs, heart and blood-vessels and are relatively thin (diameter 0.1 mm) and immature with a smooth cuticle.
2. Subgenus *Nochtiella*: *Dirofilaria (Nochtiella) repens, D. (N.) tenuis (D. (N.) conjunctivae* is a synonym of either of these), *D. (N.) striata, D. (N.) ursi.* Members of this group from humans have also been recovered from the subcutaneous or conjunctival tissues. They are usually stouter (0.2–0.5 mm in diameter) than those in the first group and have longitudinal ridges in the cuticle with transverse striations.

Dirofilaria immitis (Leidy, 1856). This is an important and common parasite of the right ventricle and pulmonary artery of the dog in most warm parts of the world and is transmitted by both anopheline and culicine mosquitoes. Immature or unfertilized adult worms have been found about 230 times in lung abscesses or in the pulmonary artery of humans, but microfilariae are not present in the peripheral blood. They usually cause a pulmonary infarct, which is seen on X-ray and often mistakenly removed as a neoplasm. In sections the parasite can be recognized by the smooth laminated cuticle, long muscle cells, broad lateral cords and, in mature females, by the typical filarial twin uteri (Fig. 112). In the dog this is a larger filaria than *D. repens* (250–300 mm × 1 mm as against 100–170 mm × 0.4–0.7 mm), but specimens from humans are usually very immature. One case of a gravid female of what was probably *D. immitis* was reported from the lung of a man who had lymphoid leukaemia (Beaver *et al.*, 1990).

Dirofilaria repens Railliet and Henry, 1911. This species is a natural parasite of the subcutaneous tissues of dogs in Europe, Asia and possibly Africa and is transmitted by mosquitoes, particularly *Aedes* (probably *A. albopictus* in Italy). It has been reported about 400 times from 30 countries, most (168) from Italy (Muro *et al.*, 1999). There are also a few cases reported each year from Spain, France and Russia

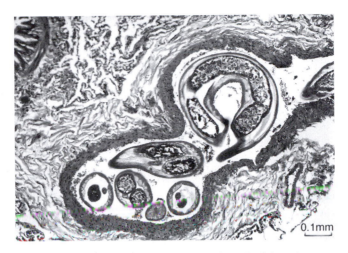

Fig. 112. Section of lung with immature *Dirofilaria immitis* in a branch of the pulmonary artery. A pulmonary infarct may follow the death of the worm.

(Pampiglione *et al.*, 1995). *D. repens* in humans produces a painful migratory subcutaneous nodule, which at biopsy shows a threadlike parasite (0.3 mm in diameter) in the centre of an inflammatory reaction with many tissue eosinophils (Fig. 113). Many cases are under the conjunctiva or around the eye, probably because these are most likely to be diagnosed. A technique using PCR amplification of DNA can differentiate between *D. immitis* and *D. repens* infections (Faria *et al.*, 1996).

Dirofilaria tenuis Chandler, 1942. About 40 human cases have been reported from the USA, mostly from women in Florida. The natural host is the racoon and 14–45% were found to be infected in Florida, with mosquito intermediate hosts. It causes subcutaneous lesions, often around or in the eye, similar to those of *D. repens* (Beaver, 1987).

Dirofilaria striata (Molin, 1858). This species is a natural parasite of various wild cats and has been found a few times in the

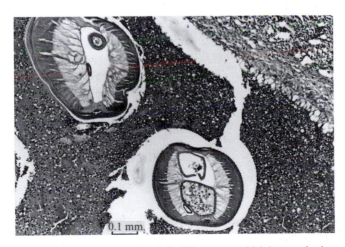

Fig. 113. Section of breast from a woman with adult of *D. repens*, which has evoked a granulomatous reaction. Note ridges on the cuticle of the worm.

subcutaneous tissues and eye of humans in the USA. It is transmitted by mosquitoes.

Dirofilaria ursi Yamaguti, 1941. This is a natural parasite of the bear and subcutaneous lesions have been found very rarely in humans in Canada and the USA. It is transmitted by the black-fly *Simulium*.

Superfamily Dracunculoidea

Dracunculus medinensis
(Linnaeus, 1758) Gallandant, 1773

SYNONYMS
Gordius medinensis Linnaeus, 1758; *Filaria medinensis* L.; *Fuellebornius medinensis* Leiper, 1926.

DISEASE AND COMMON NAMES
Dracunculiasis or dracunculosis, dracontiasis; guinea or medina worm, le dragonneu, filaire de Medine.

LOCAL NAMES
Farentit (Arabic), Mfa (Fanti and Twi), Kurkunu (Hausa), Naru (Hindi), Reshteh or Piyook (Persian), Rishta (Uzbek), Orok al Mai (Yemen), Sobiya (Yoruba).

GEOGRAPHICAL DISTRIBUTION
Dracunculus is now found only in the countries of West and Central Africa just south of the Sahara (Benin, Burkina Faso, Central African Republic, Côte d'Ivoire, Ghana, Mali, Mauritania, Niger, Nigeria, Sudan, Togo and Uganda). There are also very small foci in Cameroon and Ethiopia and possibly still in Chad, Kenya and Senegal. Infection has been officially eliminated from the formerly endemic areas in India (1999) and Pakistan (1994) in the last few years and the disease has probably now vanished from Saudi Arabia and Yemen.

LOCATION IN HOST
Adult females emerge from the subcutaneous tissues, usually of the foot or lower limbs but sometimes from any part of the body.

MORPHOLOGY
The mature female measures 500–800 mm × 1.0–2.0 mm. The mouth has a triangular oval opening surrounded by a quadrangular cuticularized plate, with an internal circle of four double papillae. The vulva opens halfway down the body but is non-functional in the mature worm. The uterus has an anterior and a posterior branch and is filled with 1–3 million embryos; it fills the entire body cavity (pseudocoel), the gut being entirely flattened.

Males recovered from experimental infections in animals measure 15–40 mm × 0.4 mm (Fig. 114). The tail has 4 (3–6)

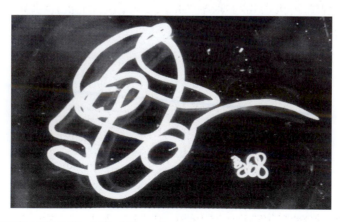

Fig. 114. Adult female and smaller male of *D. medinensis*.

pairs of preanal and 4–6 pairs of postanal papillae; the subequal spicules are 490–750 µm long, with a gubernaculum measuring about 117 µm. Males remain in the connective tissues surrounding deeper muscles, usually in the thoracic region, and are either absorbed or eventually calcify; they have only doubtfully been recovered in human infections.

LIFE CYCLE

The mature female worm moves to the surface of the skin and forms a blister, which bursts. The first-stage larvae are expelled from the ruptured uterus when the affected part of the body (usually the foot or leg) comes into contact with water. The larvae on average measure 643 (490–737) µm × 23 (18–24) µm and have a fully formed gut, although they do not feed. The tail is long and pointed and the cuticle is striated. The larvae in water are very active, their thrashing movements resembling those of a free-living nematode (Fig. 115). They live for 4–7 days in pond water and for further development have to be ingested by various predatory species of small (1–2 mm) microcrustacean cyclopoids. Intermediate hosts belong to the genera *Mesocyclops* (*M.*

aequatorialis and *M. kieferi*), *Metacyclops* (*M. margaretae*) and *Thermocyclops* (*T. crassus*, *T. incisus*, *T. inopinus* and *T. oblongatus*). The larvae penetrate the gut wall of cyclops (Fig. 116) and, after two moults in the haemocoel, reach the infective third stage in 14 days at 24°C. The infective larva measures on average 450 µm × 14 µm and has a short bilobed tail. When infected cyclops are ingested in drinking water, the released larvae burrow into the wall of the duodenum, migrate across the abdominal mesenteries and penetrate through the abdomen and thorax in about 15 days. There is no increase in size during this early migration but, after two moults, the sexually mature worms meet and mate in the subcutaneous tissue, approximately 100 days after infection. After fertilization, the males become encapsulated and eventually die. They are usually absorbed, although occasionally calcified specimens have been seen on X-ray. The females move down the muscle planes, reaching the extremities 8–10 months after infection; by 10 months the uterus contains fully formed larvae. The mature females emerge from the tissues about 1 year after ingestion of larvae.

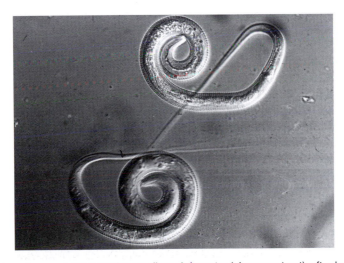

Fig. 115. First-stage larvae of *Dracunculus medinensis* in water (phase contrast) after being expelled by adult female (actual size 0.66 mm).

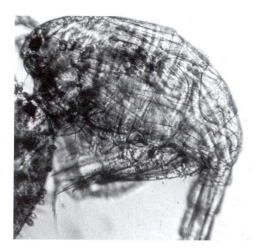

Fig. 116. Cyclops with larvae of *Dracunculus* in the haemocoel.

CLINICAL MANIFESTATIONS

There are usually none while the female worms are moving freely through the connective tissues, but when about to emerge to the surface a few larvae are released into the subdermis through a rupture at the anterior end of the worm (the uterus is non-functional). The host reaction results in the formation of a burning, painful, blister, which bursts in a few days to give a shallow ulcer, and there is then a marked inflammatory response against the cuticle of the entire worm, preventing its removal

(Fig. 117). In many patients (30–80%), urticaria, sometimes accompanied by fever, giddiness, gastrointestinal symptoms, dyspnoea and infraorbital oedema, appears the day before the blister forms but vanishes in a few hours. The blister is the first sign in about 60% of cases. It is minute when first noticed but may grow to a few centimetres in diameter before it bursts, usually in 1–3 days. The formation of the blister is accompanied by local itching and often an intense pain, which can be relieved by immersion of the affected part in cold water. A portion of the worm is extruded through the ulcer formed by the bursting of the blister, the edges of which consist of pinkish granulation tissue. In simple cases the anterior end of the worm is exposed by sloughing of the white central eschar of the ulcer and more of the worm protrudes, particularly after immersion in water; after many thousands of larvae are expelled the portion of worm outside the body becomes flaccid. Complete expulsion of the worm occurs, on average, in 4 weeks and the lesion then rapidly resolves.

Secondary bacterial infection of the track of an emerging worm occurs in about 50% of cases and patients then become seriously incapacitated (Fig. 118). In a study in an area of Nigeria, 58% of cases, almost all of whom belonged to the 14–40-

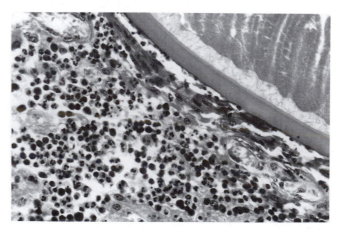

Fig. 117. Section of subcutaneous tissues with portion of an adult female. Removed just after blister formation so that there is a strong tissue reaction.

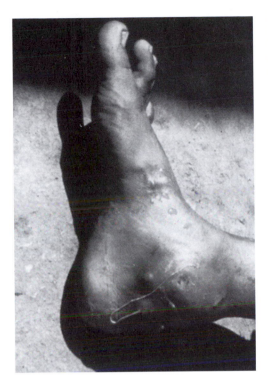

Fig. 118. Female of *D. medinensis* emerging from ankle of woman. There is secondary bacterial infection up the track of the worm.

year-old working population or were schoolchildren, were disabled for an average of 12.7 weeks during the yam and rice harvest time and about 12,000 were permanently incapacitated (Smith *et al.*, 1989). Permanent physical impairment occurs in about 0.5% of infected individuals and in one study in Ghana 28% of patients had continuing pain 12–18 months after infection (Hours and Cairncross, 1994), while in another study in Benin there was 0.3% mortality from tetanus and septicaemia (Chippaux and Massougbodi, 1991). Infection is a major cause of school absenteeism and the parasite is unusual among parasitic helminths as it does not appear to confer any immune response, so that individuals can be reinfected year after year.

Sometimes female worms fail to reach the surface, usually when unfertilized, and become encysted and calcify and are then only apparent on X-ray. This occurs in a proportion of apparently uninfected persons who live in an endemic area. Occasionally an encysted worm may cause more serious effects if in an unusual site; these include constrictive pericarditis, paraplegia, lymph node abscess and urogenital complications.

PATHOGENESIS

The blister fluid consists of a bacteriologically sterile fluid containing lymphocytes, neutrophils, eosinophils and larvae.

In a proportion of cases the female worm bursts in the tissues before emergence, releasing many thousands of larvae. This results in an intense tissue reaction, with myositis and formation of an abscess containing up to 0.5 l of pus, which can lead to chronic ulcerations, bubo or epididymo-orchitis in males. Adult females sometimes enter joints and liberate larvae into the synovial fluid, causing oedema, congestion and plasma-cell infiltration of the synovial membrane. This can lead to arthritis or fibrous ankylosis of joints and contractures of tendons, but in most cases the condition resolves eventually.

Once larvae have been released from the emerging female worm, there is a strong adhesive reaction at the cuticle along the whole length of the worm. In the early stages, the tissue reaction consists of inflammatory cells and is followed by a foreign-body giant-cell reaction. This makes extraction of the worm difficult and increases the chances of secondary bacterial infection along the track of the worm, with cellulitis.

In many endemic areas, the track of a guinea worm on the foot provides an important mode of entry for tetanus spores.

DIAGNOSIS

Clinical and parasitological. Patients in an endemic area usually have no doubt of the diagnosis as soon as, or even before, the first signs appear. Local itching, urticaria and a burning pain at the site of a small blister are usually the first signs of infection, although sometimes a palpable and sometimes moving worm may have been recognized earlier. The blister bursts in about 4 days and active larvae, obtained by placing cold water on the resulting small ulcer, can be recognized under a low-powered microscope.

Immunological. Not useful in practice. ELISA, dot ELISA and SDS-PAGE/Western blotting worked well for patent infections. The most specific reaction appears to be for detection of IgG4 antibodies and might be able to detect infections up to 6 months before patency (Saroj-Bapna and Renapurkar, 1996; Bloch and Simonsen, 1998). The fluorescent antibody test using deep-frozen first-stage larvae was shown to demonstrate prepatent infections in monkeys 30 years ago. No evidence has been found for the presence of circulating antigens (Bloch *et al.*, 1998).

TREATMENT

Surgery. Guinea worms have been wound out on sticks since antiquity (e.g. in the Rg Veda of about 1350 BC and possibly they represent the fiery serpents afflicting the Israelites in the wilderness, which Moses recommended should be set upon a pole). Provided that bacterial infection or other complications have not occurred, regular winding out of the worm on a small stick, combined with sterile dressing and acriflavine cream, usually results in complete expulsion in 3–4 weeks with little pain. This should be commenced as soon after emergence as possible.

Surgical removal of mature female worms before emergence is sometimes possible using a small incision. At this stage there is no host reaction to the cuticle of the worm, as occurs once emergence commences, but care must be taken that the worm is not wound around a ligament.

Chemotherapy. There is no evidence that any chemotherapeutic agent has a direct action against guinea worms. However, many compounds, including thiabendazole, niridazole, metronidazole, mebendazole and albendazole have been reported as hastening the expulsion of worms and may act as anti-inflammatory agents. Ivermectin had no action in one field trial or against pre-emergent *D. insignis* in ferrets.

EPIDEMIOLOGY

Dracunculiasis is typically a disease of poor rural communities and is the only infectious agent that is transmitted entirely through drinking water. In all areas transmission is markedly seasonal and in most parts of Africa (and formerly in India) the maximum incidence coincides with the planting season, resulting in great economic hardship. In semi-desert (Sahel) areas of Africa (Burkina Faso, Chad, northern Cameroon, Mauritania, Niger, northern Nigeria, Senegal and Sudan), drinking water is obtained from ponds during the rainy season but from deep wells for the rest of the year when the ponds are dry. However, in the humid (guinea) savannah regions of West Africa where rainfall exceeds 150 cm year^{-1} (Benin, Côte d'Ivoire, Ghana, southern Nigeria and Togo), there is no transmission during the rainy season, when ponds turn into streams and cyclops densities are low because of the large volume and turbidity of the water. Similarly, infection was highest during the dry season in step wells in India.

The life history of the parasite is well adapted to provide the maximum chances of transmission, as the female takes almost exactly a year to mature and release its larvae at the optimum period each year.

PREVENTION AND CONTROL

The United Nations World Health Assembly in 1991 endorsed a campaign to eradicate dracunculiasis from the world and originally set a date of the end of 1995. Although this date has had to be postponed by another 10 years, the prevalence and distribution of the infection have diminished markedly in the last few years and it has already been eliminated from Asia. The situation in most African countries is not so far advanced, but active campaigns are being carried out in all endemic countries and some are free of the disease, while most are at the stage of case containment, whereby all infected individuals can be quickly identified and stopped from entering ponds.

There are various possible interventions once active surveillance measures have been initiated, based on knowledge of the life cycle of the parasite. It has been estimated that passive surveillance identifies about 2% of cases.

The provision of safe drinking water, principally from tube-wells, is a priority in rural areas of Africa and Asia, and assistance is being provided by many aid agencies in order to prevent other water-borne diseases, such as typhoid, infantile diarrhoea, etc., as well as guinea worm. It has recently been estimated that 1100 million people (about 21% of the world's population) do not have access to clean water.

There are various interventions possible but the use of chemotherapy has no part in control, except sometimes in aiding patient compliance. Interventions which are being made include the following.

1. Filtering or boiling all drinking-water. Boiling water is not usually feasible, because wood fuel is a scarce commodity, but filters are playing an important role in all countries now mounting campaigns. The manufacturer of a monofilament nylon material has provided enough to provide filter nets for all endemic villagers. These nets are long-lasting, have a regular pore size, are easily washed and dry quickly and are being widely used.

2. Persuading or preventing infected persons with an emerging worm from entering ponds used for drinking water. The identification and bandaging of very early lesions can also help to prevent subsequent immersion. The cooperation of local teams and of schoolchildren can be useful in convincing infected persons of the need for a change in behaviour.

3. Treating water sources. The chemical treatment of ponds can prove a useful adjuvant to other measures, particularly when there is only a low level of transmission remaining. The insecticide temephos has low toxicity to mammals and fish and at 1

p.p.m. kills cyclops for 5–6 weeks but, in areas with a long transmission season, has to be added a few times a year. The amount of temephos estimated to be needed for total eradication in Africa has been donated by the manufacturer.

Health education interventions by local health workers are a very important component of any control or eradication campaign, and village development committees are able to assist in other primary health problems.

Guinea worm was eliminated from the Bokhara area of Uzbekistan in the early 1930s and from the south of Iran, where infection was confined to large covered cisterns (known as 'birkehs'), in the 1970s. It is interesting to note that infection has not returned to Bokhara in spite of the fact that still only 33% of the population has piped water (Cairncross *et al.*, 2002). It was eliminated from Pakistan in 1994, India in 1997, Kenya and Senegal in 1996 and Cameroon, Chad and Yemen by 1999. There are also very few cases left in Benin, Burkina Faso, Central African Republic, Côte d'Ivoire, Ethiopia, Mali, Mauritania, Niger, Togo and Uganda. However, there are three countries which still have appreciable numbers of cases. These are Nigeria, which had 11,617 cases in 1999 (but 650,000 cases in 1988), Ghana, with 5524 cases in 1999 (but 180,000 cases in 1989), and Sudan, with 56,226 cases reported in 1999. The apparent number of cases went up substantially in 2000 in Ghana, which demonstrates the difficulties in identifying the many hundreds of small isolated endemic villages. However, there are now intensive campaigns in both Ghana and Nigeria and it is likely that elimination will follow in the next few years. The future for elimination in Sudan is more uncertain. Because of political problems it has been difficult to actively survey, let alone treat, many infected villages and there is also the problem of migrants from Sudan reintroducing infection into neighbouring countries. Thirty-seven other countries where the disease used to be present in historical times have been certified as free by the WHO.

ZOONOTIC ASPECTS

Female worms of the genus *Dracunculus* have been reported as emerging from a wide range of mammals and reptiles from many parts of the world, both endemic and non-endemic for the human disease (Muller, 1971). Those found in reptiles clearly belong to other species but the situation in regard to those in mammals is not clear. For instance guinea worm is common in wild carnivores in North America and was named *D. insignis* by Leidy in 1858 but there is very little morphological evidence for separating this from the human species.

There have been three documented cases of human zoonotic infections, from Japan in 1986 (Kobayashi *et al.*, 1986) and from Korea and Indonesia in 1926. In both cases the patients had eaten raw freshwater fish which have been proved experimentally to be capable of acting as paratenic hosts.

In most highly endemic areas occasional infections, principally in dogs and occasionally other mammals, have been reported, but there is no evidence that they have any part in maintaining transmission. What is presumably the human parasite can still be found in dogs in the formerly endemic areas of Tamil Nadu in India and Uzbekistan, but no new human cases have been reported. Infection has also been found in dogs and cats in previously non-endemic Central Asian Republics; Azerbaijan, Kazakhstan and possibly Turkmenia (Cairncross *et al.*, 2002). There has also been a recent report of *D. medinensis* from a cat in China (Fu *et al.*, 1999) and it is very likely that in many parts of the world there are widespread but under-reported animal cycles completely independent of human infection. However, it is unlikely that zoonotic infections have any importance in human transmission.

References

Akahane, H., Sano, M. and Kobayashi, M. (1998) Three cases of human gnathostomiasis caused by *Gnathostoma hispidum*, with particular reference to the identification of parasitic larvae. *Southeast Asian Journal of Tropical Medicine and Public Health* 29, 611–614.

Akue, J.P., Egwang, T.G. and Devaney, E. (1994) High levels of parasite-specific IgG4 in the absence of microfilaraemia in *Loa loa* infection. *Tropical Medicine and Parasitology* 45, 246–248.

Amaral, G., Dreyer, G., Figueredos-Silva, J., Noroes, J., Cavalcanti, A., Samico, S.C., Santos, A. and Coutinho, A. (1994) Live adult worms detected by ultrasonography in human bancroftian filariasis. *American Journal of Tropical Medicine and Hygiene* 50, 753–757.

Ando, K. (1989) Two cases of infection with *Gnathostoma nipponicum* in humans [English summary]. *Saishin Igaku* 44, 804–806.

Ando, K., Hatsushika, R., Akahane, H., Taylor, D., Mura, K. and Chinzei, Y. (1991) *Gnathostoma nipponicum* infection in the past human cases in Japan. *Japanese Journal of Parasitology* 40, 184–186.

Andrews, J.R.H., Ainsworth, R. and Abernethy, D. (1994) *Trichinella pseudospiralis* in humans: description of a case and its treatment. *Transactions of the Royal Society of Tropical Medicine and Hygiene* 88, 200–203.

Baird, J.K. and Neafie, R.C. (1988) South American brugian filariasis: report of human infection acquired in Peru. *American Journal of Tropical Medicine and Hygiene* 39, 185–188.

Baird, J.K., Neafie, R.C., Lanoie, L. and Connor, D.H. (1987) Adult *Mansonella perstans* in the abdominal cavity of nine Africans. *American Journal of Tropical Medicine and Hygiene* 37, 578–584.

Bangs, M.J., Purnomo and Andersen, E.M. (1994) A case of capillariasis in a highland community of Irian Jaya, Indonesia. *Annals of Tropical Medicine and Parasitology* 88, 685–687.

Beaver, P.C. (1989) Intraocular filariasis: a brief review. *American Journal of Tropical Medicine and Hygiene* 40, 40–45.

Beaver, P.C., Orihel, T.C. and Leonard, G. (1990) Pulmonary dirofilariasis: restudy of worms reported gravid. *American Journal of Tropical Medicine and Hygiene* 43, 167–169.

Bessonov, A.S. (1998) Taxonomic position of nematodes of the genus *Trichinella* Railliet, 1895. [in Russian, English Summary]. *Meditsinskaya Parazitologiya I Parazitarnye Bolezni* 1, 3–6.

Bloch, P. and Simonsen, P.E. (1998) Studies on immunodiagnosis of dracunculiasis. I. Detection of specific serum antibodies. *Acta Tropica* 70, 73–86.

Bloch, P., Vennervald, B.J. and Simonsen, P.E. (1998) Studies on immunodiagnosis of dracunculiasis. II. Search for circulating antigens. *Acta Tropica* 70, 303–315.

Botero, D., Aguledo, L.M. and Uribe, F.J. (1984) Intraocular filaria: a *Loaina* species from man in Colombia. *American Journal of Tropical Medicine and Hygiene* 33, 578–582.

Boussinesq, M., Bain, O., Chabaud, A.G., Gawdon-Wendel, N., Kamno, J. and Chippaux, J.P. (1995) A new zoonosis of the cerebrospinal fluid of man, probably caused by *Meningonema peruzzii*, a filaria of the central nervous system of Cercopithecidae. *Parasite* 2, 173–176.

Bradley, J.E. and Unnasch, T.R. (1996) Molecular approaches to the diagnosis of onchocerciasis. *Advances in Parasitology* 37, 58–106.

Bradley, J.E., Atogho, B.M., Elson, L., Stewart, G.R. and Boussinesq, M. (1998) A cocktail of recombinant *Onchocerca volvulus* antigens for serological diagnosis with the potential to predict endemicity of onchocerciasis infection. *American Journal of Tropical Medicine and Hygiene* 59, 877–882.

Brooker, S. and Michael, E. (2000) The potential of geographical information systems and remote sensing in the epidemiology and control of human helminth infections. *Advances in Parasitology* 47, 246–288.

Bruschi, F. (1999) How can *Trichinella* escape host immune response? *Helminthologia* 3, 179–184.

Cairncross, S., Muller, R. and Zagarian, N. (2002) Dracunculiasis (guinea worm disease) and its eradication. *Clinical Microbiology Reviews* (in press).

Capo, V. and Despommier, D.D. (1996) Clinical aspects of infection with *Trichinella* spp. *Clinical Microbiology Reviews* 9, 47–54.

Chan, S.W. and Ko, R.C. (1990) Serodiagnosis of human trichinosis using a gel filtration antigen and indirect IgG-ELISA. *Transactions of the Royal Society of Tropical Medicine and Hygiene* 84, 721–722.

Chippaux, J.-P. and Massougbodi, A. (1991) Evaluation clinique et épidemiologique de la dracunculose au Benin. *Médecine Tropicale* 51, 269–274.

Chippaux, J.-P., Ernould, J.C., Gardon, J., Gardon-Wendel, N., Chadre, F. and Barbieri, N. (1992) Ivermectin treatment of loiasis. *Transactions of the Royal Society of Tropical Medicine and Hygiene* 86, 289.

Choe, G., Lee, H.S., Seo, J.K., Chai, J.Y., Lee, S.H., Eom, K.S. and Chi, J.G. (1993) Hepatic capillariasis: first report in the Republic of Korea. *American Journal of Tropical Medicine and Hygiene* 48, 610–625.

Davies, J.B. (1995) A rapid staining and clearing technique for detecting filarial larvae in alcohol-preserved vectors. *Transactions of the Royal Society of Tropical Medicine and Hygiene* 89, 280.

Denham, D.A. and Fletcher, C. (1987) The cat infected with *Brugia pahangi* as a model of human filariasis. *CIBA Foundation Symposium* 127, 225–235.

Dissanayake, S., Watawana, L. and Piessens, W.F. (1995) Lymphatic pathology in *Wuchereria bancrofti* microfilaraemic infections. *Transactions of the Royal Society of Tropical Medicine and Hygiene* 89, 517–521.

Dreyer, G., Amaral, F., Noroes, J., Medeiros, Z. and Addiss, D. (1995) A new tool to assess the adulticidal efficacy *in vivo* of antifilarial drugs for bancroftian filariasis. *Transactions of the Royal Society of Tropical Medicine and Hygiene* 89, 225–226 (also 1994, 88, 558).

Dreyer, G., Noroes, J. and Addiss, D. (1997) The silent burden of sexual disability associated with lymphatic filariasis. *Acta Tropica* 63, 57–60.

Dreyer, G., Noroes, J., Figueredo-Silva, J. and Piessens, W.F. (2000) Pathogenesis of lymphatic disease in bancroftian filariasis: a clinical perspective. *Parasitology Today* 16, 544–548.

Dujardin, J.P., Fain, A. and Maertens, K. (1982) Survey on the human filariasis in the region of Bwamanda in Northwest Zaire. *Annales de la Société belge de Médecine tropicale* 62, 315–342.

Dye, C. (1992) Does facilitation imply a threshold for the eradication of lymphatic filariasis? *Parasitology Today* 8, 109–110.

Eberhard, M.L., Hurwitz, H., Sun, A.M. and Coletta, D. (1989) Intestinal perforation by larval *Eustrongylides* (Nematoda: Dioctophymatoidae) in New Jersey. *American Journal of Tropical Medicine and Hygiene* 40, 648–650.

Faria, G., Lanfrancotti, A., Della Torre, A., Cancrini, G. and Coluzzi, M. (1996) Polymerase chain reaction-identification of *Dirofilaria repens* and *Dirofilaria immitis*. *Parasitology* 113, 567–571.

Freedman, D.O., de Almeida-Filho, P.J., Besh, S., Maia-e-Silva, M.C., Braga, C. and Maciel, A. (1994) Lymphoscintigraphic analysis of lymphatic abnormalities in symptomatic and asymptomatic human filariasis. *Journal of Infectious Diseases* 170, 927–933.

Fu, A.Q., Tao, J.P., Wang, Z.X., Jiang, B.L., Liu, Y.X. and Qui, H.H. (1999) Observations on the morphology of *Dracunculus medinensis* from a cat in China [in Chinese, English summary]. *Chinese Journal of Zoonoses* 15, 35–38.

Gyapong, J.O. (1998) The relationship between infection and disease in *Wuchereria bancrofti* infection in Ghana. *Transactions of the Royal Society of Tropical Medicine and Hygiene* 92, 390–392.

Hasegawa, H., Korenaga, M., Kumazawa, H. and Imamawa, K. (1996) *Mermis* sp. found from human urine in Kochi Prefecture, Japan (Nematoda: Mermithidae). *Japanese Journal of Parasitology* 45, 43–46.

Hours, M. and Cairncross, S. (1994) Long-term disability due to guinea worm disease. *Transactions of the Royal Society of Tropical Medicine and Hygiene* 88, 559–560.

Hunt, D.J., Muller, R., Hellyar, A.G. and Payne, S.R. (1984) Mermithid in man. *Transactions of the Royal Society of Tropical Medicine and Hygiene* 78, 698–700.

International Task Force (1993) Recommendations for disease eradication. *CDC Morbidity and Mortality Weekly Report* 42, 1–38.

Jelinek, T. and Loscher, T. (1994) Human infection with *Gongylonema pulchrum*: a case report. *Tropical Medicine and Parasitology* 45, 329–330.

Kapel, C.M.O., Webster, P., Lind, P., Pozio, E., Henriksen, S.A., Murrell, K.D. and Nansen, P. (1998) *Trichinella spiralis*, *T. britovi* and *T. nativa*: infectivity, larval distribution in muscle, and antibody response after experimental infection of pigs. *Parasitology Research* 84, 264–271.

Kettle, D.S. (1995) *Medical and Veterinary Entomology*. CAB International, Wallingford, UK.

Kobayashi, A., Katatura, A., Hamada, A. and Suzuki, T. (1986) Human case of dracunculiasis in Japan. *American Journal of Tropical Medicine and Hygiene* 35, 159–161.

Kraivichian, P., Kulkumthorn, M., Yingyourd, P., Akarabovorn, P. and Paireepai, C.C. (1992) Albendazole for the treatment of human gnathostomiasis. *Transactions of the Royal Society of Tropical Medicine and Hygiene* 86, 418–421.

Kumari, S., Lillibridge, C.D., Bakeer, M., Lowrie, R.C., Jr, Jayaraman, K. and Philipp, M.T. (1994) *Brugia malayi*: the diagnostic potential of recombinant excretory/secretory antigens. *Experimental Parasitology* 79, 489–505.

Lammle, P.J., Reiss, M.D., Dimock, K.A., Streit, T.G., Roberts, J.M. and Eberhard, M.L. (1998) Longitudinal analysis of the development of filarial infection and antifilarial immunity in a cohort of Haitian children. *American Journal of Tropical Medicine and Hygiene* 59, 217–221.

Lawrence, R.A. (1996) Lymphatic filariasis: what mice can tell us. *Parasitology Today* 12, 267–271.

Ljungstrom, I. (1983) Immunodiagnosis in man. In: Campbell, W.C. (ed.) Trichinella *and Trichinosis* Plenum Press, New York, USA, pp. 403–424.

Marwi, M.A., Omar, B., Mohammod, C.G. and Jeffrey, J. (1990) *Anatrichosoma* sp. egg and *Demodex folliculorum* in facial skin scrapings of Orang Aslis. *Tropical Biomedicine* 7, 193–194.

Meyer, C.G. and Kremsner, P.G. (1996). Malaria and onchocerciasis: on HLA and related matters. *Parasitology Today* 12, 179–186.

Meyers, W.M., Neafie, R.C., Moris, R. and Bourland, J. (1977) Streptocerciasis: observation of adult male *Dipetalonema streptocerca* in man. *American Journal of Tropical Medicine and Hygiene* 26, 1153–1155.

Muller, R. (1971) *Dracunculus* and dracunculiasis. *Advances in Parasitology* 9, 73–151.

Muller, R. (1987) A *Dipetalonema* by any other name. *Parasitology Today* 3, 358–359.

Murdoch, M.E., Hay, R.J., McKenzie, C.D., Williams, J.F., Ghalib, H.W., Cousens, S., Abiose, A. and Jones, B.R. (1993) A clinical classification and grading system of the cutaneous changes in onchocerciasis. *British Journal of Dermatology* 129, 260–269.

Muro, A., Genchi, C., Cordero, M. and Simón, F. (1999) Human dirofilariasis in the European Union. *Parasitology Today* 15, 386–389.

Murrell, K.D. and Bruschi, F. (1994) Trichinellosis. In: Sun, T. (ed.) *Progress in Clinical Parasitology*, Vol. 4. Norton, New York, USA, pp. 117–150.

Murrell, K.D. and Pozio, E. (2000) Trichinellosis: the zoonosis that won't go quietly. *International Journal for Parasitology* 30, 1339–1349.

Ngu, J.L., Nbenfou, C., Capuli, E., McMoli, T.E., Perler, F., Mbwagbor, J., Tume, C., Nlatte, O.B., Donfack, J. and Asonganyi, T. (1998) Novel, sensitive and low-cost diagnostic tests for 'river blindness' – detection of specific antigens in tears, urine and dermal fluid. *Tropical Medicine and International Health* 3, 339–348.

Nopparatana, C., Setasuban, P., Chaicumpa, W. and Tapchaisri, P. (1991) Purification of *Gnathostoma spinigerum* specific antigen and immunodiagnosis of human gnathostomiasis. *International Journal for Parasitology* 21, 677–687.

Noroes, J., Addiss, D., Santos, A., Medeiros, Z., Coutinho, A. and Dreyer, G. (1996) Ultrasonographic evidence of abnormal lymphatic vessels in young men with adult *Wuchereria bancrofti* infection in the scrotal area. *Journal of Urology* 156, 409–412.

Nutman, T.B. (ed.) (2000) *Lymphatic Filariasis.* Imperial College Press, London, UK.

Orihel, T.C. and Eberhard, M.L. (1998) Zoonotic filariasis. *Clinical Microbiology Reviews* 11, 366–381.

Ottesen, E.A., Duke, B.O.L., Karam, M. and Behbehani, K. (1997) Strategies and tools for the control/elimination of lymphatic filariasis. *Bulletin of the World Health Organization* 75, 491–503.

Ottesen, E.A., Ismail, M.M. and Horton, J. (1999) The role of albendazole in programmes to eliminate lymphatic filariasis. *Parasitology Today* 15, 382–386.

Pampiglione, S., Canestri-Trotti, G. and Rivasi, F. (1995) Human dirofilariasis due to *Dirofilaria* (*Nochtiella*) *repens*: a review of world literature. *Parassitologia* 37, 149–193.

Pinder, M. (1988) *Loa loa* – a neglected filaria. *Parasitology Today* 4, 279–284.

Plaisier, A.P., Stolk, W.A., van Oortmarsen, G.J. and Hobbema, J.D.F. (2000) Effectiveness of annual ivermectin treatment for *Wuchereria bancrofti* infection. *Parasitology Today* 16, 298–302.

Pozio, E. (1998) Trichinellosis in the European Union: epidemiology, ecology and economic impact. *Parasitology Today* 14, 35–38.

Pozio, E. and La Rosa, G. (2000) *Trichinella murrelli* n.sp.: etiological agent of sylvatic trichinellosis in temperature areas of North America. *Journal of Parasitology* 186, 134–139.

Pozio, E., La Rosa, G., Murrell, K.D. and Lichtenfels, J.R. (1992) Taxonomic revision of the genus *Trichinella. Journal of Parasitology* 78, 654–659.

Pozio, E., Owen, I.L., la Rosa, G., Sacchi, L., Rossi, P. and Corona, S. (1999) *Trichinella papuae* n.sp. (Nematoda), a new non-encapsulated species from domestic and sylvatic swine of Papua New Guinea. *International Journal for Parasitology* 29, 1825–1839.

Remme, J.H.F. (1995) The African Programme for Onchocerciasis Control: preparing to launch. *Parasitology Today* 11, 403–406.

Richard-Lenoble, D., Kombila, M., Bain, O., Chandenier, J. and Mariotte, O. (1988) Filariasis in Gabon: human infections with *Microfilaria rodhaini. American Journal of Tropical Medicine and Hygiene* 39, 91–92.

Samba, E.M. (1994) *The Onchocerciasis Control Programme in West Africa.* World Health Organization, Geneva, Switzerland.

Saroj-Bapna and Renapurkar, D.M. (1996) Immunodiagnosis of early dracunculiasis. *Journal of Communicable Diseases* 28, 33–37.

Schlesinger, J.J., Dubois, J.G. and Beaver, P.C. (1977) *Brugia*-like filarial infection acquired in the United States. *American Journal of Tropical Medicine and Hygiene* 26, 204–207.

Service, M.W. (ed.) (2001) *The Encyclopedia of Arthropod-transmitted Infections.* CAB International, Wallingford, UK.

Shi, Y.E., Han, J.J., Yang, W.Y. and Wei, D.X. (1988) *Thelazia callipaeda* (Nematoda: Spirurida): transmission by flies from dogs to children in Hubei, China. *Transactions of the Royal Society of Tropical Medicine and Hygiene* 82, 627.

Smith, G.S., Blum, D., Huttly, S.R.D., Okeke, N., Kirkwood, B.R. and Feachem, R.G. (1989) Disability from dracunculiasis: effect on mobility. *Annals of Tropical Medicine and Parasitology* 83, 151–158.

Sucharit, S. (1988) *Mansonella digitatum* in Thailand. *Journal of the Medical Association of Thailand* 71, 587–588.

Suntharasamai, P., Riganti, M., Chittamas, S. and Desakoru, V. (1992) Albendazole stimulates outward migration of *Gnathostoma spinigerum* to the dermis in man. *Southeast Asian Journal of Tropical Medicine and Public Health* 23, 716–722.

Taylor, M.J. (2000) *Wohlbachia* bacteria of filarial nematodes in the pathogenesis of disease and as a target for control. *Transactions of the Royal Society of Tropical Medicine and Hygiene* 94, 596–598.

Toe, L., Boatin, B.A., Adjami, A., Back, C., Merriweather, A. and Unnasch, T.R. (1998) Detection of *Onchocerca volvulus* infection by 0–150 polymerase chain reaction analysis of skin scratches. *Journal of Infectious Diseases* 178, 282–285.

Toure, F.S., Egwang, T.G., Wahl, G., Millet, R., Bain, O. and Georges, A.J. (1997) Species-specific sequence in the repeat 3 region of the gene encoding a putative *Loa loa* allergen: a diagnostic tool for occult loiasis. *American Journal of Tropical Medicine and Hygiene* 56, 57–60.

Townson, S., Hutton, D., Siemenska, J., Hollick, L., Scanlon, T., Tagboto, S.K. and Taylor, M.J. (2000) Antibiotics and *Wolbachia* in filarial nematodes: antifilarial activity of rifampicin, oxytetracycline and chloramphenicol against *Onchocerca gutturosa*, *Onchocerca lienalis* and *Brugia pahangi*. *Annals of Tropical Medicine and Parasitology* 94, 801–816.

Vanamail, P., Ramalah, K.D., Pani, S.P., Das, P.K., Grenfell, B.T. and Bundy, D.A.P. (1996) Estimation of the fecund life span of *Wuchereria bancrofti* in an endemic area. *Transactions of the Royal Society of Tropical Medicine and Hygiene* 90, 119–121.

Wahl, G. and Georges, A.J. (1995) Current knowledge on the epidemiology, diagnosis, immunology and treatment of loiasis. *Tropical Medicine and Parasitology* 46, 287–291.

Weil, G.J., Lammie, P.J. and Weiss, N. (1997) The ICT filariasis test: a rapid-format antigen test for diagnosis of bancroftian filariasis. *Parasitology Today* 13, 401–404.

Whitworth, J.A.G. and Gemade, E. (1999) Independent evaluation of onchocerciasis rapid assessment methods in Benue State, Nigeria. *Tropical Medicine and International Health* 4, 26–30.

WHO (1992) *Lymphatic Filariasis and its Control*. Technical Report Series 821, World Health Organization, Geneva, Switzerland.

WHO (1995) *Onchocerciasis and its Control*. Technical Report Series 852, World Health Organization, Geneva, Switzerland.

WHO (1999) *Building Partnerships for Lymphatic Filariasis: Strategic Plan, September 1999*. World Health Organization, Geneva, Switzerland. 61 pp.

Williams, S.A. and Johnston, D.A. (with others) (1999) Helminth genome analysis: the current status of the filarial and schistosome genome projects. *Parasitology* 118 (suppl.), 519–538.

Wittner, M., Turner, J.W., Jacquette, G., Ash, L.R., Salgo, M.P. and Tanowitz, H.B. (1989) Eustrongylidiasis – a parasitic infection acquired by eating sushi. *New England Journal of Medicine* 320, 1124–1126.

Further Reading

Cairncross, S. (1992) *Guinea Worm Eradication: a Selected Bibliography*. Bureau of Hygiene and Tropical Diseases, London, UK.

Chippaux, J.-P. (1994) *Le Ver de Guinée en Afrique: Méthodes de Lutte pour l'Èradication*. ORSTOM, Paris, France.

Cross, J.H. (1995) *Capillaria philippinensis* and *Trichostrongylus orientalis*. In: Farthing, M.J.G., Keusch, G.T. and Wakelin, D. (eds) *Enteric Infection 2: Intestinal Helminths*. Chapman and Hall, London, UK, pp. 151–163.

Daengsvang, S. (1980) *A Monograph on the Genus* Gnathostoma *and Gnathostomiasis in Thailand*. Seamic, Tokyo, Japan.

Dissanaike, A.S. (1986) A review of *Brugia* sp. with special reference to *Brugia malayi* and to zoonotic infections. *Tropical Biomedicine* 3, 67–72.

Goddard, J. (1996) *Physicians' Guide to Arthropods of Medical Importance*, 2nd edn. CRC Press, Boca Raton, Florida, USA.

Grenfell, B.T. and Michael, E. (1992) Infection and disease in lymphatic filariasis: an epidemiological approach. *Parasitology* 104 (suppl.), S81-S90.

Hinz, E. (1996) *Helminthiasen des Menschen in Thailand*. Peter Lang, Frankfurt am Main, Germany, pp. 137–141.

Hopkins, D.R. and Ruiz-Tiben, E. (1991) Strategies for dracunculiasis eradication. *Bulletin of the World Health Organization* 69, 533–540.

Muller, R. (1979) Guinea worm disease; epidemiology, control and treatment. *Bulletin of the World Health Organization* 57, 683–689.

Peters, W. (1992) *Colour Atlas of Arthropods in Clinical Medicine.* Wolfe, London, UK.

RSTM&H (2000) Elimination of lymphatic filariasis as a public health problem. *Transactions of the Royal Society of Tropical Medicine and Hygiene* 94, 589–602.

Sasa, M. (1976) *Human Filariasis.* University Park Press, Tokyo, Japan.

6

Other (Non-helminth) Groups

Included in this section are a hetero-geneous collection of endoparasites that are not strictly helminths, but which may be confused with them, particularly in biopsy tissue sections.

Pentastomes

The members of this small group of para-sites form a separate phylum (Pentastomida), usually placed somewhere between the annelids and the arthropods. Larvae of seven species have been reported from humans but only two are of any importance.

Armillifer (= Porocephalus) armillata

This is a parasite of the respiratory tract of snakes in Africa and Asia, while the larvae are found encysted in the tissues of rodents and other mammals. Human infection is presumed to be by ingestion of eggs on veg-etation or in water. The egg contains an embryo (0.2 mm in length), which bores through the intestinal wall and encysts in the mesenteries of the peritoneal cavity (particularly the liver). The coiled larva moults twice and grows until it measures 20–25 mm in length. These third-stage lar-vae have characteristic annulations, giving a beaded appearance (Fig. 119). Larvae may produce a considerable inflammatory response but usually cause no symptoms and are only seen on X-rays taken for other

reasons when calcified, or probably are absorbed and never diagnosed. Severe pathology is rare and is associated with migration of the primary larvae before they become encysted, or in a few cases consid-erable tissue damage has been caused by the third-stage larvae leaving the fibrous capsule and undergoing another migration; in both cases a form of visceral larva migrans results.

Human infection is common in some areas of the world, such as Malaysia and West Africa (Benin, Cameroon, Congo, Gabon, Nigeria and Senegal).

On X-ray *Armillifer* may be mistaken for guinea worm and in tissue sections they are superficially similar to spargana, gnathostomes, fly larvae or the chigoe flea (*Tunga penetrans*). In tissue sections penta-stomes may be differentiated by the pres-ence of a body cavity and intestine (as have all the others except spargana), chitinous tracheae (as have fly larvae and *Tunga*), striated muscle fibres and the presence of reproductive organs.

Armillifer agkistrodontis, a parasite of the viper, has been recovered once in China after treatment with mebendazole at 400 mg three times daily for 3 days in a patient with abdominal pain who had drunk snake bile and blood (Zhang *et al.*, 1997).

Linguatula serrata

Known as the 'tongue worm' this is a nat-ural parasite of the nasal passages of dogs

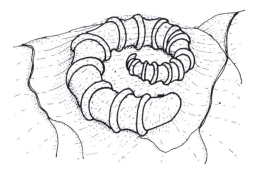

Fig. 119. Early encysted larva of *Armillifer armillata* on intestinal wall ($\times$ 6).

and other carnivores, with the larval stages occurring in herbivores. In Lebanon a type of pharyngitis known as 'halzoun' occurs in humans from ingestion of insufficiently cooked liver of sheep and goats containing larvae; in Sudan the similar 'Marrara syndrome' is found, with an allergic nasopharyngitis accompanied by itching in the throat, deafness, tinnitus and facial palsy (Yagi *et al.*, 1996). Larvae can migrate from the stomach to the tonsils and symptoms often include sneezing and coughing also. The condition usually recovers spontaneously in about a week when the parasites become dislodged. Ocular cases have been reported from Ecuador, Israel and the USA (five cases), with conjunctivitis and a larval worm in the anterior chamber. A larva has been found in the pericardial sac of a woman in Georgia, USA, two cases with larvae causing tortuous tunnels and lymphatic nodules in the abdomen in Costa Rica and larvae in the bile-duct, causing jaundice and gallstones, in a patient in Turkey.

Leeches

Leeches belong to the phylum Annelida and many species are adapted to sucking the blood of vertebrates. Most are external blood feeders and, although they may be a major nuisance in areas of Asia, are not likely to be mistaken for parasitic helminths. There are a few forms causing internal infection, of which the best known genus is *Limnatis*, reported from humans in southern Europe, North Africa, North America and Asia. *Limnatis nilotica* is a parasite of cattle and lives in water-holes and springs. Adults may measure 15 cm in length but are capable of great contraction and extension. The body is greenish-black in colour with thin orange stripes, and there are two suckers, one around the mouth, the other at the posterior end. When a very young worm is ingested in drinking water, it attaches to the mucous membranes of the mouth, pharynx, vocal cords or trachea, where it may remain attached for days or weeks. The leech feeds on blood and secretes an anticoagulant, which can cause excessive bleeding and even death. Usually, however, clinical symptoms result from the mechanical action of worms, which cause an oedematous reaction with paroxysmal coughing and dyspnoea. Various species of leeches have attached to the conjunctiva (in Turkey and the USA), causing periorbital haematomas, and invaded the nose (India), vaginal wall (India) and urethra (Malaysia).

Engorged leeches can be removed with forceps; otherwise an anaesthetic (0.5% tetracaine) or irritant substance may be necessary to induce them to detach.

Myiasis

Accidental myiasis may be caused by larvae of flies belonging to various families, such as the blowflies, flesh-flies and house-flies. The larvae or eggs are usually ingested with contaminated food or water and the larvae are found in the intestinal tract or passed out in the faeces.

The larvae of some flies are obligate parasites in the tissues of various vertebrates, the adults being known as warble flies or bot-flies. The larvae can be mistaken for helminths when causing larva migrans, although they can be recognized easily when removed. In tissue sections fly larvae can be differentiated by the chitinous tracheae, lack of reproductive organs and non-striated muscles.

Dermatobia hominis (the tropical warble

fly of South America) is the only genus that can complete its entire larval development in humans. The larvae are found in a wide range of mammalian hosts and in humans occur in unprotected parts of the body. The eggs are laid by the female fly on mosquitoes, other flies or ticks, which transport them to humans. The eggs hatch when the mosquito feeds and the larvae penetrate the skin, with a channel remaining to the surface. The posterior ends of the larvae poke out from an ulcer on the skin at intervals before they drop out in 6–12 weeks after infection and pupate in the soil. Larvae produce a severe pruritus, and a suppurating wound may result from scratching.

Cochliomyia hominovorax (the New World screw-worm) is widely distributed in cattle in the Americas. Eggs are deposited on the skin next to a wound or on mucous membranes of the nose, mouth or vagina. The hatched maggots (up to 400) tunnel deeply to produce a communal boil-like lesion, oozing pus, which often becomes secondarily infected and leads to death in about 8% of untreated cases. After 1 week of feeding the mature maggots exit and drop to the ground to pupate. One case was successfully treated with topical application of 1% ivermectin, which killed all larvae by 24 h (Victoria *et al.*, 1999). This fly was accidently introduced into Libya in 1988, but fortunately was eradicated before it spread to the rest of Africa (Hall and Wall, 1995). *Chrysomya bezziana* (the Old World screw-worm) is a similar fly in Asia and Africa.

Gasterophilus sp. (the horse bot-fly) first-stage larvae occasionally wander under the skin of humans (particularly in Russia, with a recent case in an infant in the USA). The dark transverse bands of the larvae can sometimes be seen under the skin (particularly if mineral oil is rubbed into the skin to make it transparent) inside a serpiginous tunnel. The larvae may move several millimetres a day, producing a pruritus similar to creeping eruption.

Hypoderma bovis (the cattle bot-fly) larvae may bore down deeply into the tissues, while those of *Oestrus ovis* (the sheep bot-fly) are usually found in humans in the external membranes of the eye, and those of *Rhinoestrus purpureus* (the Russian gadfly) in the nose.

Cordylobia anthropophaga (the African tumbu fly) belongs to a different group from the previous forms and has larvae that produce a boil-like swelling at the site of penetration in many animals. The eggs hatch in moist soil and penetration is usually through the feet. The larvae leave the body in 8–9 days. A recent case in the breast of a Nigerian woman appeared to be a tumour on a mammogram.

References

Hall, M. and Wall, R. (1995) Myiasis of humans and domestic animals. *Advances in Parasitology* 35, 257–334.

Victoria, J., Trujillo, R. and Barreto, M. (1999) Myiasis: a successful treatment with topical ivermectin. *International Journal of Dermatology* 38, 142–144.

Yagi, H., El Bahari, S., Mohamed, H.A., Ahmed, E.R.S., Mustafa, M., Saad, M.B.A., Sulaiman, S.M. and El Hassan, A.M. (1996) The Marrara syndrome: a hypersensitivity reaction of the upper respiratory tract and buccopharyngeal mucosa to nymphs of *Linguatula serrata*. *Acta Tropica* 62, 127–134.

Zhang, Q.Y., Wang, B.F., Huang, M. and Cheng, T.F. (1997) Viper's blood and bile. *Lancet British edition* 349, 250.

Further Reading

Hall, M. and Wall, R. (1995) Myiasis of humans and domestic animals. *Advances in Parasitology* 35, 257–334.

7

Immunology of Helminths

Introduction

Parasites, like all pathogens, elicit a wide range of immune responses in their hosts. The nature of these responses is determined both by the host and by the parasite. Even within a single host species there is variation in the capacity to express immune responses, which reflects genetic differences as well as differences in such variables as age, sex, nutrition, physiological status and the presence of concurrent infections. Parasite-determined variation in response arises from differences in the level and frequency of infection, as well as from the genetic variation that exists within widely distributed species. Much of our current knowledge of antiparasite responses has come from experimental studies in laboratory rodents, and the extent to which this can be extended to humans is sometimes controversial. However, there is no doubt that the essential principles of immune responsiveness to parasites apply to all mammalian hosts. An important principle, which has particular relevance to helminths, is that very few of the responses elicited by infection are likely to be functionally protective. Many are irrelevant to protection and some, as seen very clearly in schistosomiasis, may have severe pathological consequences. One of the important goals for immunoparasitologists is to identify those responses that are beneficial and devise ways of promoting these while reducing immunopathological responses.

The Immune Response

Immune responses to infection can be divided into two categories, innate and adaptive. In general terms, the first covers responses that are expressed immediately on exposure to infection, show little memory or enhancement on re-exposure, have broad molecular specificity (termed pattern recognition) and are associated with the activities of non-lymphoid cells. In contrast, adaptive responses depend upon the activity of lymphocytes, are induced in an antigen-specific manner, show memory and consequently are enhanced when the host is re-exposed to the same infection. The focus here will be on adaptive responses, but it should be emphasized that the distinction between the two categories is often blurred, that innate responses may be essential for the correct induction of adaptive responses, and that both can contribute to the overall response be it protective or pathological.

Adaptive Responses

Adaptive immunity is dependent upon the recognition of and the response to specific sequences (antigenic determinants or epitopes) associated with molecules that are foreign to the body (i.e. are 'non-self'). Recognition is absolutely dependent upon lymphocytes, a unique population of cells, characterized by possession of epitope-specific receptors on their cell membranes.

Lymphocytes are divided into two major populations – T (thymus-dependent) cells, which carry T-cell receptors (TCR) and B (bursa- or bone-marrow-derived) cells, in which the B-cell receptor is immunoglobulin (Ig). As far as parasitic infections are concerned most adaptive immune responses are initiated when T cells recognize epitopes, and this requires the successful completion of two distinct processes. The first is presentation of epitopes to T cells by non-lymphoid antigen-presenting cells, such as macrophages, dendritic cells and B cells, and the second is recognition of those epitopes by TCR. Recognition is a complex process that involves multiple receptor–ligand interactions between antigen-presenting cells and the T cell concerned, as well as epitope–receptor binding. These interactions involve a variety of molecules carried on each cell surface, as well as binding of receptors on the T-cell surface to soluble signalling molecules (cytokines). Once activated, T cells themselves release cytokines and interact directly and indirectly with other cells.

T cells can be categorized into a number of subsets by the surface molecules they carry (e.g. CD4+ helper cells or CD8+ cytotoxic cells) and by the cytokines they release (e.g. helper cells can be divided into at least three subsets on this basis). Different T-cell subsets regulate different components of the immune system's effector and memory responses. Key effector mechanisms are mediated via antibody production, cytotoxicity and inflammation; all three involve the coordinated activity of lymphocytes and non-lymphoid cells.

The interactions of these components in the initiation of the immune response are shown in Fig. 120.

respond directly to certain types of antigen (particularly polysaccharides), in almost all cases involving parasites B cells require T-cell help, the T cells helping to determine the class of antibody by the pattern of cytokines they produce. The specificity of the antibodies produced is the same as that of the surface receptor carried by the B cells involved initially, but plasma cells release large amounts of the molecule in a soluble form and modify the molecules to perform a variety of biological functions.

Ig molecules are formed from paired heavy and light glycoprotein chains and can be divided into two functional regions, the Fab region, which determines epitope recognition, and the Fc region, which determines other biological functions (Fig. 121). Differences in the Fc regions define the five major classes of antibodies (IgM, IgD, IgG, IgA, IgE). Binding of antibody to a target epitope may itself have protective value, e.g. if the target is carried by a crucial enzyme or sensory cell; more frequently, antibody binding serves to identify the target immunologically and thus act as a focus for other effector mechanisms. An important mechanism involves the activation of complement, a complex series of plasma proteins capable of triggering non-lymphoid effector cells, of increasing phagocytic activity and of damaging cell membranes to bring about cell lysis. Bound antibody also acts to increase interactions between the target and non-lymphoid cells that carry the appropriate Fc receptor. Antibody binding and complement activation can therefore both be involved in what is collectively termed antibody-dependent cellular cytotoxicity (ADCC), a mechanism thought to be involved in immune protection against a number of helminths (Fig. 122).

Antibody Production

Antibodies (circulating Ig) are produced by B cells that have been appropriately stimulated and have gone through a sequence of developmental steps to produce plasma cells. Although it is possible for B cells to

Cytotoxicity

In addition to ADCC, cytotoxicity can be brought about directly by T cells, particularly CD8+ cells and specialized natural killer (NK) cells These bind to targets through the TCR or other receptors and

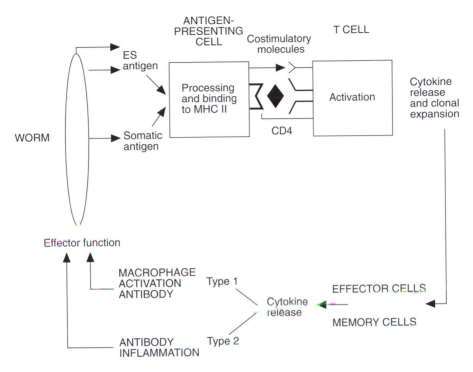

Fig. 120. Initiation of the immune response to a parasitic worm. Worms release antigens in their excretions/secretions (ES antigens), from their cuticle, and from their bodies (somatic antigens) when the worm is killed. Antigen is taken up by antigen-presenting cells and presented by major histocompatibility complex (MHC) molecules to T cells. Recognition of antigen by the T-cell receptor and ligation of accessory and costimulatory molecules activate the T cell. The activated cells release cytokines and undergo clonal expansion to produce clones of cells with identical T-cell receptors. These cells, acting through cytokines, become effector cells or memory cells. Effector cells, through release of type 1 or type 2 cytokines, coordinate a variety of effector activities against the parasite. Key to symbols: ▨ MHC molecule; ◆ Antigen; ⊵ T-cell receptor.

release a number of potent molecules that damage cell membranes or cause intracellular damage. T-cell cytotoxicity is well established as a protective mechanism in infections involving intracellular protozoans, but there is little evidence for its importance in helminths.

Inflammation

Parasites bring about inflammatory changes in a variety of ways. Their invasion and activities in tissues cause mechanical and chemical damage, and their interactions with non-lymphoid cells cause the release of potent mediators, which themselves can

damage tissues, but it is probable that immune-mediated inflammation plays a major role in a majority of infections involving helminths. This form of inflammation can be mediated by antibodies, particularly when complement is involved, and by T cells. Antibody of the IgE class is particularly important in this respect, as it binds to cells that have the potential to release powerful biological mediators (e.g. amines) when the bound antibody becomes complexed with its specific antigen. T-cell-mediated inflammation is the result of cytokine release and the increased production, or increased activity, of a wide variety of non-lymphoid cells. Again it is the release of potent mediators that initiates

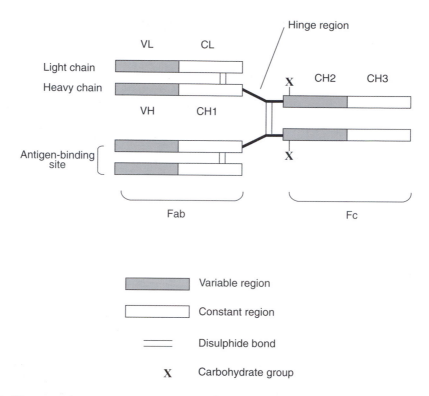

Fig. 121. Diagrammatic representation of an immunoglobulin molecule (based on IgG). The molecule is made up of two light (L) chains and two heavy (H) chains, held by disulphide bonds. The bond between the paired chains can be split by enzymes to break up the molecule into the Fab and Fc fragments. Each chain forms a number of regions (domains): the variable (V) regions form the antigen-binding site of the Fab fragments; the constant (C) regions of the Fc fragment confer the biological properties of the molecule, e.g. binding to receptors and activation of complement.

the inflammatory damage. Some of the mediators released during inflammation, however caused, can damage parasites directly; in other cases the tissue changes associated with inflammation may affect the parasite indirectly, essentially by bringing about dramatic changes in its environment.

Non-lymphoid Cells

Lymphocytes and non-lymphoid cells both arise from precursors in the bone marrow, but then follow divergent pathways of development – the lymphoid and the myeloid. The latter pathway gives rise to the two major categories of non-lymphoid cells, the macrophage–monocyte line and the granulocyte line. Monocytes circulate in the blood and mature as macrophages in the tissues. Three groups of granulocytes (neutrophils, eosinophils and basophils) mature in the bone marrow and move into tissues from the blood, while the fourth (mast cells) matures in tissues. All non-lymphoid cells can participate in innate and adaptive responses through their phagocytic activities and through their ability to release powerful mediators. Macrophages, neutrophils and eosinophils often infiltrate tissues around worms and may form granulomas when parasite stages become trapped in tissues. Basophils and mast cells – the amine-containing cells – are involved primarily through the capac-

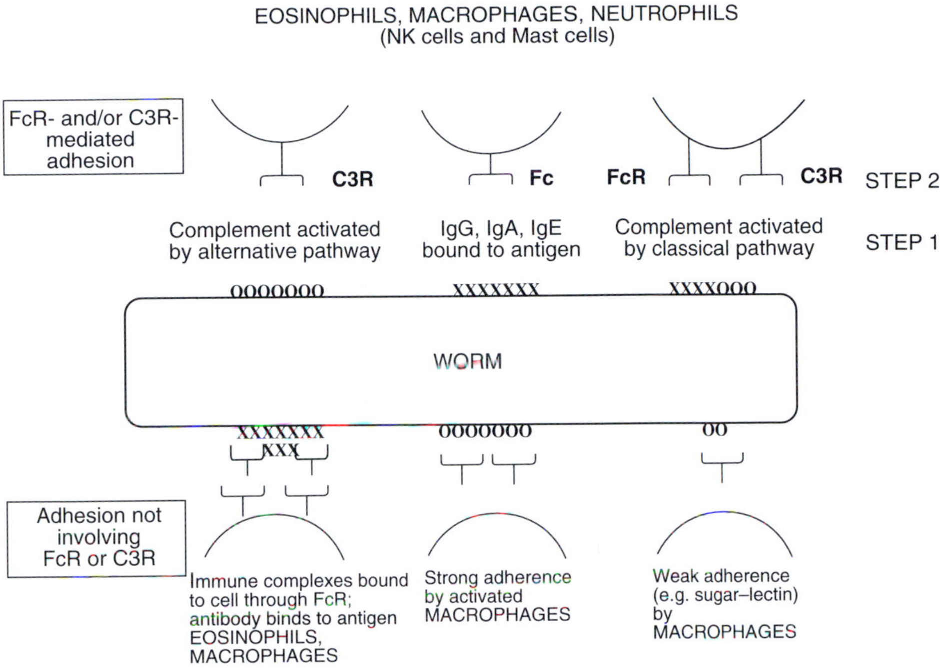

Fig. 122. Mechanisms by which cells mediate cytotoxic activity against parasitic worms. Adhesion between cells and parasites can involve cellular receptors for the Fc portion of immunoglobulin molecules (FcR), or receptors for components of complement such as C3(C3R), when these molecules are bound to the parasite's surface. Adhesion can also occur through mechanisms not involving direct binding of immunoglobulin or complement to the parasite (e.g. via immune complexes, lectin–sugar binding and intermolecular forces).

ity to release a variety of mediators. Whereas phagocytosis is an effective defence mechanism against protozoans, worms, even larvae, are too large to be taken in by single cells. A more characteristic response is for cells to bind closely to the parasite surface, through antibody- or complement-mediated mechanisms, and then to release mediators directly on to the worm surface. In that way the outer surface is damaged, often irreversibly, and the worm killed.

Parasites and their Antigens

Parasites, and helminths in particular, are complex organisms, often with complex life cycles. The presence of an infection therefore exposes the host to a battery of parasite-derived foreign molecules, which can be recognized by the immune system. These are commonly proteins, glycoproteins or carbohydrates, but molecules such as glycolipids can also be antigenic. In the case of helminths, antigens may be present on the parasite surface, released from the worm as it develops, reproduces and metabolizes (collectively referred to as excretory/secretory (ES) antigens) or released when the worm dies and is destroyed. Antigens of intracellular protozoans may be expressed on the surface of the host cell, and this also occurs in the nematode *Trichinella spiralis* during its intramuscular phase.

The antigens presented by helminths frequently change as the parasite goes through its life cycle, i.e. there is stage specificity in antigen expression. This can result in the responses raised against one life-cycle stage being ineffective against a later stage. Equally life-cycle stages may differ in their immunogenicity (their ability to generate immune responses), although this is also influenced by their location. Metabolically active stages that migrate through tissues, or remain there for long periods, are often potently immunogenic, *Ascaris* larvae and schistosome eggs being excellent examples. Resting larval stages, particularly those that become encysted or enter immunologically privileged sites, such as the central nervous system (CNS), may generate much less response – tapeworm larvae are good examples. Some parasites living in the intestine (e.g. hookworms) can stimulate strong immune responses, their antigens being taken up across the mucosa, but others, notably the tapeworms, appear much less immunogenic. Many nematodes and larval trematodes release antigens that act as allergens – i.e. stimulate the formation of IgE – and thus the host develops hypersensitivity to the parasite, allergic symptoms being common in many helminth infections.

Not all molecules released by helminths act as immunogens, in the sense of stimulating positive immune responses. Many worms are now known to release immunomodulatory molecules, which suppress, divert or inactivate components of the immune response. Good examples have been described in infections with filarial worms and with hookworms, but immunomodulation is probably a widespread phenomenon. Helminths also express, or acquire, molecules that act as immunological disguises (glycolipids in adult schistosomes, albumin in microfilaria larvae, host proteins in cestode larvae), which enable them to reduce the degree of 'foreignness' they present to the host's immune system, effectively being seen as self rather than non-self. Some molecules, although immunogenic, have been shown to elicit antibody responses (e.g. IgM antibodies to carbohydrate antigens of *S. mansoni*) that block the protective action of other antibody classes and

thus decrease protective immunity ('blocking antibodies').

Expression of Immune Responses

The detailed understanding of the immune system that we now have enables us to interpret in mechanistic terms many of the characteristics of the immune responses that parasitic infections generate. It seems a general rule that, whereas many protozoa, particularly the intracellular species, elicit lymphocyte responses dominated by the T-helper 1 (Th1) subset, helminth infections elicit Th2-dominated responses. Th1 responses are associated with cellular immunity (e.g. activation of macrophages) and production of specific classes of IgG antibodies. In contrast, Th2 cells coordinate a pattern of antibody responses, which includes IgE, and regulate the production and activity of inflammatory cells, particularly eosinophils and mast cells. The reason for this Th subset bias is not fully understood, but it reflects the nature of particular antigens, the ways in which these are presented to T cells and the cytokine environment in which T-cell responses take place. Thus T-cell responses occurring in the presence of the cytokine interleukin 12 (IL-12) (derived from previously activated NK cells) become polarized to the Th1 subset, while those occurring in the presence of IL-4 (derived from cells such as mast cells) become polarized to the Th2 subset.

The nature and degree of the immune response elicited by infection are not only dependent on the level and frequency of infection and the characteristics of the parasite concerned, they are also influenced by the location of the parasite. Helminths occupy a very wide variety of habitats in the host's body, and the capacity of these to respond to infection and the nature of the response expressed can differ quite markedly. A useful distinction in immunological terms is seen in the responses to parasites living within the intestine and those elsewhere in the body, i.e. between parasites living in mucosal and systemic locations. Although the mucosal and systemic immune systems are clearly interconnected, the populations of lymphocytes in each and their patterns of migration are distinct. The responses occurring within the intestinal wall itself are similar in many respects to those elsewhere in the body, but a major difference is seen in the predominant class of Ig produced there and secreted into the gut lumen (IgA), whereas the systemic immune system is dominated by IgG and IgM antibodies. The mucosal tissues are readily infiltrated by inflammatory cells, characteristically including a discrete population of mast cells. Interactions between these cells and IgE can trigger hypersensitivity reactions, which lead to major changes in intestinal structure and function. The mucosal immune system operates not only in the intestine, but also in the lungs and urogenital tissues. Systemic immunity has different characteristics in different locations, and these influence the antiparasite responses generated by infection. Important differences are seen, for example, between responses in the CNS, usually regarded as an immunologically privileged site (i.e. with reduced responsiveness), and those in the skin, where a separate population of antigen-presenting cells (Langerhans cells) operates and where cellular inflammatory responses are readily generated. In contrast to protozoans, relatively few helminths live for any length of time in the blood, adult schistosomes and microfilaria larvae being exceptions. Despite being bathed in antibodies and complement and potentially exposed to a variety of non-lymphoid cells, both survive for prolonged periods, because they possess effective evasion mechanisms which prevent them from being recognized.

Protective Immune Responses in Infected Hosts

Although it is easy to demonstrate that parasitic infections elicit immune responses in their human hosts, it is more difficult to demonstrate the relation of these responses to protective immunity. Immune responses in parasitized humans can be measured in a variety of ways. These include tests that demonstrate the presence of specific antiparasite antibody, lymphocyte responses and cytokine production, skin sensitivity to antigen, increased production of 'non-specific' IgM and increased numbers of eosinophils, as well as histopathological demonstration of the presence of immune cells in infected tissues. In addition, the capacity of antibodies and cells taken from infected individuals to kill parasites or parasite-infected cells can be tested *in vitro*. Demonstrable protection against reinfection, in individuals or in populations (e.g. *Leishmania major*), is clear evidence of immunity, but is relatively rare in helminth infections. Evidence of age-related declines in infection rates in endemic areas (e.g. in malaria and in helminth infections) suggests the operation of host-protective immunity, as does protection against the pathological effects of infection (e.g. malaria), but neither is necessarily conclusive. 'Experiments of nature' – i.e. study of infections in individuals with compromised immune systems – can indicate the importance of immune competence in preventing the consequences of infection (e.g. giardiasis, cryptosporidiosis or strongyloidiasis). However, these lines of evidence can often only be deduced from detailed and extensive population studies and sophisticated statistical analysis. More direct evidence that host-protective immunity can operate effectively against parasites can be gained from studies in experimental models, although it is often not possible to use in such models (particularly rodents) the species of parasite that are of interest in humans.

There are experimental models for most of the major human helminth infections, the majority of these being in rodent hosts. Under controlled conditions, it is possible to show that, in many cases, infections elicit strong immune responses and that these may confer substantial protection on the host. Protection developing during an initial infection can be quantified by determining the numbers of worms recovered at intervals after infection or by the levels and duration of larval and egg output. In other cases protection is not seen, and worms persist for long periods in the presence of specific immune responses. Good examples from work with mouse models include the long-term survival of schistosomes, larval cestodes, liver flukes, microfilariae and certain intestinal nematodes. Immunity to reinfection can be seen in models where there is no resistance to the primary infection, but the nature of this reinfection immunity needs to be examined carefully. For example, the resistance of mice to reinfection with *Schistosoma mansoni* reflects the pathological changes that the primary infection has brought about in the liver, rather than specific immune destruction of the incoming worms. Resistance to reinfection with *Taenia taeniaeformis* in mice carrying mature cysticerci reflects the operation of immune responses against the penetrating oncospheres and early cysticerci before these have developed resistance to complement-mediated damage. Resistance of mice to reinfection with *Heligmosomoides polygyrus* (an intestinal nematode widely used as a model of chronic infection) is expressed only if the previous adult infection and its associated immunosuppressive effects have been removed by anthelminthic treatment. Once the existence of host-protective immunity has been established, potential mechanisms of immune-mediated resistance and the response components involved can be studied using *in vitro* approaches. Good examples include analysis of ADCC mechanisms against schistosomula and microfilariae. However, the demonstration of effective immune killing under *in vitro* conditions does not necessarily correlate with *in vivo* patterns of response. The capacity of hosts to become immune can also be studied in experimental models by using attenuated parasites or isolated parasite molecules as vaccine antigens. For example, mice can be effectively vaccinated against *S. mansoni* using irradiated cercariae, rats against the same species with defined recombinant antigens (e.g. glutathione-S-transferase) and mice against intestinal nematodes with defined antigens or synthetic peptides from these antigens.

Demonstration of protective immunity in human populations that are naturally exposed to helminth infections is much more difficult than it is in the laboratory, because of the number of confounding factors that have to be taken into account. Unlike experimental animals, individual humans are exposed to varying intensities and frequencies of infection and differ from one another in factors that are known to influence immunity (e.g. age, sex, infection, nutritional and physiological status and genetics), as well as access to anthelminthic treatment. What was a general view that there is little immunologically mediated resistance to helminths, despite abundant evidence of immune responses as such, has been considerably modified as a result of immunoepidemiological and *in vitro* studies. For example, it now seems quite clear, from detailed treatment/reinfection studies, that humans do develop protective immunity to infection with *S. mansoni* and *S. haematobium*. Correlative studies have linked resistance to levels of parasite-specific IgE and to eosinophil activity, data that are supported by *in vitro* work. Although the picture is much less clear with the major gastrointestinal nematodes, there are data suggesting that a level of protective immunity is acquired, at least in hookworm and *Trichuris* infections. Knowledge of the cellular and molecular mechanisms underlying immune responses has increased the predictive value of studies that attempt to correlate infection status with particular immune components. This is best seen with the many studies that now use T-cell and cytokine data as analytical tools. The various clinical categories found in populations exposed to lymphatic filariasis (from the putatively immune, parasite-negative endemic normals to infected individuals with obstructive disease) have been correlated with particular patterns of Th-cell response and cytokine production, although the relationship is clearly complex. Epidemiological and genetic studies on populations exposed to *S. mansoni* have pinpointed a major gene that controls the expression of protective immunity, and have revealed positive correlations between resistance and the genetic control of Th2-related cytokines. For many helminth infections, however, evidence for protective immunity is slight, and there is little information about the underlying basis of the immune responses that infection elicits.

Exploitation of Immune Responses

Diagnosis

Whether or not immune responses confer any protection against helminths their presence can be used as a means of diagnosing infection. A majority of diagnostic tests make use of antibody responses, and these can be measured by many techniques. Perhaps the most widespread at present is the ELISA, which can be used with very small quantities of serum, can be automated for large-scale surveys and is read using colorimetric assays. One drawback of antibody-based tests is that the presence of antiparasite antibody does not necessarily imply the presence of a current infection, although measurement of particular classes of antibody (e.g. IgG4) is a good indicator. The ELISA can be adapted to test for antigen rather than antibody, and of course this is a positive indicator of parasites in the body. Antigen detection has been widely used in schistosome and filarial infections. An exciting new development is the development of non-invasive detection of ES antigens by an antigen-capture ELISA in faeces (coproantigens), urine and perhaps saliva (e.g. see p. 24 for schistosomiasis in urine and p. 77 for cestodes in faeces).

Conventionally, ELISA tests have used multiwell plates to provide the solid-phase substrate on which antigen or antibody can be bound, and they require spectrophotometric readouts. Recent development of the dipstick technique, where reagents are bound to a nitrocellulose strip and coupled with built-in controls, allows immediate identification of a positive or negative response and can be used in the absence of sophisticated laboratory equipment. A lim-

iting factor in all diagnostic tests is the availability of purified antigens to give high levels of both sensitivity and specificity. The use of recombinant and synthetic techniques for antigen production is overcoming this limitation.

A number of older diagnostic tests used cellular responses to injected antigen as an indicator of infection. These have largely been phased out, largely because of low specificity and the danger of adverse reactions.

The immunology of trematodes is discussed on p. 23 and p. 41, of cestodes on p. 93, of intestinal nematodes on p. 121 and of filarial nematodes on pp. 196 and 217.

Vaccination

As with all infectious diseases, vaccination against helminths is seen as one of the most effective ways in which infections could be controlled. Until quite recently, success in this field has been negligible compared with the progress made with viral and bacterial vaccines. Although many of the latter were initially developed quite empirically, this approach has not been successful with helminths, where the problems of eliciting the required protective responses are much greater. Experimental vaccines using attenuated larval stages have proved effective in rodents against parasites such as schistosomes, hookworms and some filarial nematodes. Attenuated larvae have also been used to reduce disease in schistosome-exposed cattle, but the ethical problems involved with the use of live vaccines in humans have prevented further development. Most progress has been achieved with the development of recombinant vaccines, which were first used successfully against larval cestodes in sheep, show promise against gastrointestinal nematodes in sheep and are being tested in trials for use against *S. mansoni* in humans. The latter vaccine is based on the use of recombinant glutathione-*S*-transferase, a molecule that also has protective value against other schistosome species.

8

Epidemiological Aspects of Helminth Infections

Epidemiology may be defined as the study of the factors influencing the occurrence and distribution of infection. In general, it is concerned with populations rather than with individual cases.

Epidemiological studies serve two main functions: first, they provide the necessary data for determining the medical, economic and social importance of an infection, in order to evaluate and plan the effort and funds that should be devoted to it; secondly, they can help to discover the relevant factors whose manipulation could lead to prevention or control of disease. There have been many recent studies that have provided important findings on the relative importance of helminth infections as causes of the morbidity discussed in the various sections and these are helping in the evaluation of the benefits (including economic) of control campaigns.

Unlike microorganisms, such as viruses, bacteria and protozoa, in which a few organisms can multiply quickly and cause serious disease, helminths are large parasites which, in most cases, do not multiply directly within the body of their hosts. For this reason the number of parasites present at any one time can be of great importance in determining the likelihood of morbidity, and thus helminth infections tend to be chronic and insidious, with increase in the intensity of infection possible through repeated reinfection. For microorganisms the infected host provides the most convenient unit of study in epidemiological surveys, while the individual helminth provides the most convenient basic unit of study, and measurements of worm burden (e.g. directly by counting worms in faeces after chemotherapy, or indirectly, by egg counts or recently by immunological estimates of circulating worm antigens) can be very important.

Epidemiological studies can be divided into two main categories. Descriptive studies can be used in order to determine the frequency and intensity of infections, where and when they occur and what kind of people become infected; repeated studies over a period of time (longitudinal cross-sectional studies) are often more useful than studies at one period in time (horizontal cross-sectional studies) and are essential for determining the rate of acquiring infection (incidence).

In general, epidemiology is a quantitative science and properly designed and statistically valid techniques are of critical importance and there should be standardization of the methods employed. Changes in technique can often make it difficult to compare older with more recent figures. For instance, newer serological techniques are often considerably more sensitive than older parasitological methods (e.g. microfilarial counts compared with the immunochromatographic (ITC) test in lymphatic filariasis).

Attempts to control or eradicate human helminth infections are usually aimed at breaking the life cycle by manipulating one or more of the various transmission factors. However, with a well-established endemic parasite, this might be very difficult to accomplish. Helminths are almost invariably overdispersed or aggregated (a negative binomial distribution) within their hosts, so that many hosts harbour just a few parasites while a small proportion (about 15% in the case of ascariasis) have heavy infections. Thus large sample sizes are necessary in order to obtain accurate figures of intensity of infection.

The regulation of the abundance and prevalence of helminth infections is mostly by density-dependent (or negative-feedback) factors in the host population or individual host, so that herd immunity, degree of input of susceptibles and fluctuations in transmission rates do not tend to regulate the number of parasites present and infections can be long-lived and stable. While the likelihood of heavy infections is obviously affected by differences in host behaviour, there is also clear evidence, at least for the schistosomes, that it is genetically determined. The age of the host is often an important factor in the occurrence and severity of infection and age prevalence and age intensity curves can be calculated (see Fig. 55).

The basic reproductive rate or, more accurately, number (R_0) determines the ability of the parasite to perpetuate itself. It can be defined as the average number of offspring (or of female offspring in the the case of dioecious parasites) produced throughout the lifetime of a female parasite, which themselves achieve maturity in the absence of density-dependent constraints. R_0 must be > 1 for the parasite to maintain itself, while, if there were no constraints, the numbers of parasites would increase exponentially (provided R_0 was > 1). In practice, helminth populations tend to remain stable over time (Anderson, 1998), although R_0 will vary within the host population from one geographical locality to another.

The search for a more quantitative expression of the factors involved in the transmission of parasitic diseases has continued since Ronald Ross applied a system of differential equations (known as a mathematical model) to the description of malaria transmission. A model can be constructed based on the life cycle of the parasite and, provided that the parasite population is at equilibrium, the net reproductive rate should equal unity. For instance, with the schistosomes, this rate can be expressed as the product of various factors:

net reproductive = (net reproductive rate
rate of parasite   of parasite in snail
                       population) ×
                       (probability of infecting a
                       definitive host) × (net
                       reproductive rate of
                       parasite in definitive
                       host) × (probability of
                       infecting a snail)

Provided that figures are available in order to calculate these various components, it should be possible to predict the effect of variations in each on the overall transmission picture. Preferably any model should include all the factors that have a significant influence on transmission, even if this complicates the analysis.

The transmission threshold is the level of parasite transmission, reproduction and mortality rates that maintain infection and below which the parasite will die out (R_0 < 1) and, by manipulation of various parameters in the model, the effect of each on the likely ease of elimination of the parasite can be forecast.

References and Further Reading

Anderson, R.M. (1998) Epidemiology of parasitic infections. In: Cox, F.E.G., Kreier, J.P. and Wakelin, D. (eds) *Topley and Wilson's Microbiology and Microbial Infections,* 9th edn, Vol. 5. Arnold, London, UK, pp. 39–55.

Anderson, R.M. and May, R.M. (1985) Helminth infections of humans: mathematical models, population dynamics, and control. *Advances in Parasitology* 24, 1–101.

Bundy, D.A.P. and Medley, G.F. (1992a) Epidemiology and population dynamics of helminth infection. In: Moqbel, R. (ed.) *Allergy and Immunity to Helminths: Common Mechanisms or Divergent Pathways.* Taylor and Francis, London, UK, pp. 17–37.

Bundy, D.A.P. and Medley, G.F. (1992b) Immuno-epidemiology of human geohelminthiasis: ecological and immunological determinants of worm burden. *Parasitology* 104 (suppl.), S105-S110.

Giesecke, J. (1994) *Modern Infectious Disease Epidemiology.* Arnold, London, UK.

Woolhouse, M.E.J. (1992) On the application of mathematical models of schistosome transmission dynamics. II. Control. *Acta Tropica* 50, 189–204.

9

Helminthological Techniques

The most important laboratory techniques in medical helminthology are those concerned with the diagnosis of infection. Routine diagnostic techniques include the recovery of eggs or larvae in faeces or, for the filarial worms, identification of microfilariae in blood or skin snips.

Immunodiagnostic methods are advancing at a rapid rate and are now the methods of choice for the diagnosis of fascioliasis, cysticercosis, echinococcosis, aberrant tissue helminths and lymphatic filariasis, although not, as yet, for the diagnosis of intestinal helminths. Immunodiagnostic tests are discussed on page 250 and in the diagnosis sections of various helminths and details of relevant texts (such as Walls and Schantz, 1986; Garcia and Bruckner, 1997; Garcia, 1999) are given in the general references.

While not strictly a helminthological technique, it is often useful to stain eosinophils and mast cells in tissues and the methods of Ball and Hay or Kermanizadeh and colleagues (see Cassella and Hay, 1995) can be used.

Faecal Examination

The eggs of helminths commonly encountered in the faeces of humans are shown in Fig. 123 and those of rarer or spurious parasites in Fig. 124. The eggs most commonly found in spurious infections (i.e. when no adults are present) are those of the sheep liver flukes, *Dicrocoelium* and *Fasciola*, which are passed after eating infected liver, those of free-living or plant-parasitic nematodes, such as *Heterodera*, which are ingested in or on vegetables, and mite eggs.

The inexperienced operator needs to exercise caution in identifying helminth eggs. Provided eggs are present and are seen, it is usually a comparatively simple matter to recognize them for what they are. However, when eggs are absent, all too frequently other objects serve as acceptable substitutes. Particularly popular are mite eggs, starch grains, pollen grains and plant cells; but sometimes even air bubbles are mistaken for eggs. Starch grains and plant cells can be differentiated from eggs by their lack of internal structures and by their irregular outlines and great size range. Pollen grains are more difficult to distinguish, as they appear to have an operculum, but they are kidney-shaped and much denser than the *Clonorchis* type of egg, with which they are usually confused. An expert system has been devised for identification of helminth eggs (Esterre *et al.*, 1987).

In order to minimize mistakes, the size of objects seen under the microscope should always be considered. As a rough guide, an egg measures about 1/15 (*Clonorchis*) to 1/3 (*Fasciolopsis*) of the diameter of the microscope field at a magnification of ×400 (×40 objective and ×10 objective).

Any larvae found in fresh faeces will be those of *Strongyloides* (Fig. 125), but it is possible for larvae of hookworms to be

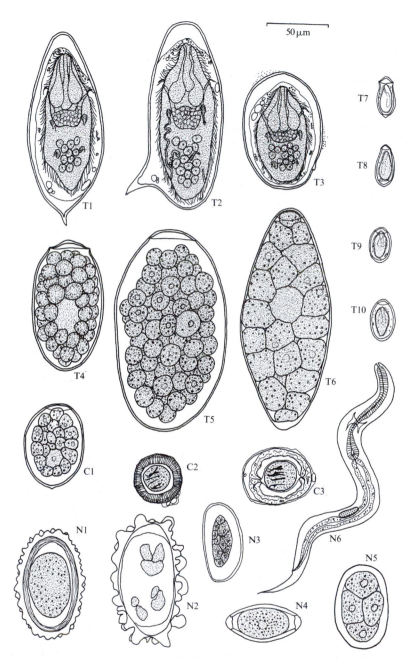

Fig. 123. Helminth eggs and larva commonly found in human faeces. T1. *Schistosoma haematobium* (in urine); T2. *S. mansoni;* T3. *S. japonicum;* T4. *Paragonimus westermani;* T5. *Fasciolopsis buski* (egg of *Fasciola hepatica* is identical); T6. *Gastrodiscoides hominis;* T7. *Clonorchis sinensis;* T8. *Opisthorchis felineus* (egg of *O. viverrini* is identical); T9. *Metagonimus yokogawai;* T10. *Heterophyes heterophyes;* C1. *Diphyllobothrium latum;* C2. *Taenia saginata* or *T. solium* ; C3. *Hymenolepis nana;* N1. *Ascaris lumbricoides;* N2. *A. lumbricoides* (infertile); N3. *Enterobius vermicularis;* N4. *Trichuris trichiura;* N5. Hookworms (eggs of *Necator* and *Ancylostoma* are identical); N6. Larva of *Strongyloides stercoralis.*

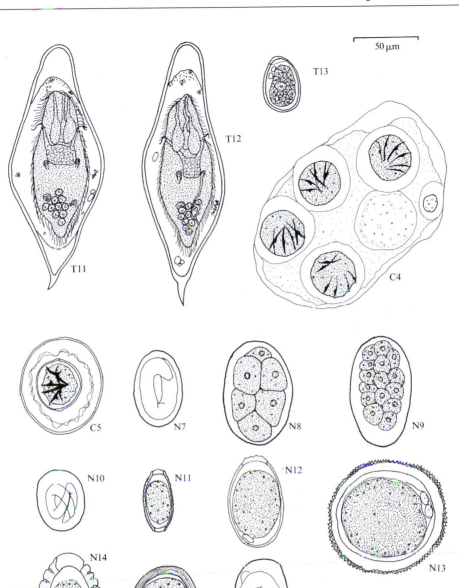

Fig. 124. Rarer eggs found in human faeces. T11. *Schistosoma intercalatum*; T12. *S. mattheei*; T13. *Dicrocoelium dendriticum* (often spurious from eating infected liver); C4. *Dipylidium caninum* egg mass; C5. *Hymenolepis diminuta*; N7. *Strongyloides fuelleborni*; N8. *Ternidens deminuta* (egg of *Oesophagostomum bifurcum* is similar); N9. *Trichostrongylus* spp.; N10. *Physaloptera* sp.; N11. *Aonchotheca philippinensis*; N12. *Gnathostoma spinigerum* (rarely reaches adult stage in humans); N13. *Toxocara canis* (not found in human faeces, although the similar egg of *T. cati* has been found a few times); N14. *Dioctophyma renale*; N15. *Ascaris lumbricoides* (decorticated); N16. Hookworms (embryonated as sometimes found in very old faeces); N17. *Meloidogyne* sp. (root-knot nematodes, spurious infection from eating root vegetables).

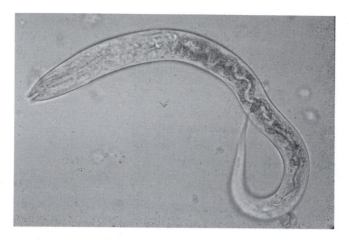

Fig. 125. First-stage larva of *Strongyloides stercoralis* as found in human faeces (actual size 250 μm).

present in old faeces or even adults of coprophilic nematodes in old stools collected from the ground.

Freshly passed stool specimens should be collected in waxed paper or plastic stool containers (although the latter are often found very useful for other purposes and not returned), using a wooden applicator, and can be stored for a few days in the refrigerator or preserved in 10% formalin. Alternatively large numbers of samples can be collected in sealed polyethylene tubing (12.5 cm × 7.6 cm × 0.1 mm thickness) and preserved in merthiolate/iodine/formalin (MIF) stain and preservative (200 ml of 1:1000 merthiolate, 25 ml of 40% formaldehyde solution, 5 ml of glycerol and 250 ml of distilled water; 0.15 ml of 5% Lugol's iodine can be added just before use for the detection of protozoal cysts (great care should be taken with formaldehyde as it is an irritant and can be carcinogenic). The simplest method for the detection of eggs is direct microscopical examination of a smear of about 5 mg of faeces, diluted with freshly filtered tap water or saline, on a slide covered with a coverslip.

The use of small disposable polyethylene envelopes 7 cm × 4 cm × 0.03 mm thick and a single microscope slide has been advocated for mass surveys to save expense of slides and coverslips. With this method a larger 100 mg sample can be smeared. However, these direct methods are not very sensitive.

Sodium acetate/acetic acid/formalin (SAF) fixative can also be used for preserving eggs and protozoa in faeces (sodium acetate 1.5 g, glacial acetic acid 2.0 ml, 40% solution of formaldehyde 4.0 ml and distilled water 92.0 ml).

Kato–Katz cellophane thick-smear technique

In this method, a faecal sample on scrap paper is pressed through a small screen and, with a spatula, a roughly 50 mg sample of sieved faeces is placed on a microscope slide (Fig. 126a, b, c and d). For a quantitative measurement, the faeces sample is placed on a template with a central hole over the slide, excess faeces removed with the spatula and the template carefully removed, leaving a cylinder of faeces (Fig. 126e). The template should be 1 mm thick, with a hole of 9 mm, which will deliver 50 mg of faeces, and it can be made of metal, plastic or cardboard; many should be made. A cellophane square (obtainable from cigarette packets, etc.) measuring 25 mm × 30 or 35 mm which has been soaked in a mixture of 100 ml glycerine, 100 ml of distilled water and 1 ml of 3% aqueous malachite green or 3% methylene blue is placed over it as a coverslip (Fig. 126f and g). The microscope slide can be turned over and pressed against a hard surface until newsprint can

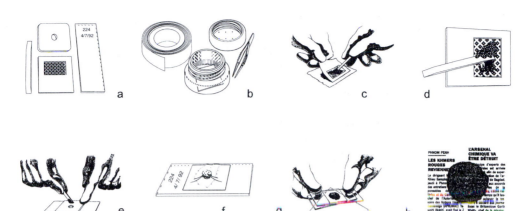

Fig. 126. Illustrations of Kato–Katz technique: (a) Equipment, (b) Strips of hydrophilic cellophane and a jar with lid, (c, d, e, f, g. and h). Pressing faeces through sieve so that an amount above sieve can be put into template, covered with cellophane and compressed so that a newspaper can be read through it.

be read through the faecal sample (Fig. 126h); alternatively, a rubber bung can be used. Carefully remove the slide by gently sliding it sideways and leaving it for 20–30 min at 37°C or 1 h at room temperature for the faeces to clear progressively. Hookworm eggs clear first and will not be visible by 2 h, while *Ascaris*, *Trichuris* and schistosome eggs will still be visible weeks or even months later. The slide can be turned over on to filter-paper to prevent drying temporarily. In a modification to allow almost immediate observation and long storage, a mixture of 100 ml polyethylene glycol, 100 ml formalin and 200 ml saturated saline (plus 2 ml colour, as above, if desired) can be substituted.

The smear should be examined in a systematic manner and the number of eggs of each species recorded. Multiply by 20 to give eggs per gram. (A hole of 6.5 mm in a 0.5 mm thick template will give a sample size of 20 mg, which should be multiplied by 50. This has the advantage that clearing time is reduced to 15 min.) Naturally, if quantitative measurements are not required, the template is unnecessary.

Concentration methods

Concentration methods are useful for prevalence surveys, but are not always use-ful for measuring the intensity of an infection because so many eggs may be present in a sample that they cannot be easily counted.

Formol–ether technique

The advantage of this method is that it is quick and can be used to search for protozoal cysts and *Strongyloides* larvae, as well as helminth eggs. Using an applicator stick, 1 or 2 g of faeces is emulsified in a centrifuge tube with 10 ml of 10% formalin. The suspension is then passed through a metal or plastic sieve (400 μm mesh) or two layers of gauze (for single use) into a beaker, evaporating dish or another centrifuge tube. Replace into another centrifuge tube (if necessary). Add more 10% formalin to bring up to 10 ml again, and 3 ml of ether or ethyl acetate (or even petroleum, if the others are unavailable). Ether is very volatile and can explode in the refrigerator so great care is needed. The tube is then stoppered and shaken vigorously for at least 30 s. It is then centrifuged at 300–500 r.p.m. for 1–3 min until there are four layers: a top layer of ether or ethyl acetate, a second layer consisting of a fatty deposit, a third layer of formalin and a small deposit containing the eggs at the bottom. The fatty deposit at the interface of the liquids is loosened with a glass rod and the centrifuge tube quickly inverted at an angle of 45° to the ground so that the liquids run out (Fig. 127). Drops of water from a tap can be run down the glass tube while the debris is being cleaned off from the tube with the rod (the liquid from many samples can be poured into a small beaker, centrifuged and the ether recovered and used again if in short supply). Some water will run up the rod by capillary action and the deposit at the bottom of the tube is shaken and an aliquot removed with a Pasteur pipette when the tube is upright and placed on a microscope slide, covered with a large coverslip and examined using a ×10 objective. If there is no tap handy, the debris at the interface can be loosened with an applicator stick and the contents of the tube carefully poured away, allowing one or two drops to return to the bottom. For protozoal cysts, a drop of 1% Lugol's iodine, or Sergeaunt's stain for amoebae, can be added and the sample examined under a higher power.

Zinc sulphate centrifugal flotation method

This method is not suitable for trematode or *Diphyllobothrium* eggs, as they become very distorted.

1. A faecal suspension is made by emulsifying 5–10 g of faeces with about ten times

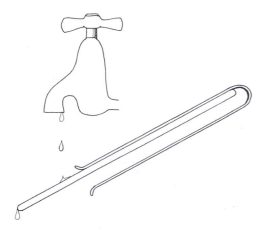

Fig. 127. Running supernatant off down a glass rod, leaving sediment behind at bottom of centrifuge tube (a conical tube is often used).

its volume of tap water, using a pestle and mortar.
2. About 10 ml is strained through a gauze or sieve (350 µm pore size) into a round-bottomed centrifuge tube.
3. After centrifugation for 1 min the supernatant is discarded and 2–3 ml of water added. After breaking up the deposit by tapping the bottom of the tube, more water is added to fill the tube.
4. The previous step is repeated until the supernatant is clear.
5. The last supernatant is poured off and 2–3 ml of 33% zinc sulphate (or saturated salt solution) added. The sediment is broken up by tapping the tube and then this is filled with more of the zinc sulphate solution.
6. The tube is centrifuged rapidly for 1 min and brought to a stop.
7. A loopful of the material floating on the surface is taken up and placed on a slide for examination. The loop should be about 6 mm in diameter and of wire that is stiff enough not to bend in routine handling. The loop is bent at right angles to the wire and must not be dipped below the surface of the liquid.

Quantitative techniques in faecal examinations

For the schistosomes and most of the intestinal nematodes, figures have been given of the average egg production per female per 24 h. Thus, in theory at least, by estimating the number of eggs in the faeces, a measure of the number of adults present can be obtained. An estimate of the number of worms present can be of importance in determining the success of chemotherapy and in epidemiological studies. The most commonly used quantitative egg-counting techniques are given below.

Kato–Katz and formol–ether techniques

Kato–Katz can detect as few as 100 eggs g^{-1} of faeces and is now regarded as the standard. As is true for all such methods, it assumes that eggs are randomly dispersed in the faeces, which appears to be true in most cases; allowance could be made for the state of the faeces, as shown below for the Stoll method, but this is not usually done. The formol–ether method can be used as a semi-quantitative estimate and has the advantage that it is quick, many samples being treated simultaneously, and that it also picks up protozoal cysts. The faecal sample size should be 0.2 g and all the deposit counted (or a specified number of drops of the total in the pipette). Fig. 128 shows good correlation between the two techniques.

The Stoll dilution egg-counting technique

The method was originally devised in 1926 for the study of hookworm infection and is still one of the best available today.

However, it is not suitable for less than about 200 eggs g^{-1} of faeces.

1. Add 0.1 N sodium hydroxide solution up to the 56 ml mark in a Stoll diluting flask. The diluting flask is made from a Ehrlenmeyer flask with a neck of 20 mm diameter glass tube fused on the top and graduated at 56 and 60 ml (Fig. 129). They are closed with a rubber stopper.
2. Faeces is carefully added with an applicator stick until the meniscus has been displaced to the 60 ml mark. For greater accuracy 4 g of faeces can be weighed out.
3. A few glass beads are added, a rubber stopper inserted and the flask well shaken. It is set aside for several hours preferably overnight, and then shaken again to thoroughly comminute the specimen.

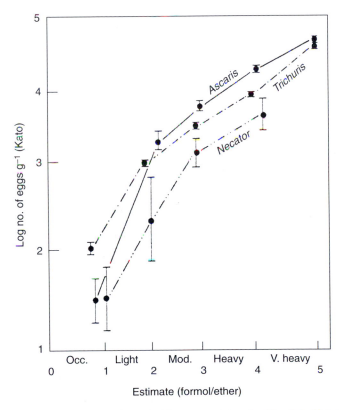

Fig. 128. Comparison of eggs per gram (e.p.g.) of faeces as determined by Kato–Katz technique and estimate by formol–ether method on the same 40 faecal samples (occasional = 1–500 e.p.g.; light = 501–2500; moderate = 2501–10,000; heavy = 10,001–20,000; very heavy = 20,000 +). The good correlation shows that a quick approximate procedure is likely to be satisfactory in many surveys.

4. The flask is shaken well to resuspend the specimen and 0.075 ml removed with a wide-bore Pasteur pipette graduated at this level. This must be done with one squeeze of the bulb to prevent loss of eggs.

5. The drop is expelled on to a microscope slide and covered with a 22 mm × 40 mm coverslip. All the eggs in the preparation are counted, using a low-powered objective. It is desirable to count several drops to obtain an average count from each specimen.

6. The stool samples can be classified as formed (F), soft formed (SF), mushy (M) or diarrhoeic (D) and the egg counts multiplied by the following factors – SF × $1\frac{1}{2}$, M × 2 and D × 3 – to compensate for the amount of fluid in these types of specimen. The results are multiplied by 200 for expression as eggs per gram. Also 24 h faecal samples can be weighed and the total output per 24 h obtained.

McMaster counting chamber

The chamber is commercially available and consists of two glass slides kept 1.5 mm apart by glass bridges at the ends and in the centre. A 1 cm² square is ruled on the underside of the top slide of the two chambers. The volume beneath each ruled area is therefore 0.15 cm³. It is used principally in veterinary studies and is not suitable for heavy eggs such as those of *Fasciola*.

1. 2 g of the well-mixed faecal sample is weighed out and placed in a glass jar containing a few glass beads. Alternatively, a pestle and mortar can be used to mix the faeces.

2. 58 ml of a saturated salt solution (or a 40% sugar solution or a 33% salt solution) is added and the faeces mixed to form a smooth emulsion.

3. The suspension is passed through a 400 µm metal or plastic sieve or gauze and a sample removed with a wide-bore Pasteur pipette.

4. The suspension is run into the counting chamber, which is then set aside for 1–2 min to allow the eggs to float to the surface.

5. The eggs come to rest against the undersurface of the top slide and are in the same focal plane as the two ruled areas. They are counted using a low-power objective.

Macdonald pipette

This is an extremely rapid and simple field procedure provided there is a glass-blower who can make lots of the special pipettes (Fig. 130).

Five grams of faeces are weighed out and 45 ml of tap water measured out. The faeces is mixed with some of the water in a pestle and mortar, transferred to a closable jar and washed out with more water. The total volume is made up to 45 ml, the jar closed and shaken vigorously and 0.1 ml samples are withdrawn using a Macdonald pipette and examined on a microscope slide under low power. The mean figure is multiplied by 100 to give eggs per gram. With freshly passed faeces the pestle and mortar can be replaced by shaking with 45 ml of water and some glass beads.

Diagnosis of Larvae in Human Faeces by Culturing to the Infective Stage

It is necessary to culture larvae to the infective third stage before a differential diagno-

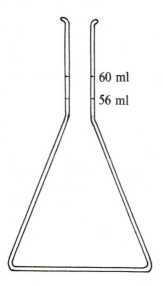

Fig. 129. Stoll flask.

60 ml

56 ml

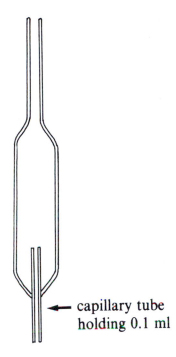

← capillary tube
holding 0.1 ml

Fig. 130. Macdonald pipette.

sis of hookworm species (and possibly *Oesophagostomum*, *Ternidens* and *Trichostrongylus* in some areas) can be made. A simple method of accomplishing this is the Harada–Mori test-tube filter-paper method.

1. Test tubes are filled with 7 ml of distilled water and placed in a rack.
2. About 0.5 g of the fresh faecal sample is smeared along the length of a strip of filter-paper (15 cm × 1.5 cm) creased longitudinally, leaving 5 cm clear at one end. The strip is placed in the test-tube with the unsmeared portion reaching to the bottom of the tube.
3. The top of each is covered with a cellophane strip, held in place by a rubber band and the rack of tubes incubated at 28°C for 10 days.
4. The top and filter-paper are removed with forceps and both destroyed (use caution in handling as the larvae are now infective).
5. The larvae will be in the water at the bottom of the tube and can be seen with the aid of a magnifying glass.

6. The tube can be placed in water at 50°C for about 15 min in order to kill the larvae without distorting them.
7. When cool, the tubes are shaken and the contents transferred to a centrifuge tube, which is spun gently for 2 min.
8. The supernatant is pipetted off and the sediment examined on a microscope slide, using a coverslip.

Alternative methods for *Strongyloides* larvae are given on p. 121 and the differential features used in identification are shown in Table 9 (p. 131).

Methods in Filariasis

Staining of microfilariae

Wet preparations made from a drop of blood under a coverslip can first be examined for the presence of microfilariae under the microscope and are easily seen moving under the low power (×100 magnification). This method avoids the lengthy process of staining negative material, but many light infections will be missed.

Method A: Giemsa

There are various Romanowsky stains that may be used for staining blood parasites (Wright, Leishman and May-Grunwald), but Giemsa is one of the best for microfilariae.

The sheaths of *Loa loa* microfilariae never stain by this method. The sheaths of *Wuchereria* stain faintly, while those of *Brugia malayi* stain an intense pink colour.

1. A large drop of blood (20 mm^3) from a Sahli-type pipette is spread out to form a thick smear (25 mm × 7 mm) on a grease-free microscope slide by means of a needle.
2. The smear is dried overnight (be careful of cockroaches and ants in the tropics), dehaemoglobinized in distilled water for about 2 min and, when completely colourless, left to dry.
3. The smear is preserved with absolute or methyl alcohol by flushing for 30 s and allowed to dry.

4. Ten drops of concentrated Giemsa stain are added to 10 ml of distilled water (pH 7.2) and placed into a staining dish. The blood film is left in the stain for 30 min.
5. The slide is removed from the stain, flushed briefly and very gently under running water and left to dry.
6. When completely dry, the film can be mounted in a neutral mounting medium (DPX or euparol) with a cover glass.

Method B: haematoxylin

1. A thick drop made from peripheral blood is spread over an area of about 2 cm^2 on a microscope slide and allowed to dry in air, preferably overnight. (For special purposes or if it is necessary to measure microfilariae, a sequestrinated blood film can be left in a humid chamber overnight at 10°C and then left to dry. Alternatively, a thin smear can be fixed while wet in three parts of methyl alcohol to one part of glacial acetic acid.) It is important when reporting measurements of microfilariae to state the method of preparation and fixation.
2. The smear is dehaemoglobinized in tap water and again dried. It is then fixed for a few minutes in methanol or absolute alcohol (fixed smears can be stored for months).
3. When dry, the slide is stained with hot haematoxylin (Mayer, Delafield, Ehrlich or Harris). The staining time is variable, depending on the batch of stain and on the age of the film, but 10–15 min is usually sufficient.
4. The slide is rinsed in tap water and examined under the low power of a microscope. If understained, more hot haematoxylin can be applied and, if overstained, the slide can be differentiated in acid alcohol (1% hydrochloric acid in 70% alcohol). It is better to slightly overstain and then differentiate as this removes the blue background from the film.
5. The slide is blued in tap water (add drop of ammonia if not alkaline) for 15 min and allowed to dry.
6. The slide can be mounted in a neutral resin mountant.

Microfilarial counting techniques

1. For quantitative studies, 20 mm^3 of blood can be taken in a haemoglobin pipette to make a thick film, stained as above and the result expressed in microfilariae per millilitre of blood. However, this is time-consuming and a proportion of microfilariae are lost during the staining procedure.
2. One of the simplest and most sensitive methods of detecting microfilariae (down to one microfilaria 100 mm^3) is to mix a measured quantity of blood with about ten times its volume of distilled water in a simple slide counting chamber and then to examine immediately. The chamber can be made by sticking thin strips of a glass slide with an adhesive to form a rectangle on another slide at about ×30 magnification. It is difficult to identify microfilariae by this method and, if necessary, stained preparations may need to be made as well.
3. If very few microfilariae are expected, as in cases of amicrofilaraemic filariasis, 1–10 ml of blood can be filtered through a Nuclepore or Millipore membrane filter (pore size 5 μm) fitted to a hypodermic syringe by a Swinney adaptor and the membrane examined either fresh or stained as above. Using the Nuclepore membrane (General Electric Company, Pleasanton, California), sequestrinated or citrated blood is passed through the filter on a syringe, followed by 0.85% saline solution. Finally, air is passed through to partially dry the membrane, which can be examined directly under a coverslip using ×50–70 magnification, or fixed in methanol, stained in hot haematoxylin, blued, dried and a drop of chloroform added in order to make the membrane transparent before viewing. This method can detect microfilariae in a concentration 1/50 that of a thick film.
4. Knott's concentration technique has been widely used for the last 60 years but is not as sensitive as the previous techniques. In a quick modification, 1 ml of blood is lysed with 10 ml of 1% formalin in a centrifuge tube, centrifuged at 500 g for 1 min and the supernatant poured off. The sediment is then spread out on microscope slides and dried and stained as above.

5. Another modification of the Knott technique involves spinning in QBC® tubes and examining the buffy layer under fluorescent light (Bawden *et al.*, 1994).

Staining of filarial larvae in insects before dissection

1. Insects are killed and identified and placed in 80% alcohol, where they can be kept indefinitely.
2. They are taken through descending dilutions of alcohol to distilled water and are then stained for 3 days at room temperature in Mayer's acid haemalum stain.
3. Insects are removed and differentiated in distilled water for 3 days. They are then stored in glycerol until required for dissection; 100–200 mosquitoes can be stored in a McCartney bottle.
4. Insects are dissected under the stereoscopic microscope (×35 magnification) by reflected light, using fine needles. All stages of developing larvae are stained and can be easily detected.
5. Larvae should be mounted in glycerol for detailed morphological study.

Technique for mass dissection of filarial vectors and mounting of filarial larvae obtained

1. Insects are immobilized by cold or by a pyrethrum spray and then sorted into separate species. All females of one species are crushed by gently rolling with a test-tube on a glass or Perspex plate in physiological saline. This is repeated for each species separately.
2. Insects are transferred to sieves (bolting silk with a pore size of 50 μm is suitable), glued across the bottom of the top half of a cut plastic cup and suspended in a clamped glass funnel containing physiological saline. Care must be taken that there are no air bubbles below the sieve. Each sieve is left for 3 h at room temperature (the procedure can also be used for obtaining larvae for infection experiments, when a tissue culture medium should be used, with incubation at 37°C).

3. About 1 ml is run into a Syracuse watch-glass (these can be made by a glass-blower by pressing in the end of a heated test tube and cutting the end off) and examined for larvae under a stereoscopic microscope.
4. Most of the saline is removed with a Pasteur pipette under the microscope and replaced by fixative. TAF (7 ml of 10% formalin, 2 ml of triethanomaine and 2 ml of distilled water) is excellent but 70% alcohol containing 10% glycerol can be used. Fixation is for 5 min.
5. Fixative is removed with a fine pipette and replaced by 96% alcohol containing 5% glycerol and the watch-glass is left in an incubator for 30 min at 37°C (or overnight at room temperature) until only pure glycerol is left. Larvae can be stained with new fast blue R or examined when mounted under phase contrast.
6. Larvae are transferred with a mounted cat's whisker to a small drop of anhydrous glycerol on a clean 22 mm square coverslip. Excess glycerol is removed with a very fine pipette, leaving only a smear.
7. The coverslip is turned over on to a cavity slide and sealed around and under the edge with mounting medium. For cheapness, three short pieces of glass wool can be used instead of using a cavity slide or a small chamber can be made.

Caution needs to be exercised when this technique is used for *Onchocerca volvulus* in *Simulium* as larvae may be of the morphologically indistinguishable *O. ochengi*.

Preservation and Examination of Adult Helminths

Before fixing, specimens should preferably be washed in 0.85% saline.

Trematodes and cestodes

For examining the various organ systems in whole mounts of these organisms, some degree of flattening is usually necessary but, as this causes distortion, material should also be fixed unflattened for subsequent sectioning. Extension of trematodes can be obtained by constant shaking and of cestodes by suspension or by winding around a test-tube, while fixing in hot 5–10% formalin.

Staining trematodes or tapeworm segments

METHOD
1. The trematode or proglottides should be flattened between glass microscope slides held at the ends with rubber bands or, for smaller specimens, with a dab of petroleum jelly at each end of the slide. They are fixed in 80% alcohol or 10% formol saline (a few drops of acetic acid added to either of these fixatives improves the staining) or Carnoy's fixative.
2. The flattened specimen is taken from between the slides when fixed and immersed in the diluted aceto alum carmine stain in a small glass dish. The staining time depends in each case on the size of the specimen – from 20–30 min for a small trematode to several hours for larger specimens.
3. Specimens are washed in 50% alcohol to remove excess stain and examined under the microscope.
4. If understained the specimen can be returned to the stain, and if overstained it can be differentiated in acid alcohol (100 ml 70% alcohol and 2 ml hydrochloric acid).
5. When stained, the specimen is washed well in water to remove acid, dehydrated in several changes of alcohol, cleared in beechwood creosote and mounted in Canada balsam or another mounting medium.

RESULT
The internal structures of the specimens are stained in precise shades of red against a clear to pink background of the connective tissues.

The above technique may be carried out using alum haematoxylin instead of the carmine. Ehrlich's haematoxylin diluted with an equal volume of water has proved satisfactory for this method.

ACETO ALUM CARMINE STAIN
Boil together:

Potassium aluminium sulphate	27 g
Carmine	17 g
Distilled water	200 g

These should be gently heated in a large flask, as the mixture is liable to froth when boiling. The mixture is boiled until the colour changes from the bright red of the carmine to a deep red colour. When cool, 20 ml of glacial acid is added. For use the stain is diluted to a rose-pink colour (1 in 5 to 1 in 10).

Nematodes

If possible, nematodes should be looked at alive and measurements made; small specimens can often be immobilized by adding a drop of propylene phenoxetol or tetramisole.

Fixation

1. Hot 70% alcohol with constant shaking. Simple and usually satisfactory.
2. Hot formol–acetic 4:1 (formalin 40% 10 ml; glacial acetic acid 1 ml; distilled water up to 100 ml) over a boiling water-bath.
3. TAF (formalin 40% 7 ml; triethanolamine 2 ml; distilled water to 100 ml). Hygroscopic so prevents drying of specimens.

Storage

Storing in 70% alcohol with 10% glycerol or pure glycerol will prevent drying up; 10% formalin is not as satisfactory, as specimens go mushy after a time.

Mounting

1. Temporary (these mounts are probably the most satisfactory).
(a) Glycerine. Worms are left overnight in a partly opened Petri dish or solid watch glass in 70% alcohol plus 10% glycerol in an oven at about 40°C, mounted in pure glycerol and returned to the bottle after examination. Specimens can be turned over for examination of all sides and examined under phase contrast.
(b) Lactophenol. Some lactophenol is added to the specimen in 70% alcohol and slowly replaced with pure lactophenol over a few hours until specimen clears (hot lactophenol

at 65°C may be used for rapid clearing). Worms are replaced in 70% alcohol after examination.

2. Permanent.

(a) Mounts are made in Canada balsam or DPX after dehydration slowly through alcohols and xylene. Specimens can be stained with haematoxylin if desired; however, the results often leave much to be desired because of distortion.

(b) Specimens are transferred to polyvinyl lactophenol from lactophenol. However, specimens go on clearing until completely transparent. Cotton blue can be dissolved in the polyvinyl lactophenol for staining.

(c) Glycerine. A tiny drop of glycerol on a coverslip with a cavity slide is used for larvae, and ringed slides for adults. Results are good but the preparations are rather fragile.

(d) Glycerine jelly. A tiny warmed drop on a coverslip is used for *en face* mounts of the anterior end on a cavity slide (Aquamount needs no heat).

Recognition of Helminths in Sections

Before a tentative diagnosis is made of possible helminth material seen in a section, it is important that the size of the specimen is considered. It is useful first to look at the slide against the light before placing it on the microscope stage; the cysticercus larva of *Taenia*, for instance, can often be recognized in this way.

The descriptions given below are based on sections stained in haematoxylin and eosin.

Trematodes

In sections of living trematodes an outer tegument, often with spines, is always present. Depending on the region of the worm cut through, one or more of the following organs should also be seen embedded in a loose ground tissue (parenchyma): vitellaria; gut caeca (usually double); ovaries; testes; suckers; uterus, probably filled with eggs. The diagram of a complete fluke (Fig.

2) should be consulted in order to understand which organs will be present in cross-sections cut at different levels (there is some variation in different species, particularly in the relative positions of the ovaries and testes).

If the organism in the tissues is dead and surrounded by a host reaction, then identification is more difficult. However, a parasite can usually be identified as a platyhelminth or nematode even if no organs are recognizable.

Cestodes

Larval cestodes in humans may be found in any tissue. The most important larvae encountered in sections are the hollow cysts of taeniid tapeworms, which include the cysticercus of *Taenia solium*, the coenurus of *Multiceps* spp. and the hydatid of *Echinococcus* spp. In sections the protoscolex (or protoscolices) will usually show clearly demarcated suckers and possibly hooks (the latter are birefringent and show up well under a polarizing microscope). The characteristic structure of each type of cyst can be seen from Fig. 32. Two solid larvae may also be found in tissues (ignoring the cysticercoid of *Hymenolepis nana*, which occurs only in the villi of the ileum): the tetrathyridium of *Meocestoides* and the sparganum (plerocercoid) of *Spirometra*. These may show few diagnostic features, but the former have many large calcareous corpuscles and perhaps suckers and the latter the circular muscles which separate the parenchyma into inner and outer zones, typical also of adult tapeworms.

Nematodes

Adults encountered in sections can usually be easily recognized as belonging to the phylum. In cross-section they are seen to have an outer acellular cuticle, enclosing a thin hypodermis layer, which often consists of longitudinal cords that separate the somatic muscles into longitudinal fields and contain the excretory canals (when present). The number and form of the muscle cells are an important feature in determining to which order a specimen belongs. The gut is separated from the outer layers by a body cavity (pseudocoel).

The characteristic structures seen in cross-sections of the various groups of nematodes are shown in Fig. 131. The most common adult nematodes recovered from the tissues are filariae; females of non-human species are usually not fertilized but have the double uterus typical of the group. A key for differentiating the larvae of *Ascaris*, *Toxocara*, *Necator*, *Ancylostoma* and *Strongyloides* in tissue sections can be made based on their relative diameters, the structure of the excretory cells and the presence or absence of lateral alae.

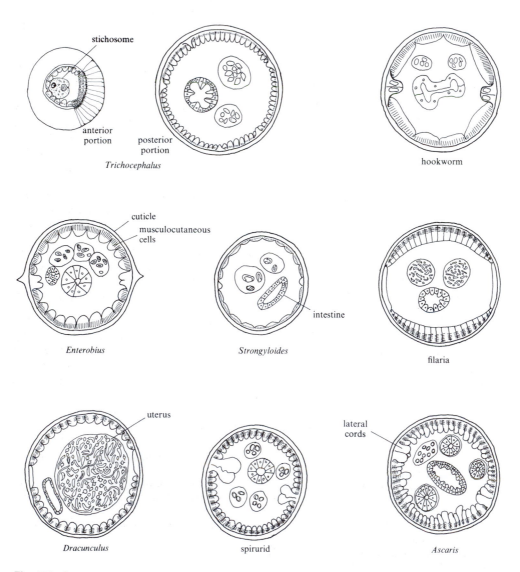

Fig. 131. Cross-sections of females belonging to the various groups of nematodes. The dorsal and ventral cords are not shown (*Trichocephalus* = *Trichuris*).

Identification Key for Sections of Nematodes

1. **A.** Hypodermal cords few to many arranged asymmetrically. Lateral excretory canals absent. In the ovaries and testes the germinal region extends the entire length of the gonad and gametes at various stages of development can be found at any level. Oesophagus non-muscular. TRICHURIDS
(*Aonchotheca, Calodium, Eucoleus, Trichinella, Trichuris*)

    B. Hypodermal cords 2–4 arranged symmetrically. Excretory canals in lateral cords except at extremities. In the ovaries and testes the germinal region confined to proximal extremity of gonad and gametes at uniform stage of development at any one level. **2**

2. **A.** Intestine composed of a few large multinucleate cells rarely with more than two cells in a cross-section. Anterior paired excretory gland cells present. STRONGYLIDS
(hookworms, trichostrongyles, *Oesophagostomum, Ternidens*)

    B. Intestine composed of few to many small uninucleate cells. Excretory glands single, paired or absent. **3**

3. **A.** Somatic muscle cells few, large and flat. Lateral alae present or absent. **4**

    B. Somatic muscle cells many, U-shaped in cross-section. Lateral alae usually absent. **5**

4. **A.** Lateral alae present. Vagina long and muscular. Oesophagus has posterior bulb. Many eggs in uterus. Excretory gland cells absent. *Enterobius*

    B. Lateral alae absent. Vagina very short. Ova large. Ovoviviparous, with eggs developing into larvae. Excretory cells single or paired. Very small and often larvae (or eggs) in tissues. *Strongyloides*

5. **A.** Somatic musculature divided by large lateral cords (often very wide and flattened) into two crescent-shaped fields. **6**

    B. Somatic musculature divided into four fields. **7**

6. **A.** Females have double uterus often containing microfilariae. Diameter less than 0.5 mm. FILARIIDS
(*Brugia, Dirofilaria, Loa, Mansonella, Wuchereria*)

    B. Females with single uterus containing larvae with long pointed tails. Diameter more than 1 mm. *Dracunculus*

7. **A.** Lateral cords very large, stalked and project into body cavity; frequently unequal in size. SPIRURUDS
(*Gnathostoma, Thelazia*)

    B. Lateral cords large and project into body cavity but not stalked; usually unequal in size . ASCARIDS
(*Anisakis, Ascaris, Toxascaris, Toxocara*)

References and Further Reading

Ash, L.R. and Orihel, T.C. (1991) *Parasites: a Guide to Laboratory Procedures and Identification.* ASCP Press, Chicago, USA.

Bawden, M., Slaten, D. and Malone, J. (1994) QBC®: rapid filaria diagnoses from blood. *Mansonella ozzardi* and *Wuchereria bancrofti. Transactions of the Royal Society of Tropical Medicine and Hygiene* 88, 66.

Cassella, J.P. and Hay, J. (1995) Tissue eosinophil and mast cell staining in helminth infections. *Parasitology Today* 11, 464–465.

Chitwood, M.B. and Lichtenfels, J.R. (1972) Identification of parasitic metazoa in tissue sections. *Journal of Parasitology* 32, 407–519.

Esterre, P., Vignes, R. and Lebbe, J. (1987) Identification assistée par ordinateur de principaux oeufs d'helminthes en coprologie humaine. *Bulletin de la Société Française de Parasitologie* 5, 241–244.

Gillespie, S.H. and Hawkey, P.M. (eds) (1995) *Medical Parasitology: a Practical Approach.* IRL Press, Oxford, UK.

Petithory, J.C. and Ardoin-Guidon, F. (1995) *Parasitologie: vrais et faux parasites en coprologie microscopique.* Cahier de Formation – Biologie Médicale no. 3. Bioforma, Paris, France.

Price, D.L. (1993) *Procedure Manual for the Diagnosis of Intestinal Parasites.* CRC Press, Boca Raton, USA.

WHO (1991) *Basic Laboratory Methods in Medical Parasitology.* World Health Organization, Geneva, Switzerland.

Appendix 1

Summary of Some Landmarks in Medical Helminthology

1500 BC	Ebers papyrus possibly described various helminth diseases.
400 BC–AD 1200	*Taenia, Ascaris, Enterobius* and *Dracunculus* described in Greek, Roman, Arabic and Chinese writings.
AD 1379	Jehan de Brie illustrated *Fasciola hepatica* from sheep.
1674	Textbook by Velschius on *Dracunculus*.
1684	Redi described many new helminths from domestic and wild animals.
1700	Textbook by Andry on human helminths.
1835	Paget discovered larval *Trichinella spiralis* in a man, which was described by Owen.
1845	Dujardin elucidated the relationship between adult and cycticercus of *Taenia saginata*.
1851	Küchenmeister, Van Beneden, etc. described the life cycle of *Taenia solium*.
1851	Adult *Schistosoma haematobium* were found in the vesical veins by Bilharz in Cairo.
1852	Life cycle of *Echinococcus granulosus* determined by Von Siebold.
1857–1898	Textbooks by Küchenmeister (1857), Davaine (1860), Cobbold (1864), Leuckart (1867) and Manson (1898).
1865	The life cycle of *Enterobius* was worked out by Leuckart.
1870	Fedchenko observed larval development of *Dracunculus* in Cyclops.
1876	Adult *Wuchereria bancrofti* found in lymph glands by Bancroft; surprisingly in Australia.
1878	Life cycle of *Wuchereria bancrofti* shown to involve mosquito by Manson.
1882–1883	Leuckart and Thomas showed that the life cycle of *Fasciola hepatica* involves a snail.
1887	*Hymenolepis nana* shown not to need an intermediate host by Grassi and Rovelli.
1896	Looss demonstrated the active penetration of hookworm larvae through the skin (by accidentally infecting himself).
1897	Eosinophilia first associated with *Trichinella spiralis* infection by Brown.
1900	*W. bancrofti* infective larvae shown to enter through the puncture wound of mosquito by Low.
1901–1913	Weinland's studies on *Ascaris* biochemistry and physiology.
1904	Adult *Schistosoma japonicum* found by Katsurada.
1907	*Schistosoma mansoni* differentiated from *S. haematobium* by Sambon.
1909	Rockefeller Sanitary Commision established to combat hookworm disease.
1911	An intradermal test for the diagnosis of hydatid disease described by Casoni.

1912	Complement fixation test used for diagnosis of *Trichinella*.
1911–1919	Role of snail and fish in the transmission of *Clonorchis* and of snail and crab in that of *Paragonimus* determined in Japan.
1913	Life cycle of *S. japonicum* involving snail discovered by Miyagawa.
1914–1921	Life cycle of *Loa loa* involving *Chrysops* shown by Leiper, Kleine and Connal.
1915	Leiper elucidated the life cycle of *S. haematobium*.
1918	Connection between blindness and onchocerciasis recognized by Pacheco-Luna and Robles in Guatemala.
	Antimony tartrate advocated for treatment of schistosomiasis by Cristopherson.
1918	Life cycle of *Diphyllobothrium latum* determined by Rosen and Janicki.
1920	Chandler suggested copper sulphate for the control of snail intermediate hosts of trematodes.
1921	Migration of *Ascaris* larvae through body discovered by Koino and Koino. Life cycle of *Fasciolopsis buski* worked out by Nagagawa.
1926	The vector of *Onchocerca volvulus* shown to be *Simulium* by Blacklock.
1927	Brug found microfilariae of *Brugia malayi* in blood.
1928	Stoll described 'self-cure' phenomenon in gastrointestinal nematodes of domestic stock.
1929	Faust's *Human Helminthology* published.
1930s–1950s	Work of Culbertson, Taliaferro, Vogel and Minning on mechanisms of immunity to helminth infections.
1932	Löffler described pulmonary lesions and eosinophilia due to larval migration of *Ascaris*.
1934	Development of *Mansonella* in *Culicoides* shown by Buckley.
1947	Diethylcarbamazine (DEC) first used in treatment of filariasis.
1951	Piperazine used for treatment of *Ascaris* and *Enterobius*.
	Role of *Angiostrongylus cantonensis* in causation of eosinophilic meningitis elucidated by Alicata and by Rosen and coworkers.
1952	Importance of *Toxocara* larvae in visceral larva migrans shown by Beaver.
1954	Onchocerciasis eradicated from Kenya by McMahon.
	Increasing use of new synthetic insecticides (chlorinated hydrocarbons and organophosphates) in control of filariasis.
	Discovery of new synthetic molluscicides for the control of schistosomiasis.
1956	Work by Buckley and Edeson on tropical pulmonary eosinophilia and zoonotic aspects of *Brugia* infection (genus *Brugia* erected by Buckley in 1959).
1964	Discovery of intestinal capillariasis in the Philippines.
1971	Discovery of abdominal capillariasis in Costa Rica.

For a much fuller account the book by Grove (1990) (see p. 284) should be consulted.

It is not always easy to assess the importance of recent work but some of the most notable advances in medical helminthology have been in the fields of immunity, immunodiagnosis and immunopathology, the search for human vaccines, the action of broad-action anthelminthics, such as praziquantel, the benzimidazoles and ivermectin, the importance of strain differences in many human helminths, such as *Echinococcus*, *Trichinella* and *Onchocerca*, the epidemiology and medical importance of soil-transmitted nematodes, molecular biology, including the sequencing of the complete genome of the free-living nematode *Caenorhabditis elegans*, and the global control campaigns, whether under way or envisaged, for onchocerciasis, dracunculiasis, lymphatic filariasis, schistosomiasis and geohelminths.

Appendix 2
Glossary of Helminthological Terms

These terms should be regarded as explanations rather than as strict definitions and do not necessarily apply to all other helminths not found in humans.

aberrant parasite A parasite that is never transmitted between humans and which develops abnormally in humans (e.g. *Echinococcus multilocularis, Parastrongylus, Toxocara*).

accidental parasite One that is not usually transmitted between humans but which develops in a similar manner to that in its normal host (e.g. *Fasciola, Dipylidium, Taenia solium* cysticerci, *Trichinella*).

aggregation See **overdispersal**.

alae ('wings') Extensions of the cuticle of nematodes (e.g. in *Enterobius*); sometimes present only at the head (cervical alae, e.g. *Toxocara*) or tail end (caudal alae, e.g. male *Dirofilaria*).

amphid One of a pair of receptors situated at the anterior end of nematodes.

anthelminthic Any chemotherapeutic substance directed against a helminthic infection.

antibody An immunoglobulin molecule that recognizes a specific antigen.

antigen A molecule that is foreign to the body and is recognized. Because of the large size of helminths in relation to invading microorganisms, most functional antigens of helminths are excretory or secretory. The tegument of Platyhelminthes is also a site for attack by host defences, but the tough cuticle of nematodes is largely resistant.

autoinfection Reinfection without exposure from the environment; self-infection

(e.g. *Strongyloides, Aonchotheca* and *Hymenolepis nana*).

carrier A host that harbours a particular pathogen without manifestations of disease.

caudal bursa (= bursa copulatrix) Umbrella-like expansion of the caudal end of the male in strongylid nematodes, used to clasp the female when mating.

cercaria The free-living larva, usually possessing a tail, which escapes from a sporocyst or redia generation of a trematode within the snail host, and constitutes the transfer stage to the next (usually definitive) host.

cirrus Retractile muscular organ at the terminal end of the male reproductive system of Platyhelminthes, which serves as a penis during fertilization.

coenurus Larval cystic stage of the tapeworm *Multiceps*, containing an inner germinal layer producing multiple scolices within a single fluid-filled cavity (see **cysticercus** and **hydatid cyst**).

commensal A symbiotic relationship in which one individual gains without having beneficial or detrimental effects on its partner.

concomitant immunity A state of immunity that prevents establishment of a new infection but is ineffective against any existing parasites that may be present (e.g. as in schistosomiasis).

control Attack on an infection so that it will no longer be clinically or economically important (e.g. projected global campaigns against lymphatic filariasis or schistosomiasis plus intestinal helminths. See **elimination** or **eradication**).

cuticle The outer chitinous body layer of nematodes (see **tegument**).

cysticercoid The solid second larval stage of tapeworms containing an invaginated scolex. Usually tailed and found in invertebrates (e.g. *Dipylidium* and *Hymenolepis*).

cysticercus (= bladderworm) The hollow fluid-filled second larval stage of *Taenia*, containing a single invaginated scolex (see **coenurus**, **hydatid cyst** and **metacestode**).

digenetic Three or more generations (literally two) required for completion of one life cycle, as in digenetic trematodes.

dioecious Having female and male reproductive organs in different individuals (e.g. schistosomes and nematodes).

domestic cycle (= pastoral or synanthropic cycle) Life cycle of a zoonotic parasite involving domestic stock or pets, with a high risk of infecting humans (e.g. usually in *Echinococcus granulosus* and *Trichinella spiralis*).

ectoparasite Living upon or in the superficial tissues of a host.

ectopic site Outside the normal location, as in the position of a parasite that lodges in an atypical part of the body.

egg count A quantitative measure of the number of eggs present in the faeces, usually expressed as eggs per gram, in order to estimate the number of adults present.

ejaculatory duct The muscular terminus of the male genitalia of nematodes, opening into the cloaca.

elimination Campaign resulting in the complete absence of an infection in a country or region (e.g. *Dracunculus* in Asia). Can also refer to absence of disease rather than of the causative parasite (e.g. intention of global elimination of lymphatic filariasis campaign). (See **control** and **eradication**.)

embryo The stage in development following cleavage of the zygote up to, but not including, the first larval stage.

embryophore In tapeworms, the envelope immediately around the oncosphere and derived from it. In taeniids it forms a thick protective layer composed of a keratin type of protein.

endoparasite Living within another organism, including the digestive and respiratory tract of the latter.

eradication Complete elimination of a helminth infection throughout the world (e.g. hopefully *Dracunculus* soon. (See **control** and **elimination**.)

evasion of the immune response Mechanisms by which helminths avoid the immune response of the host either by occupying a privileged site or by covering themselves with host or host-like antigens (e.g. schistosomes).

feral cycle (= sylvatic cycle) Life cycle of a zoonotic parasite involving wild animals and having a low risk of infecting humans (except hunters) (e.g. *Echinococcus multilocularis*) (see **domestic cycle**).

filariform larva A non-feeding nematode larva characterized by its delicate elongate structure and by its slim, capillary oesophagus without a posterior bulb (e.g. in hookworms, *Strongyloides* and filariae).

flame cell See **solenocyte**.

furcocercous cercaria Fork-tailed, as in the cercaria of schistosomes.

genital atrium In Platyhelminthes, the chamber collecting the terminal ends of the genital tubules and opening to the exterior by the genital pore.

geohelminth A term applied to any nematode that is transmitted to humans after development in the soil (e.g. *Strongyloides*, hookworms, *Ascaris* and *Trichuris*).

gonotyl Genital sucker, retractile and associated with or incorporated into the ventral sucker, in some genera of trematodes (e.g. *Heterophyes*).

gravid Filled with eggs, as in the terminal proglottides of a cyclophyllidean tapeworm or *Enterobius*.

gubernaculum A small, sclerotinized, accessory structure in male nematodes, which serves to guide the spicules out of the cloaca.

gymnocephalous cercaria Literally naked-headed; refers to cercariae without ornamentation of body or tail, as in that of *Fasciola hepatica*.

gynaecophoric canal In male schistosomes, the ventral incurved fold of the body extending from the ventral sucker to the caudal extremity, for carrying the female.

hermaphroditic Containing both male and female organs in the same individual; monoecious (e.g. cestodes and trematodes except schistosomes).

heterogonic Development in which both males and females are present in a colony (see **hologonic**).

hexacanth embryo 'Six-hooked' embryo, the mature embryo containing six hooklets within the egg of many tapeworms, including all species that parasitize humans.

hologonic Development in which only one sex (usually the female) is present in a colony, as in parasitic *Strongyloides*.

host An organism that harbours and nourishes a parasite.

definitive host One that harbours the sexually mature stage of the parasite (e.g. humans are the only definitive hosts for *Taenia saginata*).

intermediate host An obligate host that alternates with the definitive host and harbours the larval stage of the parasite (e.g. snails are intermediate hosts for all human trematodes).

paratenic host A carrier or transport host. One in which the parasite remains viable but does not develop.

reservoir host An animal host in which infection usually resides; also one which harbours the infection when humans are not infected (e.g. ruminants are reservoir hosts for many *Trichostrongylus* species).

hydatid cyst Larval cystic stage of the tapeworm *Echinococcus granulosus*, containing an inner germinal layer producing many protoscolices, which when set free into the cystic cavity, develop into daughter cysts and usually have a thick laminated wall surrounded by an outer fibrous capsule of host origin (see **coenurus** and **cysticercus**).

hydatid cyst, alveolar (= multilocular) Larval cystic stage of the tapeworm *Echinococcus multilocularis* (AE), similar to the **hydatid cyst** (above) but in which budding is external (exogenous) as well as internal (endogenous), so that many small cysts are formed. There is no thick outer capsule.

hyperendemic High prevalence of infection in a human community.

hypodermis In helminths, the layer of tissue immediately below the tegument (trematodes and cestodes) or cuticle (nematodes).

immunomodulation An alteration, either negative or positive, of the immune response (see **immunosuppresion**).

immunopathology Damage to tissues caused directly or indirectly by immune mechanisms (the importance of this in helminth infections is being increasingly recognized).

immunosuppression A down-regulation of the immune response.

incidence of infection The number of new cases of an infection reported in an area in a unit of time (taken to be a year if not given) (see **prevalence of infection**).

infestation Existence of parasitic organisms on the outside of the body of a host or in the superficial tissues; ectoparasitism (e.g. lice and fleas).

intensity of infection Number of parasites harboured by a host. The mean intensity is calculated for the whole host population (including those uninfected).

larva The postembryonic stage of a helminth, in which internal organs are developing or are developed and are at least partially functional.

Laurer's canal In trematodes, a tubule leading from the dorsal surface to the region of the ootype and seminal receptacle; it may be patent, vestigial or lacking. It probably functions as a copulatory canal.

LD_{50} (= lethal dose 50) and LC_{50} (= lethal concentration 50). The dose or concentration of a chemotherapeutic, insecticidal or molluscicidal agent estimated statistically to kill 50% of the helminths, insects or snails being treated (also LD_{90} and LC_{90}).

Mehlis' glands In Platyhelminthes, the glands surrounding the ootype. They produce mucus to lubricate the uterus and probably participate in eggshell formation.

metacercaria The stage of trematodes following the cercaria, with loss of tail, which becomes encysted and awaits passive transfer to the definitive host (present in all trematodes of humans except schistosomes).

metacestode A collective term for any of the various larval stages of cestodes which are found in the intermediate host (e.g. oncosphere, procercoid, plerocercoid, tetrathyridium, cysticercus, cysticercoid, coenurus, hydatid).

microcercous cercaria Cercaria with a short, stumpy tail (e.g. cercaria of *Paragonimus westermani*).

microfilaria The first prelarval stage of a filaria, which either escapes from the eggshell (i.e. is unsheathed) or stretches the shell into an elongated sac (i.e. is sheathed) and is found in the blood or skin.

miracidium The ciliated free-living first-stage larva hatched from the eggs of trematodes.

nosogeography Knowledge concerning the geographical distribution of diseases.

oncosphere The stage that hatches from the eggshell and later escapes from the embryophore of tapeworms; in human tapeworm infections it is six-hooked (i.e. a hexacanth embryo).

ootype The chamber in the reproductive system of Platyhelminthes where the several components of the eggs are assembled.

ovejector A muscular organ in some female nematodes that forces eggs from the uterus into the vagina.

overdispersal Situation where most hosts harbour a few parasites while a few hosts harbour many parasites. Gives a negative binomial distribution.

oviparous Producing and laying eggs (see **ovoviviparous**).

ovoviviparous Discharging living young rather than eggs (e.g. *Dracunculus*, filariae, *Strongyloides* and *Trichinella*) (see **oviparous**).

papillae Small sensory knobs, either at the anterior end (dierids) or at the posterior end in the male, where their number and position may be of taxonomic importance.

parasite An organism that lives at the expense of another larger organism, its host; which is physiologically dependent on its host, has a higher reproductive capacity than it and may kill the host in heavy infections.

   facultative One that may employ either a free-living or a parasitic mode of life. e.g. *Strongyloides*.

obligate One that necessarily lives a parasitic existence, e.g. all the other human helminths.

parasitocoenosis (= parasite mix) The assemblage of parasites associated with a host population.

parenchyma In Platyhelminthes, the loose, usually undifferentiated tissue that forms a matrix in which the viscera are embedded.

parthenogenesis Production of progeny from the ovum without fertilization (e.g. parasitic female of *Strongyloides*).

pastoral cycle See **domestic cycle**.

patent infection Open or apparent, as indicated by unmistakable signs, like eggs in the faeces or microfilariae in circulating blood (see **prepatent period**).

pathogen A parasite causing injury to a host (see **commensal** and **parasite**).

phasmid One of a pair of caudal organelles (sensory receptors?) found in most parasitic nematodes (i.e. the Phasmidia), including all those in humans except *Aonchotheca*, *Dioctophyma*, *Trichinella* and *Trichuris*.

pipestem fibrosis (Symmer's) A fibrotic reaction formed around a vein in schistosomiasis, so called because of its resemblance in section to the stem of an old-fashioned clay pipe.

plerocercoid larva A second larval stage of pseudophyllid tapeworms in which the scolex is embedded in a greatly enlarged tail (e.g. larva of *Dyphyllobothrium latum*) (see **sparganum** and **procercoid larva**).

prepatent period The period that a parasite is present in the body before it gives rise to parasitological evidence of its presence (e.g. eggs in the faeces or microfilariae in the blood).

prevalence of infection The number of cases of an infection present in an area (actually per unit of population) at a fixed point in time. Prevalence = incidence × average duration (see **incidence of infection**).

proboscis In acanthocephalans and in the dog tapeworm *Dipylidium caninum* an anterior protrusible organ, typically studded with hooklets.

procercoid larva The first larval stage of pseudophyllidean tapeworms, which develops from the oncosphere; it consists of a body proper and a caudal vestige of the oncosphere containing the hooklets called a cercomer (see **plerocercoid larva**).

proglottid One complete unit of a tapeworm, commonly called a segment. In cyclophyllideans the most anterior are immature; further back they are mature, containing the male and female sex organs; and the posterior proglottides are gravid, being filled with eggs.

pseudocoel Body cavity of nematodes, not lined completely with mesothelium and not equivalent to a coelomic cavity.

pseudotubercle A foreign-body reaction resembling a tubercle but not provoked by tubercle bacilli (e.g. by schistosome eggs).

refractory host One that is not readily infectible by a particular parasite (see **susceptible host**).

retrofection A variety of autoinfection in which larvae hatch from eggs in the anal region, migrate up the large bowel and develop into adults (e.g. *Enterobius*).

rhabditiform larva A feeding first-stage nematode larva (of strongylids and *Strongyloides*) in which the oesophagus is functional, is usually muscular and has an enlarged posterior bulb.

rostellum The somewhat protuberant apical portion of the scolex of certain tapeworms, frequently bearing a circle of hooklets, as in *Taenia solium*.

schistosomulum Immature stage of schistosomes, from the time of entry into the definitive host until the worm reaches sexual maturity.

scolex Attachment end of a tapeworm, commonly referred to as the anterior end or holdfast, which often bears suckers and hooks.

seminal receptacle (= *Receptaculum seminis*) The storage reservoir for spermatozoa in the female.

seminal vesicle (= *Vesicula seminalis*) The storage reservoir for spermatozoa in the male.

sensitivity (of diagnostic procedure) The probability that the procedure will diagnose a real positive reaction.

sign Objective evidence of disease (see **symptom**).

solenocyte Literally canal cell. In Platyhelminthes, the cell with a tuft of cilia at the head of each capillary in the excretory system; commonly called a flame cell.

sparganum The second plerocercoid larval stage of the pseudophyllidean tapeworm *Spirometra*, which occurs in mammals (particularly when in humans), characterized by its elongated shape and lack of a cystic cavity.

specificity (of an immunodiagnostic test) The probability that a real negative host is recognized by the test to be negative (i.e. number of real negatives divided by number of real negatives plus number of false positives).

spicules (copulatory) Two (or sometimes, in aphasmids, one) bristle-like, lanceolate sclerotinized structures in the outer genital chamber of male nematodes, introduced into the vulva or vagina of the female during copulation to guide the sperm.

strobilization The production of proglottides from the neck region of tapeworms.

superinfection New infection superimposed on an existing one of the same species.

susceptible host A host that is readily infected by a particular parasite (see **refractory host**).

sylvatic cycle See **feral cycle**.

symbiosis State of two organisms living together for mutual advantage, the relationships being so intimate that the participating species rely on one another for their existence. Mutualism is similar but the two organisms can live apart.

symptom Any subjective evidence of disease in a patient (see **sign**).

tegument The outer layer of the body wall of helminths.

tetrathyridium In the tapeworm genus *Mesocestoides*, the second larval stage, in which the scolex with its four suckers is invaginated into the anterior end of a plerocercoid type of body.

uterus The tubule in helminths containing the fully formed eggs before they are voided.

vagina An outer chamber of the female genitalia in nematodes; also the tubule leading from the genital atrium to the ootype in cestodes (see **vulva**).

vas deferens The common male duct arising from one or more vasa efferentia and leading into the seminal vesicle.

vas efferens The male duct conveying spermatozoa from the testis to the vas deferens.

vector An intermediate host that carries the parasite to the definitive host.

  biological vector A host essential to the development and transmission of a parasite, in which the parasite undergoes development (e.g. insects and filariae).

  mechanical vector A non-essential disseminator of parasites, in which the parasite does not develop (e.g. flies sometimes carrying the eggs of *Taenia* or *Ascaris*).

vermicide Therapeutic agent producing the death of a helminth (see **anthelminthic**).

vermifuge Therapeutic agent producing evacuation of a helminth from the intestine without necessarily causing its death (e.g. the action of piperazine against *Ascaris* and *Enterobius*).

vitellaria (= vitelline glands) The glands in Platyhelminthes which produce yolk material and the shell of the egg.

vulva The outermost, unpaired chamber of the female genitalia in nematodes.

worm burden The number of worms present in the host (this is often estimated from the **egg count**).

xiphidiocercaria Cercaria with a stylet, median dorsal in position in the oral sucker; having associated penetration glands with duct openings on either side of the stylet (as in *Paragonimus*).

zoonosis Infection or disease naturally transmitted between humans and other vertebrates.

zooprophylaxis The prevention or amelioration of disease in humans by prior exposure to a heterologous infection of animals.

Appendix 3
Location of Helminths in the Human Body

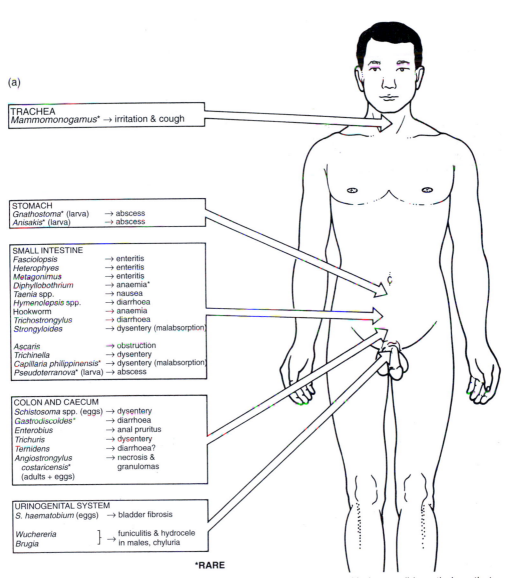

(a)

TRACHEA
*Mammomonogamus** → irritation & cough

STOMACH
*Gnathostoma** (larva)   → abscess
*Anisakis** (larva)   → abscess

SMALL INTESTINE
Fasciolopsis	→ enteritis
Heterophyes	→ enteritis
Metagonimus	→ enteritis
Diphyllobothrium	→ anaemia*
Taenia spp.	→ nausea
Hymenolepsis spp.	→ diarrhoea
Hookworm	→ anaemia
Trichostrongylus	→ diarrhoea
Strongyloides	→ dysentery (malabsorption)
Ascaris	→ obstruction
Trichinella	→ dysentery
*Capillaria philippinensis**	→ dysentery (malabsorption)
*Pseudoterranova** (larva)	→ abscess

COLON AND CAECUM
Schistosoma spp. (eggs)	→ dysentery
*Gastrodiscoides**	→ diarrhoea
Enterobius	→ anal pruritus
Trichuris	→ dysentery
Ternidens	→ diarrhoea?
*Angiostrongylus costaricensis** (adults + eggs)	→ necrosis & granulomas

URINOGENITAL SYSTEM
S. haematobium (eggs) → bladder fibrosis

Wuchereria ⎤
Brugia   ⎦ → funiculitis & hydrocele in males, chyluria

*RARE

Fig. 132. Location in the human body of helminths and other metazoa with the possible pathology that may result. Organs through which a parasite passes without causing any pathology are ignored. Not included: *Oesophagostomum bifurcum* in the colon and caecum causing nodules. (Name changes: *Angiostrongylus* = *Parastrongylus*; *Capillaria philippinensis* = *Aonchotheca philippinensis*; *Capillaria hepatica* = *Calodium hepaticum*.) (After Muller and Baker, 1990.)

(b)

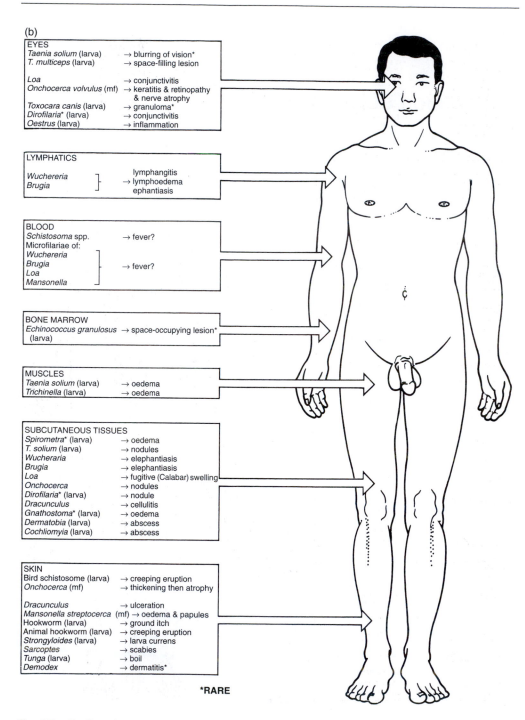

EYES
Taenia solium (larva)	→ blurring of vision*
T. multiceps (larva)	→ space-filling lesion
Loa	→ conjunctivitis
Onchocerca volvulus (mf)	→ keratitis & retinopathy & nerve atrophy
Toxocara canis (larva)	→ granuloma*
*Dirofilaria** (larva)	→ conjunctivitis
Oestrus (larva)	→ inflammation

LYMPHATICS
Wuchereria	lymphangitis
Brugia	→ lymphoedema ephantiasis

BLOOD
Schistosoma spp.	→ fever?
Microfilariae of:	
Wuchereria	
Brugia	→ fever?
Loa	
Mansonella	

BONE MARROW
Echinococcus granulosus (larva)	→ space-occupying lesion*

MUSCLES
Taenia solium (larva)	→ oedema
Trichinella (larva)	→ oedema

SUBCUTANEOUS TISSUES
*Spirometra** (larva)	→ oedema
T. solium (larva)	→ nodules
Wucheraria	→ elephantiasis
Brugia	→ elephantiasis
Loa	→ fugitive (Calabar) swelling
Onchocerca	→ nodules
*Dirofilaria** (larva)	→ nodule
Dracunculus	→ cellulitis
*Gnathostoma** (larva)	→ oedema
Dermatobia (larva)	→ abscess
Cochliomyia (larva)	→ abscess

SKIN
Bird schistosome (larva)	→ creeping eruption
Onchocerca (mf)	→ thickening then atrophy
Dracunculus	→ ulceration
Mansonella streptocerca (mf)	→ oedema & papules
Hookworm (larva)	→ ground itch
Animal hookworm (larva)	→ creeping eruption
Strongyloides (larva)	→ larva currens
Sarcoptes	→ scabies
Tunga (larva)	→ boil
Demodex	→ dermatitis*

*****RARE**

Fig. 132. *Continued.*

(c)

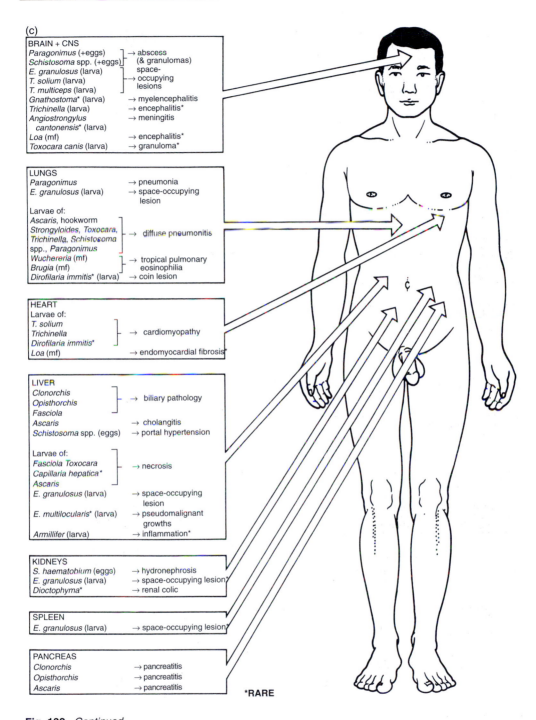

BRAIN + CNS
Paragonimus (+eggs)   ⎤ → abscess
Schistosoma spp. (+eggs) ⎦   (& granulomas)
E. granulosus (larva)   ⎤ space-
T. solium (larva)   ⎬→ occupying
T. multiceps (larva)   ⎦ lesions
*Gnathostoma** (larva)   → myelencephalitis
Trichinella (larva)   → encephalitis*
Angiostrongylus   → meningitis
   *cantonensis** (larva)
Loa (mf)   → encephalitis*
Toxocara canis (larva)   → granuloma*

LUNGS
Paragonimus   → pneumonia
E. granulosus (larva)   → space-occupying
   lesion
Larvae of:
Ascaris, hookworm   ⎤
Strongyloides, Toxocara,   ⎬→ diffuse pneumonitis
Trichinella, Schistosoma   ⎦
spp., *Paragonimus*
Wuchereria (mf)   ⎤→ tropical pulmonary
Brugia (mf)   ⎦ eosinophilia
*Dirofilaria immitis** (larva)   → coin lesion

HEART
Larvae of:
T. solium   ⎤
Trichinella   ⎬→ cardiomyopathy
*Dirofilaria immitis**   ⎦
Loa (mf)   → endomyocardial fibrosis*

LIVER
Clonorchis   ⎤
Opisthorchis   ⎬→ biliary pathology
Fasciola   ⎦
Ascaris   → cholangitis
Schistosoma spp. (eggs)   → portal hypertension

Larvae of:
Fasciola Toxocara   ⎤
*Capillaria hepatica**   ⎬→ necrosis
Ascaris   ⎦
E. granulosus (larva)   → space-occupying
   lesion
*E. multilocularis** (larva)   → pseudomalignant
   growths
Armillifer (larva)   → inflammation*

KIDNEYS
S. haematobium (eggs)   → hydronephrosis
E. granulosus (larva)   → space-occupying lesion
*Dioctophyma**   → renal colic

SPLEEN
E. granulosus (larva)   → space-occupying lesion

PANCREAS
Clonorchis   → pancreatitis
Opisthorchis   → pancreatitis
Ascaris   → pancreatitis

*RARE

Fig. 132. *Continued.*

General References and Further Reading

Abdi, Y.A. (1994) *Handbook of Drugs for Tropical Parasitic Diseases*, 2nd edn. Taylor and Francis, London, UK.

Ash, L.R. and Orihel, T.C. (1990) *Atlas of Human Parasitology*. American Society of Clinical Pathologists, Chicago, USA.

Ashford, R.W. and Crewe, W. (1998) *The Parasites of* Homo sapiens. Liverpool School of Tropical Medicine, Liverpool, UK.

Barnard, C.J. and Behnke, J.M. (eds) (1990) *Parasitism and Host Behaviour*. Taylor and Francis, London, UK.

Bennet, E.-M., Behm, C. and Bryant, C. (eds) (1989) *Comparative Biochemistry of Parasitic Helminths*. Chapman and Hall, London, UK.

Bogitsch, B.J. and Cheng, T.C. (1998) *Human Parasitology*, 2nd edn. Academic Press, San Diego, USA.

Boothroyd, J.C. and Komuniecki, R. (1995) *Molecular Approaches to Parasitology*. Willey-Liss, New York, USA.

Brooker, S. and Michael, E. (2000) The potential of geographical information systems (GIS) and remote sensing in the epidemiology and control of human helminth infections. *Advances in Parasitology* 47, 246–288.

Bryant, C. and Behm, C. (1989) *Biochemical Adaptation in Parasites*. Chapman and Hall, London, UK.

Campbell, W.C. and Rew, R.S. (1986) *Chemotherapy of Parasitic Diseases*. Plenum, New York, USA.

Chowdhury, N. and Tada, I. (eds) (1994) *Helminthology*. Springer-Verlag, Berlin, Germany.

Combes, C. (1995) *Interactions durables: Écologie et évolution du parasitisme*. Masson, Paris, France.

Cook, G.C. (1990) *Parasitic Disease in Clinical Practice*. Springer-Verlag, Berlin, Germany.

Cook, G.C. (ed.) (1996) *Manson's Tropical Diseases*. Saunders, London, UK.

Coombs, I. and Crompton, D.W.T. (1991) *A Guide to Human Helminths*. Taylor and Francis, London, UK.

Cox, F.E.G., Kreier, J.P. and Wakelin, D. (eds) (1998) *Topley and Wilson's Microbiology and Microbial Infections*. Vol. 5 *Parasitology*, 9th edn. Arnold, London, UK.

Dailey, M.D. (1996) *Meyer, Olsen and Schmidt's Essentials of Parasitology*, 6th edn. Brown, Dubuque, Iowa, USA.

Despommier, D.D., Gwadz, R.W. and Hotez, P.J. (1994) *Parasitic Diseases*, 3rd edn. Springer-Verlag, New York, USA.

Esch, G.W. and Fernández, J.C. (1993) *A Functional Biology of Parasitism: Ecological and Evolutionary Implications*. Chapman and Hall, London, UK.

Euzeby, J. (1981) *Diagnostic expérimental des helminthoses animales (animaux domestiques – animaux de laboratoire – primates)*, 2 vols. Ministère de l'Agriculture, Paris, France.

Farthing, M.J.G. and Keusch, G.T. (eds) (1995) *Enteric Infections 2: Intestinal Helminths*. Chapman and Hall, London, UK.

Freedman, D.O. (1997) *Immunopathogenic Aspects of Disease Induced by Helminth Parasites*. Chemical Immunology, Vol. 66, S. Karger, Basle, 236 pp.

Garcia, L.S. (1999) *Practical Guide to Diagnostic Parasitology*. American Society for Microbiology, Washington, USA.

Garcia, L.S. and Bruckner, D.A. (1997) *Diagnostic Medical Parasitology*. American Society for Microbiology, Washington, USA.

Gentilini, M. (1993) *Médecine Tropicale*. Flammarion, Paris, France.

Gillespie, S.H. and Hawkey, R.M. (1995) *Medical Parasitology: a Practical Approach*. Oxford University Press, New York, USA.

Goldsmith, R. and Heyeman, D. (1989) *Tropical Medicine and Parasitology*. Appleton and Lange, Hemel Hempstead, UK.

Gutterierrez, Y. (2000) *Diagnostic Pathology of Parasitic Infections with Clinical Correlations*, 2nd edn. Oxford University Press, New York, USA.

Hall, A. (1982) Intestinal helminths of man: the interpretation of egg counts. *Parasitology* 85, 605–613.

Halton, D.W., Behnke, J.M. and Marshall, I. (eds) (2001) *Practical Exercises in Parasitology*. Cambridge University Press, Cambridge, UK.

Hugh-Jones, M.E., Hubbert, W.T. and Hagstad, H.V. (1995) *Zoonoses: Recognition, Control and Prevention*. Iowa State University Press, Ames, USA.

Hyde, J.E. (1990) *Molecular Parasitology*. Open University, Buckingham, UK.

Hyde, J.E. (1993) *Protocols in Molecular Parasitology*. Humana Press, Totowa, New Jersey, USA.

James, D.M. and Gilles, H.M. (1985) *Human Antiparasitic Drugs: Pharmacology and Usage*. John Wiley & Sons, Chichester, UK.

Kassai, T., Cordero del Campo, M., Euzeby, J., Gaafar, S., Hiepe, Th. and Himonas, C.A. (1988) Standardized nomenclature of animal parasitic diseases (SNOAPAD). *Veterinary Parasitology* 29, 299–326.

Leventhal, R. and Cheadle, R. (1996) *Medical Parasitology: a Self-instructional Text*. Davis, Philadelphia, USA.

Littlewood, T. and Bray, R. (eds) (2001) *Interrelationships of the Platyhelminthes*. Taylor and Francis, London, UK.

Macpherson, C.N.L. and Craig, P.S. (eds) (1991) *Parasitic Helminths and Zoonoses in Africa*. Unwin Hyman, London, UK.

Maizels, R.M., Blaxter, M.L., Robertson, B.D. and Selkirk, M.E. (1991) *Parasite Antigens, Parasite Genes. A Laboratory Manual for Molecular Parasitology*. Cambridge University Press, Cambridge, UK.

Markell, E.K., John, D.T. and Krotoski, W.A. (1999) *Markell and Voge's Medical Parasitology*, 8th edn. Saunders, Philadelphia, USA.

Marquardt, W.C., Demaree, R.S. and Grieve, R.B. (2000) *Parasitology and Vector Biology*. 2nd edn. Academic Press, Orlando, Florida, USA.

Marr, J.J. and Muller, M. (1995) *Biochemistry and Molecular Biology of Parasites*. Academic Press, London, UK.

Meyers, W. (2000) *Pathology of Infectious Diseases*. Vol. 1. *Helminthiases*. Armed Forces Institute of Pathology, Washington, USA.

Miyazaki, T. (1991) *An Illustrated Book of Helminthic Zoonoses*. International Medical Foundation of Japan, Tokyo, Japan.

Muller, R. (1997) Parasitology. In: Wyatt, H.V. (ed.) *Information Sources in the Life Sciences*, 4th edn. Bowker-Sauer, East Grinstead, UK, pp. 195–202.

Muller, R. and Baker, J.R. (1990) *Medical Parasitology*. Lippincott, Philadelphia, USA.

Neva, F.A. and Brown, H.W. (1994) *Basic Clinical Parasitology*, 6th edn. Appleton and Lange, Norwalk, Connecticut, USA.

Nokes, C. and Bundy, D.A.P. (1994) Does helminth infection affect mental processing and educational achievement? *Parasitology Today* 10, 14–18.

Orihel, T.C. and Ash, L.R. (1995) *Parasites in Human Tissues*. American Society of Clinical Pathologists, Chicago, USA.

Palmer, P.E.S. and Reeder, M.M. (2000) *The Imaging of Tropical Diseases*, 2 vols. Springer, Heidelberg, Germany.

Palmer, S.R., Lord Soulsby and Simpson, D.I.H. (eds) (2000) *Zoonoses*. Oxford University Press, New York, USA.

Peters, W. and Gilles, H.M. (1999) *A Colour Atlas of Tropical Medicine and Parasitology*, 5th edn. Mosby, London, UK.

Price, D.L. (1993) *Procedure Manual of the Diagnosis of Intestinal Parasites*. CRC Press, Boca Raton, USA.

Rogan, M.T. (ed.) (1997) *Analytical Parasitology*. Springer-Verlag, Berlin, Germany.

Salfelder, K., Liscans, T.R. and de Sauerleig, E. (1992) *Atlas of Parasitic Pathology*. Kluwer, Dordrecht, The Netherlands.

Schmidt, G.D. and Roberts, L.S. (1989) *Foundations of Parasitology*. Mosby, Missouri, USA.

Scott, M.E. and Smith, G. (eds) (1994) *Parasitic and Infectious Diseases: Epidemiology and Ecology*. Academic Press, New York, USA.

Smyth, J.D. (ed.) (1990) In vitro *Cultivation of Parasitic Helminths*. CRC Press, Boca Raton, Florida, USA.

Smyth, J.D. (ed.) (1994) *Introduction to Animal Parasitology*. Cambridge University Press, Cambridge, UK.

Soulsby, E.J.L. (ed.) (1987) *Immune Responses in Parasitic Infections*. CRC Press, Boca Raton, USA.

Spicer, W.J. (2000) *Clinical Bacteriology, Mycology and Parasitology*. Harcourt, London, UK.

Stephenson, L.S. (1987) *The Impact of Helminth Infections on Human Nutrition: Schistosomes and Soil-transmitted Helminths*. Taylor and Francis, London, UK.

Strickland, T. (ed.) (2000) *Hunter's Tropical Medicine and Emerging Infectious Diseases*, 8th edn. Saunders, Philadelphia, USA.

Sun, T. (1993) *Progress in Clinical Parasitology*, Vol. 3. Field and Wood, New York, USA.

Taylor, A.E.R. and Baker, J.R. (eds) (1987) In vitro *Methods for Parasite Cultivation*. Academic Press, London, UK.

Thienpont, D., Rochette, F. and Vanparijs, O.F.G. (1979) *Diagnosing Helminthiasis through Coprological Examination*. Janssen Research Foundation, Beerse, Belgium.

Ubelaker, J.E. (1993) *Stedman's ASP Parasite Names*. Williams and Wilkins, Baltimore, USA.

Urquhart, G.M., Armour, J., Duncan, J.L., Dunn, A.M. and Jennings, F.W. (1987) *Veterinary Parasitology*. Churchill Livingstone, New York, USA.

Van den Bossche, H. (1995) Principles of anthelmintic chemotherapy. In: Farthing, M.J.G., Keusch, G.T. and Wakelin, D. (eds) *Enteric Infections 2: Intestinal Helminths*. Chapman and Hall, London, UK, pp. 267–286.

van Lichtenberg, F. (1991) *Pathology of Infectious Diseases*. Raven Press, New York, USA.

Wakelin, D.M. (1988) Helminth infections. In: Wakelin, D.M. and Blackwell, J.M. (eds) *Genetics of Resistance to Bacterial and Parasitic Infection*. Taylor and Francis, London, UK, pp. 83–100.

Walls, K. and Schantz, P. (eds) (1986) *Immunodiagnosis of Parasitic Diseases. I. Helminthic Diseases*. Academic Press, Orlando, USA.

Whitfield, P.J., Molyneux, D.H., Anderson, R.M., Bryant, C., Hart, D.T., Chappell, L.H., Gutteridge, W.E. and Cox, F.E.G. (1993) *Modern Parasitology: a Textbook of Parasitology*, 2nd edn. Blackwell Scientific Publications, Oxford, UK.

WHO (1987) *Prevention and Control of Intestinal Parasitic Diseases*. World Health Organization, Geneva, Switzerland.

WHO (1990) *WHO Model Prescribing Information: Drugs Used in Parasitic Diseases*. World Health Organization, Geneva, Switzerland.

Working Group on Parasite Control – The Hashimoto Intitiative (1998) *The Global Parasite Control for the 21st Century*. Government of Japan, Kobe, Japan.

Wyler, D.J. (1990) *Modern Parasite Biology: Cellular, Immunological and Molecular Aspects*. W.H. Freeman, New York, USA.

Trematodes

Kumar, V. (1999) *Trematode Infections and Diseases of Man and Animals*. Kluwer, Dordrecht, The Netherlands.

Smyth, J.D. and Halton, D.W. (1983) *The Physiology of Trematodes*, 2nd edn. Cambridge University Press, Cambridge, UK.

Cestodes

Adams, A.M. and Rausch, R.L. (1999) Diphyllobothriasis. In: Connor, D.H., Chandler, F.W., Schwartz, D.A., Manz, H.J. and Lack, E.E. (eds) *Pathology of Infectious Diseases*. Vol. 2. Appleton and Lange, Norwalk, Connecticut, USA, pp. 1377–1390.

Arai, H.P. (ed.) (1980) *Biology of the Tapeworm* Hymenolepis diminuta. Academic Press, New York, USA.

Smyth, J.D. and McManus, D.P. (1989) *The Physiology and Biochemistry of Cestodes.* Cambridge University Press, Cambridge, UK.
Wardle, R.A., McLeod, J.A. and Radinovsky, S. (1974) *Advances in the Zoology of Tapeworms, 1950–1970.* University of Minnesota Press, Minneapolis, USA.

Nematodes

Anderson, R.C. (2000) *Nematode Parasites of Vertebrates – their Development and Transmission,* 2nd edn. CAB International, Wallingford, UK.
Bird, A.F. and Bird, J. (1991) *The Structure of Nematodes.* Academic Press, New York, USA.

Immunology

Allen, J.E. and Maizels, R.M. (1997) Th1–Th2 paradigm: reliable paradigm or dangerous dogma? *Immunology Today* 18, 387–392.
Bancroft, A.J., Grencis, R.K. and MacDonald, T.T. (1998) Th1 and Th2 cells and immunity to intestinal helminths. *Chemical Immunology* 71, 198–208.
Capron, A. (1998) Schistosomiasis: forty years' war on the worm. *Parasitology Today* 14, 379–384.
Finkelman, F.D., Shea-Donahue, T., Goldhill, J., Sullivan, C.A., Morris, S.C., Madden, K.B., Gause, W.C. and Urban, J.F., Jr (1997) Cytokine regulation of host defense against parasitic gastrointestinal nematodes: lessons from studies with rodent models. *Annual Review of Immunology* 15, 505–533.
Janeway, C. and Travers, P. (1999) *Immunobiology,* 4th edn. Churchill-Livingstone, London.
Kennedy, M.W. and Harnett, W. (eds) (2001) *Parasitic Nematodes – Molecular Biology, Biochemistry and Immunology,* CAB International, Wallingford, UK.
Kierszenbaum, F. (ed.) (1994) *Parasitic Infections and the Immune System.* Academic Press, San Diego, USA.
Liew, F.Y. and Vickerman, K. (eds) (1997) Immune effector mechanisms in parasitic infections. *Philosophical Transactions of the Royal Society B* 352, 1293–1394.
Moqbel, R. (ed.) (1992) *Allergy and Immunity to Helminths: Common Mechanisms or Divergent Pathways.* Taylor and Francis, London, UK.
Parham, P. (2000) *The Immune System.* Elsevier Science, London, UK.
Prichard, D.I. (1995) The survival strategies of hookworms. *Parasitology Today* 11, 255–259.
Roitt, I., Brostoff, J. and Male, D. (1998) *Immunology,* 5th edn. Mosby, London, UK.
Röllinghof, M. and Rommel, M. (1994) *Immunologische und molekulare Parasitologie.* Gustav Fischer, Berlin, Germany.
Wakelin, D. (1994) Host populations: genetics and immunity. In: Scott, M.E. and Smith, G. (eds) *Parasitic and Infectious Diseases.* Academic Press, London, UK, pp. 83–100.
Wakelin, D. (1996) *Immunity to Parasites: How Parasitic Infections are Controlled.* Cambridge University Press, Cambridge, UK.
Wakelin, D. (1997) Parasites and the immune system: conflict or compromise? *Bioscience* 47, 32–40.
Wang, C.C. (ed.) (1991) *Molecular and Immunological Aspects of Parasitism.* American Association for the Advancement of Science, Washington, USA.
Warren, K.S. (ed.) (1993) *Immunology and Molecular Biology of Parasitic Infections,* 3rd edn. Blackwell Scientific Publications, Boston, USA.

History

Cox, F.E.G. (ed.) (1996) *The Wellcome Trust Illustrated History of Tropical Diseases.* Wellcome Trust, London, UK.
Dunlop, R.H. and Williams, D.I. (1996) *Veterinary Medicine: an Illustrated History.* Mosby Year Book, St Louis, USA.
Farley, J. (1991) *Bilharzia. A History of Imperial Tropical Medicine.* Cambridge University Press, Cambridge, UK.

Foster, W.D. (1965) *A History of Parasitology.* Livingstone, Edinburgh, UK.

Garnham, P.C.C. (1971) *Progress in Parasitology.* Athlone Press, London, UK.

Grove, D.I. (1990) *A History of Human Helminthology.* CAB International, Wallingford, UK (available on-line at www.red-e2.com).

Hoeppli, R. (1959) *Parasites and Parasitic Infections in Early Medicine and Science.* University of Malaya Press, Singapore.

Kean, B.H., Mott, K.E. and Russell, A.J. (eds) (1978) *Tropical Medicine and Parasitology: Classic Investigations,* Vols 1 and 2. Cornell University Press, Ithaca, USA.

Index

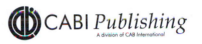
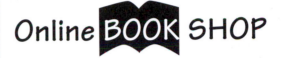
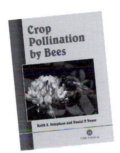
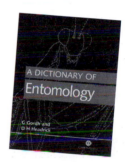
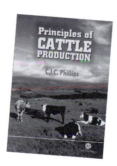
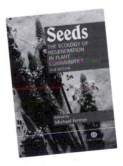
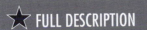
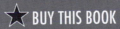
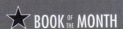